D0851526

An introduction to nutrition and metabolism

An introduction to nutrition and metabolism

DAVID A. BENDER

University College London

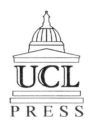

UCL

PRESS

First published in 1993 by UCL Press

UCL Press Limited
University College London
Gower Street
London WC1E 6BT

The name of University College London (UCL) is a registered
trade mark used by UCL Press with the consent of the owner.

ISBN:
1-85728-078-4 HB
1-85728-079-2 PB

A CIP catalogue record for this book
is available from the British Library.

Typeset in Times Roman.
Printed and bound by
Biddles Ltd, King's Lynn and Guildford, England.

CONTENTS

PREFACE

The food we eat has a major effect on our physical health and psychological wellbeing. An understanding of the way in which nutrients are metabolized, and hence of the principles of biochemistry, is essential for an understanding of the scientific basis of what we would call a prudent or healthy diet.

My aim in the following pages is both to explain the conclusions of the many expert committees which have deliberated on the problems of nutritional requirements, diet and health over the years, and also the scientific basis on which these experts have reached their conclusions. Much information now presented as "facts" will be proven to be incorrect in years to come. This book is intended to provide a foundation of scientific knowledge and understanding from which to interpret and evaluate future advances in nutrition and health sciences.

Nutrition is one of the sciences which underlie a proper understanding of health and human sciences and the ways in which human beings interact with their environment. In its turn, the science of nutrition is based on both biochemistry and physiology on one hand, and the social and behavioural sciences on the other. This book therefore contains a great deal of biochemistry, which is essential to an understanding of the basic science of nutrition. You do not have to "know" a metabolic pathway in order to be able to follow, and contribute to, a debate about how nutritional and metabolic factors interact with health. What is necessary is the ability to read a metabolic pathway like any other map or flow chart, and to follow the development of biochemical concepts and arguments. Many of the diagrams in this book are, perforce, complex, since they represent complex metabolic pathways. They are included for completeness and reference; the text gives an overview of the relevant and important features of the various pathways discussed.

In a book of this kind, which is an *introduction* to nutrition and metabolism, it is neither possible nor appropriate to cite the original scientific literature which provides the (sometimes conflicting) evidence for the statements made. The bibliography in Appendix IV lists some sources of more detailed information. In turn, these will lead the reader into research review essays, and thence the original research literature.

I am grateful to those of my students whose perceptive questions have helped me to formulate and organize my thoughts. This book is dedicated to those who will use it as a part of their studies, in the hope that they will be able, in their turn, to advance the frontiers of knowledge, and help their clients, patients and students to understand the basis of the advice we offer.

DAVID A. BENDER   London, October 1992

ix

CHAPTER ONE

Why eat?

An adult eats about a tonne of food a year. This book attempts to answer the question *why?* – by exploring the need for food and the uses to which that food is put in the body. Some discussion of chemistry and biochemistry is obviously essential if we are to investigate the fate of food in the body, and why there is a continuous need for food throughout life. Therefore, in the following chapters, various aspects of biochemistry and metabolism will be discussed. This should provide not only the basis of our present understanding, knowledge and concepts in nutrition, but also – possibly more important – a basis from which to interpret future research findings and evaluate new ideas and hypotheses as they are formulated.

We eat because we are hungry. Why have we evolved complex physiological and psychological mechanisms to control not only hunger but also our appetite for different types of food? Why are meals such an important part of our life?

The need for energy

We can see an obvious need for energy in order to perform measurable physical work. Work has to be done to lift a load against the force of gravity, and we require a source of energy to perform that work. As discussed in Chapter 6, we can measure the energy used in various activities, and we can measure the metabolic energy yield of the foods which are the fuel for that work. This means that we can calculate the balance between the intake of energy, as metabolic fuels, and the body's energy expenditure. Obviously, energy intake has to be adequate to meet energy

1

expenditure; as discussed in Chapters 6, 7 and 8, neither deficit nor excess intake is desirable.

Quite apart from this visible work output, the body has a considerable requirement for energy, even at rest. Only about one-third of the average person's energy expenditure is for obvious work. The remainder is required for maintenance of the body's functions, homeostasis of the internal environment and metabolic integrity. We can measure this energy requirement by the production of heat when the subject is completely at rest, in an environment at a temperature where the body is neither gaining nor losing heat. The result is called the **basal metabolic rate** (abbreviated to BMR) – the energy requirement for maintenance of body functions and metabolic integrity.

Part of this basal energy requirement is obvious: the heart beats to circulate the blood; respiration continues; there is considerable electrical activity in nerves and muscles, whether they are "working" or not; and the kidneys use a great deal of energy during the filtration of waste products from the bloodstream. All of these processes require a metabolic energy source. Less obviously, there is also a requirement for energy for the wide variety of biochemical reactions going on all the time in the body: laying down reserves in the form of fat and carbohydrate; a continuous turnover of tissue proteins and other compounds; transport of substrates into, and products out of, cells; and the production and secretion of hormones and neurotransmitters.

Units of energy

We measure energy expenditure by the production of heat (see p. 157). The unit of heat used in the early studies was the **calorie**: the amount of heat required to raise the temperature of 1 gram of water by 1°C. The calorie is sometimes still used, although because of the relatively large amounts of energy involved in human metabolism we talk in **kilocalories** (kcal, sometimes written as Calories with a capital C). One kcal is 1,000 calories (10^3 cal), and hence the amount of heat required to raise 1 kg of water through 1°C.

Correctly, we use the **joule** as the unit of energy. The Joule is an SI unit, named after James Prescott Joule, who first showed the equivalence of heat, mechanical work and other forms of energy. One joule is a very small amount of energy, and in biological systems we talk in **kilojoules** ($1\,kJ = 10^3\,J = 1,000$ joules) and **megajoules** ($1\,MJ = 10^6\,J = 1,000,000\,J$).

To convert between calories and joules:

$$1\,\text{kcal} = 4.186\,\text{kJ}$$
$$1\,\text{kJ} = 0.239\,\text{kcal}.$$

As discussed in Chapter 6, the average energy expenditure of adults is 7.5–10MJ/day for women and 8–12MJ/day for men.

Metabolic fuels

The dietary sources of metabolic energy (the metabolic fuels) are carbohydrates, fats, protein and alcohol. The metabolism of these fuels in the body results in the production of carbon dioxide and water (and also urea in the case of proteins, see p. 203). We can convert them to these same end-products chemically, by burning them in air. Although the process of metabolism in the body is more complex, it is a basic law of chemistry that, if the starting material and end-products are the same, the energy yield is the same, regardless of the route taken. Therefore we can determine the energy yield of foodstuffs by measuring the heat produced when they are burnt in air, making allowance for the extent to which they are digested and absorbed from foods. The energy yields of the metabolic fuels are shown in Table 1.1.

Table 1.1 The energy yield of metabolic fuels.

	kJ/g
Carbohydrate	17
Protein	16
Fat	37
Alcohol	29

1 kcal = 4.186 kJ or 1 kJ = 0.239 kcal

The need for carbohydrate, fat and protein Although we have a requirement for energy sources in the diet, it does not matter unduly how that requirement is met. There is no requirement for a dietary source of carbohydrate; as discussed on p. 153, the body can make as much carbohydrate as it requires from proteins. Similarly, there is no requirement for a dietary source of fat, apart from the essential fatty acids (see p. 81). There is certainly no requirement for a dietary source of alcohol!

Although there is no requirement for fat in the diet, fats do have nutritional importance:

(a)   It is difficult to eat enough of a very low-fat diet to meet energy requirements. As shown in Table 1.1, the energy yield of 1g of fat is more than twice that of 1g of carbohydrate or protein. It would be necessary to eat a considerably larger amount of a very low-fat diet to meet energy needs from carbohydrate and protein alone. However, as discussed in Chapter 2, the problem in Western coun-

3

tries is generally a high intake of fat from the diet, contributing to the development of both obesity and the so-called diseases of affluence.

(b)   Four of the vitamins – A, D, E and K (see Ch. 11) – are fat-soluble, and are found in fatty and oily foods. More importantly, their absorption from the gut requires an adequate amount of fat in the diet, since they are absorbed dissolved in fats. On a very low-fat diet the absorption of these vitamins will be much reduced.

(c)   There is a requirement for small amounts of the essential fatty acids. These are constituents of fats which are required for specific functions and which cannot be formed in the body, so that they must be provided in the diet (see p. 81).

(d)   In many foods a great deal of the flavour (and hence the pleasure of eating, see below) is carried in the fat.

(e)   Fats lubricate food, and make chewing and swallowing easier.

The need for protein

Unlike fats and carbohydrates, there is a requirement for protein in the diet. In a growing child this need is obvious. As the child grows, and the size of its body increases, so there is an increase in the total amount of protein in the body.

Adults also require protein in the diet. There is a continuous small loss of protein from the body, for example in hair, shed skin cells, enzymes and other proteins secreted into the gut and not completely digested, etc. More importantly, there is turnover of body proteins. Tissue proteins are continuously being broken down and replaced. Although there is no change in the total amount of protein in the body, an adult with an inadequate intake of protein will be unable to replace this loss, and will lose tissue protein. Protein turnover and requirements are discussed in Chapter 9.

Minerals and vitamins

In addition to metabolic fuels and protein, the body has a requirement for a variety of **mineral salts**, in very much smaller amounts. Obviously, if a metal or ion has a function in the body, it must be provided by the diet, since the different chemical elements cannot be interconverted. Again, the need is obvious for a growing child; as the body grows in size, so the total amount of the various minerals in the body will increase. In adults there is a turnover of minerals in the body, with losses that must be replaced from the diet.

There is a requirement for a different group of nutrients, also in very small amounts: the **vitamins**. These are relatively complex organic compounds that have essential functions in metabolic processes. They cannot be synthesized in the body, and so must be provided by the diet. There is turnover of the vitamins, so there must be replacement of the losses. Vitamins and minerals are discussed in Chapter 11.

Hunger and appetite

Human beings have evolved a complex system of physiological and psychological mechanisms to ensure that the body's needs for metabolic fuels and nutrients are met.

There are hunger and satiety centres in the hypothalamus, which stimulate us to begin eating (the **hunger centres**) or to stop eating when we have satisfied our needs (the **satiety centres**). We are beginning to understand the rôle of these brain centres in controlling food intake, and there are drugs which modify responses to hunger and satiety. Such drugs can be used to reduce appetite in the treatment of obesity, or to stimulate it in people with anorexia (see p. 181).

These hypothalamic appetite centres control food intake very precisely. Most people can regulate their food intake, quite unconsciously, to match their energy expenditure very closely; they neither waste away from lack of metabolic fuels for physical activity nor lay down excessively large reserves of fat. Indeed, even people who have excessive reserves of body fat, and can be considered to be so overweight or obese as to be putting their health at risk, balance their energy intake and expenditure relatively well. We are talking about an intake of a tonne of food a year, while the record obese people weigh about 250 kg (compared with average weights between 55 and 80 kg), and it takes many years to achieve such a weight.

In addition to hunger and satiety, which are basic physiological responses, we have to consider **appetite**, which is related not only to physiological need but also to the pleasure of eating: flavour and texture, and a host of social and psychological factors.

Taste and flavour

Five basic tastes can be distinguished by the tongue: salt, sweetness, bitterness, sourness and savouriness. Two of these, salt and sweetness, are pleasurable sensations, while bitterness and sourness are instinctively perceived as unpleasant, and presumably evolved as a means of protection. The sensation of **savouriness** is distinct from that of saltiness, and is sometimes called "*umami*" (Japanese for savory). It is largely due to the presence of free amino acids (and especially glutamate) in foods. Stimulation of the *umami* receptors of the tongue is the basis of flavour enhancers such as **monosodium glutamate**, which is an important constituent of traditional oriental condiments and is widely used in manufactured foods.

Salt (correctly the mineral sodium chloride) is essential to life, and wild animals will travel great distances to a salt lick. Like other animals, we have evolved a pleasurable response to salty flavours; this ensures that we meet our physiological need for salt. However, there is no shortage of salt in developed countries, and we can now indulge this pleasure to excess. As discussed on p. 25, average intakes of salt are considerably greater than requirements, and may be high enough to pose a hazard to health.

The other instinctively pleasurable taste is **sweetness**. The evolutionary reason for this is less easy to work out, but we can argue that ripe fruits are sweet – indeed the process of fruit ripening is largely one of converting starches to sugars – and, in general, ripe fruits are better sources of vitamins and minerals than unripe fruits.

Sourness and **bitterness** are instinctively unpleasant sensations. We can learn to enjoy some sour and bitter foods, but this is a process of learning or acquiring tastes, not an innate or instinctive response. We can hypothesize that the instinctive aversion to bitter flavours evolved as a protection against poisonous compounds found in some plants, many of which are bitter. The aversion to sourness is presumably the converse of the pleasurable reaction to sweetness: if we wait until the fruit is ripe it will not have the sour flavour, and will have a greater nutritional value.

In addition to the basic taste sensations provided by the taste-buds on the tongue, we can distinguish a great many flavours by the sense of smell. Again some flavours and aromas (fruity flavours, fresh coffee and, at least to a non-vegetarian, the smell of roasting meat) are pleasurable. They tempt us to eat and, if we can smell the food but not yet eat it, they stimulate our appetite. Other flavours and aromas are repulsive and tell us not to eat the food. In many cases this again can be seen as a warning of possible danger: the smell of decaying meat or fish tells us that it is not safe to eat.

Like the acquisition of a taste for bitter or sour foods, we can acquire a taste for foods with what would seem at first to be an unpleasant aroma or flavour. Here, things become more complex; a smell pleasant to one person may be repulsive to another. Some enjoy the smell of cooked cabbage and sprouts, while others can hardly bear to be in the same room.

The durian fruit is a highly prized delicacy in Southeast Asia, yet to the uninitiated it smells of sewage or faeces – hardly an appetizing aroma.

Why do people eat what they do?

People have different responses to the same taste or flavour. Sometimes we can explain this in terms of childhood memories, pleasurable or otherwise. An aversion to the smell of a food may protect someone who has a specific allergy or intolerance (although sometimes people have a craving for the foods to which they are intolerant). Most often we simply cannot explain why some people dislike foods that others eat with great relish.

Factors influencing the choice of particular foods include:

The availability of food In developed countries the simple availability of food is not likely to be a constraint on choice. We have a wide variety of foods available. When fruits and vegetables are out of season at home they are imported; frozen, canned or dried foods are widespread. By contrast, in developing countries the availability of food is a major constraint on what people choose. Little food is imported, and what is available will depend on the local soil and climate. Even in normal times the choice of foods may be very limited, while in times of drought there may be little or no food available at all, and what little is available will be very much more expensive than most people can afford.

The cost of food Even in developed countries the cost of foods may limit the choices available to some people. Among the most disadvantaged members of the community, poverty may impose severe constraints on the choice of foods. In developing countries, cost is the major problem. Indeed, even in times of famine, food may be available, but it is so expensive that few people have the money to buy it.

Habit and tradition Foods which are commonly eaten in one area may be little eaten elsewhere, even though they are available, simply because people have not been used to eating them. To a very great extent, our eating habits as adults continue the habits we learned as children.

Haggis and oat cakes are rarely eaten outside Scotland, except as specialty items; black pudding is a staple of northern British breakfasts, but is rarely seen in the southeast of England. Until the 1960s, yoghurt was almost unknown by people in Britain, apart from a few health food "cranks" and immigrants from eastern Europe; many British children believe that fish comes only as rectangular "fish fingers", while children in inland Spain may eat fish and other sea-food three or four times a week. The French mock the British habit of eating lamb with mint sauce, and the average British reaction to such French delicacies as frogs' legs and snails in garlic sauce is one of horror. The British eat their cabbage well boiled; the Germans and Dutch ferment it to produce sauerkraut.

This regional and cultural diversity of foods provides one of the pleasures of travel. As people travel more frequently, and become (perhaps grudgingly) more adventurous in their choice of foods, so they create a demand for different foods at home, and there is an increasing variety of foods available in shops and restaurants.

A further factor which has increased the range of foods available has been the migration of people from a variety of different backgrounds, all of whom have, as they have become established, introduced their traditional foods to their new homes. It is difficult to appreciate that in the 1960s there was only a handful of Tandoori restaurants in the whole of Britain, or that pizza was something you saw only in southern Italy or a few specialist restaurants.

Some people are naturally adventurous, and will try a new food just because they have never eaten it before. Others are more conservative, and will try a new food only when they see someone else eating it safely and with enjoyment. Others are yet more conservative in their food choices; the most conservative eaters "know" that they do not like a new food because they have never eaten it before.

Luxury status of scarce and expensive foods Foods that are scarce or expensive have a certain appeal of fashion or style; they are (rightly) regarded as luxuries for special occasions rather than everyday meals. Conversely, foods that are widespread and cheap have less appeal. In the 19th century, salmon and oysters (which are now relatively expensive luxury foods) were so cheap that the Articles of apprentices in London specified that they should not be given salmon more than three times a week, while oysters were eaten by the poor. Conversely, chicken and trout, which were expensive luxury foods in the 1950s, are now widely available, as a result of changes in farming practice, and they form the basis of inexpensive meals. As farming practices change, so salmon is again becoming an inexpensive meal, and venison is no longer the exclusive preserve of the wealthy landed gentry or poachers.

The social functions of food Human beings are essentially social animals, and meals are important social functions. People eating in a group are likely to eat better, or at least to have a wider variety of foods and a more lavish and luxurious meal, than people eating alone. We may well use the excuse of entertaining guests to eat foods which we "know" to be nutritionally undesirable, and we eat more at a "feast" than we really need. Indeed, the greater the variety of courses and dishes offered, the more we are likely to eat. As we reach satiety with one food, so another, different, flavour is offered to tempt appetite. Studies have shown that, faced with only one food, people tend to reach satiety sooner than when a variety of different foods is on offer. Here again we see the difference between hunger and appetite. Even when we are satiated, we can still "find room" to try something different.

Conversely, and more importantly, many lonely single people (and especially the bereaved elderly) have little stimulus to prepare meals. While poverty may be a factor in limiting their choice of foods, apathy (and frequently, in the case of widowed men, ignorance) is more important in limiting the range of foods eaten, and may result in undernutrition. There is often little or no incentive to prepare a meal, and no stimulus to appetite. When these problems are added to those of infirmity, ill-fitting dentures (which make eating painful) and arthritis (which makes handling many foods difficult), and the difficulty of carrying food home from the shops, it is not surprising that we include the elderly among those vulnerable groups of the population who are at risk of undernutrition.

The attractiveness (or otherwise) of food In hospitals and other institutions, we face a further problem. In hospitals we are dealing with people who are unwell, whose physical energy expenditure is low, but who have higher than normal requirements for energy, protein and other nutrients, as a part of the process of replacing tissue in convalescence, or as a result of fever or the metabolic effects of cancer (see p. 184). At the same time, illness impairs appetite, and a side-effect of many drugs is to distort the sense of taste, depress appetite or cause nausea. It is difficult to provide a range of exciting and attractive foods under institutional conditions, yet this is what is needed to tempt the patient's appetite.

Summary

Food serves many purposes. At the basic level it provides a metabolic fuel and meets a physiological need. However, it also serves social and psychological functions, and good food can be a source of pleasure.

We have to consider whether the foods that tempt us are nutritionally desirable, and whether our choice of foods may affect our general health. In order to understand the rôle of diet in health, and the rôle of modifications of diet in treating or controlling diseases, we have to understand the functions of the nutrients in the body, and hence the way in which the body maintains its functions and metabolic integrity.

CHAPTER TWO

Diet and health: the diseases of affluence

The World Health Organization defines health as "a state of complete mental, physical and social wellbeing, and not, merely, the absence of disease or infirmity". One of the factors essential for the attainment of health is an adequate and appropriate diet.

An adequate diet is one which provides adequate amounts of metabolic fuels and nutrients to meet physiological needs and to prevent the development of deficiency diseases. To achieve an adequate diet is a minimum objective, albeit one to which many in developing countries aspire. An appropriate diet not only meets physiological needs, but does so in a balanced way, without causing any health problems which may be associated with an excessive intake of one or more nutrients or types of food.

Human beings have evolved in a hostile environment in which food has always been scarce. It is only in the past half-century or less that food has become available in large amounts; and even then it is only in western Europe, North America and Australasia that there is a surplus of food. Food is still desperately short in much of Africa, Asia and Latin America, and indeed much of eastern Europe has inadequate food. Even without all too frequent droughts, floods and other disasters, there is scarcely enough food produced worldwide to feed all the people of the world.

This means that if we are to consider problems of diet and health we have to make a distinction between the problems of undernutrition and those associated with affluence and the ready availability of plentiful supplies of food at prices that people can afford.

On a global scale, overall lack of food is the problem. Up to 300 million people (mainly children) are at risk from protein–energy malnutrition in developing countries; this is discussed in Chapter 8. Deficiency of individual nutrients is also a major problem. Here the total amount of food may be adequate to satisfy hunger, but the quality of the diet is inadequate. Vitamin A deficiency (see p. 236) is the single most important cause of childhood blindness in the world; perhaps 100,000 children in Southeast Asia are at risk. Deficiency of vitamins B_1 (see p. 255) and B_2 (see p. 257) continues to be a major problem in large areas of Asia and Africa. Deficiency of iodine affects many millions of people living in upland areas over limestone soil; in some areas of central Brazil and the Himalayas more than 90% of the population may have goitre due to iodine deficiency (see p. 279). Iron deficiency anaemia affects many millions of women in both developing and developed countries (see p. 284). Deficiency of other vitamins and minerals also occurs, and can still be an important cause of ill health and disease, as discussed in Chapter 11. Sometimes this is the result of an acute exacerbation of a marginal food shortage, as in the new outbreaks of the niacin deficiency disease, pellagra, reported in eastern and southern Africa during the 1980s (see p. 259); sometimes it is a problem of immigrant populations living in a new environment, as with the incidence of rickets and osteomalacia among Asians living in northern Europe (see p. 242).

The problems of undernutrition are discussed in Chapter 8, protein deficiency in Chapter 9 and vitamin and mineral deficiencies in Chapter 11. In this chapter we will consider the rôle of diet and nutrition in the so-called "diseases of affluence"; the health problems of developed countries, associated with a superabundant availability of food. Diet is, of course, only one of the differences between life in the developed countries of western Europe, North America and Australasia; there are a great many other differences in environment and living conditions. Despite the problems we will discuss in this chapter, which are major causes of premature death, people in developed countries have a greater life expectancy than those in developing countries.

We must assume that human beings and their diet have evolved together. Certainly, we have changed our crops and farm animals by selective breeding over the past 10,000 years, and it is reasonable to assume that we have evolved by natural selection to be suited to our diet. The problem is that evolution is a slow process, and there have been major changes in food availability in developed countries during the past century. As recently as the 1930s (only two generations ago, and hence very recently in evolutionary terms) it was estimated that up to one-third of households in Britain could not afford an adequate diet. Malnutrition was a serious problem, and the provision of 200 ml of milk daily to schoolchildren had a significant, beneficial, effect on their health and growth.

11

Foods which were historically scarce luxuries are now commonplace and available in surplus. Sugar was an expensive luxury until the middle of the 19th century; traditionally fat was also scarce, and every effort was made to save and use all the fat (dripping) from a roast joint of meat.

Together with this increased availability of food, we have seen an increase in average life span in the developed countries over the past century. This can be attributed to: increased medical knowledge and better medical treatment; reliable supplies of clean drinking water and improved sewage disposal; and eradication of the diseases of hunger.

The diseases of affluence

Superimposed on this improvement, we have also seen the rise of "new" diseases: the major causes of death in developed countries today are heart disease, high blood pressure, strokes and cancer. These are not just diseases of old age, although it is true to say that the longer people live, the more likely they are to develop cancer. It is not simply a matter that people who have not died from infectious diseases must die from something. Heart disease is a major cause of premature death, striking a significant number of people aged under forty. This is not solely a Western phenomenon. As developing countries reach an increasing level of affluence, so people in the prosperous cities show a "Western" pattern of premature death from these same diseases.

There is a considerable body of evidence that diet is a significant factor in the development of these diseases of affluence. Not the sole cause, since they are all due to interactions of multiple factors, including heredity, a variety of environmental factors, smoking and exercise (or the lack of it). None the less, diet is a factor which is readily amenable to change. Individually we can take decisions about our diet, smoking and exercise, whereas we can do little about the stresses of city life, environmental pollution or the other problems of industrial society. We can do nothing, of course, to change our heredity.

The major change in our diet over the past century or so has been the increase in the total amount of food available, and particularly in the amount of fat and sugar we eat. We eat less dietary fibre than 100 years ago; in general we eat more highly refined cereal products, and are less reliant on cereals and vegetables. Meat is now eaten most days of the week, rather than being a "Sunday treat". At the same time, we no longer suffer from deficiency diseases, seasonal hunger is a thing of the past in developed countries, and in general we can rely on our food being wholesome and fit to eat.

We have to consider whether the changes over the past century may be a factor in the development of the diseases of affluence, and whether increased consumption of some foods or nutrients may be beneficial, protecting us against these and other diseases.

The epidemiological evidence linking dietary factors with the diseases of affluence shows that in countries or regions with, for example, a high intake of saturated fat, there is a higher incidence of cardiovascular disease and some forms of cancer than in regions with a lower intake of fat. It does not show that people who have been living on a high-fat diet will necessarily benefit from a relatively abrupt change to a low-fat diet. Indeed, the results of intervention studies over a period of 10–20 years, in which large numbers of people have been persuaded to change their diets, have been disappointing. Overall, premature death from cardio-vascular disease is little reduced, and the total death rate remains unchanged, with an increase in suicide, accidents and violent death. Nevertheless, the epidemiological data are irrefutable. People who have lived on what we can call a prudent diet, as discussed below, are significantly less at risk of death from the diseases of affluence than those whose intakes of fat (and especially saturated fat), salt and sugar are higher, and of dietary fibre, fruit and vegetables lower. Our aim must therefore be to inculcate what we consider to be prudent and appropriate dietary habits into people at an early age.

Food safety – additives and contaminants

The first general food laws anywhere in the world were passed in Britain in 1860. They were intended to stamp out widespread adulteration of common foods: diluting flour with chalk dust; mixing sugar with "sugar of lead" (lead acetate, a poisonous compound) – added because it was cheap and sweet tasting, while sugar was expensive; adding water to milk and alcoholic beverages.

Since then we have progressed considerably, and there are comprehensive regulations on food safety and hygiene, covering all aspects of food production, manufacture, sale, preparation and serving. We have compiled lists of those compounds which may legally be added to food during manufacture or processing, based on exhaustive testing for safety. Compounds not included in the list of permitted additives may not be added to foods.

Food additives may be colours and flavours, preservatives or processing aids to maintain the texture of the food, maintain stable emulsions, prevent fat from going rancid, or to prevent cooking oil spattering dangerously in the frying pan. They may be naturally occurring compounds, such as colours extracted from various plants, or they may be synthetic chemicals, or chemically synthesized compounds which are identical to those occurring in nature. What they all have in common is that they have been tested, and found to be safe, as far as anyone can tell, causing no adverse effects in experimental animals or human beings. On the very few occasions when potentially hazardous effects of a food additive have been suspected, it has been withdrawn from use with great haste, sometimes even before the hazard has been established as a real one.

Contamination of foods poses a more serious problem, because it occurs accidentally. Where we know or believe that specific compounds which might enter the food chain are hazardous, strict limits are set on the concentration which may be permitted in foods. This is generally based on estimates of the amounts likely to consumed from foods, and the **acceptable daily intake** is set at one-hundredth of the lowest level at which any adverse effect can be detected. Food manufacturers, the Ministry of Agriculture, Fisheries and Food (and equivalent government departments in other countries) and the public health services maintain a close watch on possible contamination of foods, and there are mechanisms to ensure that contaminated foods are withdrawn and destroyed rapidly. Foods being imported are subject to inspection and checks at ports to ensure safety and freedom from contamination.

Similarly, the Central Public Health Laboratory in Britain (and equivalent laboratories in other countries) monitors all reported cases of infectious **food poisoning**, and provides, together with Medical Officers of Health and Trading Standards Officers, a system for tracing, withdrawing and ordering the destruction of foods found to be contaminated with harmful bacteria. Where particular foods are especially likely to contain potentially dangerous numbers of harmful bacteria (for example the presence of *Salmonella* spp. in eggs and poultry, or *Listeria* spp. in soft cheeses), the Department of Health issues special advice. Thus eggs should be cooked, not eaten raw or partially cooked. Frozen poultry should be thoroughly defrosted before cooking, so as to ensure adequate heating of the interior, and hence destruction of the bacteria. The developing fetus is especially susceptible to infection with *Listeria*, and pregnant women are specifically advised to avoid soft cheeses which may carry an unacceptable burden of these bacteria.

Guidelines for healthy eating, and nutritional goals

There is general agreement among nutritionists and medical scientists about changes in the average "Western" diet that would be expected to

14

reduce the prevalence of the diseases of affluence, and most countries have now published nutritional guidelines and dietary advice. Changing our diet in the way suggested here is not a guarantee of immortality, and indeed some of the evidence is conflicting. As new data are gathered, old data reinterpreted and the results of long-term intervention studies of changing peoples' diets become available, it is inevitable that opinions and judgements as to what constitutes a prudent or desirable diet will change. It will be essential to have an understanding of the underlying physiology and biochemistry of nutrition, the way in which nutrients are metabolized and interact with each other and with a host of metabolic and regulatory systems in the body, in order to be able to evaluate this new information.

We have a set of generally agreed goals for what we can call a "prudent diet" for adults, which is a pattern and style of eating which is associated with the lowest risk of premature death from the diseases of affluence. The guidelines given in this chapter are based on those in the Department of Health report on *Dietary reference values for food energy and nutrients for the United Kingdom* (1991). This represents the most recent compilation and assessment of the many studies and reports by expert committees over the past 2–3 decades.

We will consider the guidelines here; in later chapters we will explore their biochemical basis.

Energy intake

Obesity involves both an increased risk of premature death from a variety of causes and increased morbidity from conditions such as varicose veins and arthritis (see Ch. 7). On the other hand, people who are significantly underweight are also at increased risk of illness and premature death. We can therefore define a range of **desirable or ideal weight** (relative to height), based on life expectancy (see p. 164).

For people whose body weight is within the desirable range, energy intake should be adequate to maintain a reasonably constant body weight, with an adequate amount of exercise. Energy expenditure in physical activity and appropriate levels of energy intake are discussed in Chapter 6.

The metabolic fuels are fats, carbohydrates, protein and alcohol. Table 2.1 shows the average percentage of energy intake from each of them in the diets of adults in Britain in the 1990s, compared with the guidelines for a prudent diet.

Calculation of the percentage of energy intake derived from the various metabolic fuels requires knowledge of both the energy yield/g of each fuel (see Table 1.1 on p. 3), and the subject's intake, based on recording the amounts of food eaten and calculating the nutrient intake from tables of

15

food composition (see Appendix II). The way the calculations are performed is shown in Table 2.2.

Table 2.1 The percentage of energy from different metabolic fuels in the average diet, compared with dietary guidelines.

	Average	Range	Guidelines
Carbohydrate	42	30–55	55
Fat	39	27–50	30
Protein	15	9–20	15
Alcohol	men 7	0–28	see Table 2.10
	women 3	0–16	

Table 2.2 Calculation of total energy intake and the percentage of energy from different metabolic fuels.

Total energy intake = energy from
    carbohydrate   = g carbohydrate × 17kJ/g
  + fat   = g fat × 37kJ/g
  + protein   = g protein × 16kJ/g
  + alcohol   = g alcohol × 29kJ/g

Percentage of energy from different metabolic fuels:

Carbohydrate

$$\frac{\text{g carbohydrate} \times 17\text{kJ/g}}{\text{total energy intake (kJ)}} \times 100\%$$

Fat

$$\frac{\text{g fat} \times 37\text{kJ/g}}{\text{total energy intake (kJ)}} \times 100\%$$

Protein

$$\frac{\text{g protein} \times 16\text{kJ/g}}{\text{total energy intake (kJ)}} \times 100\%$$

Alcohol

$$\frac{\text{grams alcohol} \times 29\text{kJ/g}}{\text{total energy intake (kJ)}} \times 100\%$$

Dietary fat intake

Discussion of fat intake means both solid fats and oils, which are simply fats that are liquid at room temperature. It involves a consideration of not only the obvious fat in the diet (the visible fat on meat, cooking oil, butter or margarine spread on bread), but also the "hidden" fat in foods. This "hidden" fat may be either the fat naturally present in foods (e.g. the fat between the muscle fibres in meat, the oils in nuts, cereals and vegetables) or fat used in the cooking and manufacture of foods.

Table 2.3 shows the average intakes of fat as a percentage of energy intake in the average diet. As well as the total amount of fat (the first line of the table), it also shows intakes of saturated and unsaturated fats separately. The chemical difference between saturated and unsaturated fats is discussed on p. 79; it is relevant here since, as discussed below, both the total amount of fat in the diet and the proportion of that fat which is saturated or unsaturated are important in considering the rôle of diet in the diseases of affluence. As a general rule, animal foods (meat, eggs and milk products) are rich sources of saturated fats, while oily fish and vegetables are rich sources of unsaturated fats (see Table 2.5).

Table 2.3 Average intakes of different types of fat. The figures show the percentage of food energy intake (i.e. excluding that from alcohol), derived from different types of fats. The guideline is that 30% of energy should be from fat, with only 10% from saturated fats (see p. 79 for a discussion of saturated and unsaturated fats).

	Average	Range
Total fat	39	30–50
Saturated fat	17	10–23
Polyunsaturated fat	6	3–12
Mono-unsaturated fat	12	8–17

There are two problems associated with a high intake of fat:
(a) The energy yield of fat (37kJ/g) is more than twice that of protein (16kJ/g) or carbohydrate (17kJ/g). This means that foods which are high in fat are also concentrated energy sources. It is easier to have an excessive energy intake on a high-fat diet, and hence a high-fat diet can be a factor in the development of obesity (see Ch. 7).
(b) Studies in many countries have shown that the average intake of fat is statistically correlated with premature death from a variety of conditions, including especially atherosclerosis and ischaemic heart disease and cancer of the colon, breast and uterus.

The concentration of cholesterol (see p. 84) in plasma, and specifically cholesterol in plasma low-density lipoproteins (LDL) is related to the development of atherosclerosis and ischaemic heart disease. The main dietary factor which affects the concentration of cholesterol in plasma is the intake of fat. Both the total amount of fat and also the relative amounts of saturated and unsaturated fats affect the concentration of cholesterol in LDL. High intakes of total fat, and especially saturated fat, are associated with undesirably high concentrations of LDL cholesterol. Relatively low intakes of fat, with a high proportion as unsaturated fat, are associated with a desirable lower concentration of LDL cholesterol.

From the results of epidemiological studies, it seems that diets providing about 30% of energy from fat are associated with the lowest risk of ischaemic heart disease. Above 35% of energy intake from fat there is an increase in serum cholesterol to above what is regarded as the normal or desirable range (above about 5.2mmol/l). There is no evidence that a fat intake below about 30% of energy intake confers any additional benefit, although a very low-fat diet is specifically recommended as part of treatment for some types of hepatitis, malabsorption and hyperlipidaemias.

As shown in Table 2.3, the average intake of fat in Britain is about 39% of energy. This means that we are aiming at a fairly considerable decrease in fat intake to meet the goal of 30% of energy from fat. Table 2.4 shows the foods which are especially high in fat. From this table, it is relatively easy to work out which foods we should eat less of in order to reduce our total intake of fat.

Table 2.4 Foods which are especially high in fat (excluding obvious fats such as butter, margarine, lard and cooking oils, and assuming that foods have not been fried in oil or fat).

		g/100g
Nuts	(depending on variety)	50–64
Meat	bacon rashers (grilled)	30–36
	duck (roast)	25
	pork (depending on joint and cooking)	20–24
	lamb (depending on joint and cooking)	19–30
	sausages (depending on type)	17–25
	bacon joint	19
	beef (depending on joint and cooking)	11–23
	chicken (roast)	14
Milk products	double cream	48
	Cheddar cheese	34
	Stilton cheese	26
	Edam cheese	24
	single cream	21
	full-cream milk	3.8
Fish *	herring	20
	salmon	20
	halibut	4
	cod	1
Eggs		11

* The fat content of canned fish will depend on whether it is canned in oil, water or a sauce.

As an aid to reducing fat intake, low-fat versions of foods which are traditionally high in fat are available. Some of these are meat products which make use of leaner (and more expensive) cuts of meat for the preparation of sausages, hamburgers and pies. Low-fat minced meat (containing about 10% fat by weight, instead of the more usual 20%) is widely available in supermarkets, although it is, of course, more expensive, and low-fat cheeses and patés are also available, as are salad dressings made with little or no oil. Some low-fat spreads can replace butter or margarine; these are listed in Table 2.5. Skimmed and semi-skimmed milk are now widely available, providing very much less fat than full-cream milk, although full-cream milk is an important source of vitamins A and D, especially for children.

Table 2.5 Types of fat spreads.

		% fat
Butter	Traditional churned butter, sometimes called sweetcream butter; may be salted or unsalted	80–82
Lactic butter	Made from cream with the addition of lactic bacteria to give a sharp taste; usually unsalted or lightly salted	80–82
Hard margarine	Hardened animal and vegetable oils, mainly used for baking	80
Soft margarine	Mainly vegetable oils, spreads easily	80
pufa margarine	Mainly sunflower, corn or soya bean oils, for a high content of polyunsaturated fatty acids (pufa)	80
Dairy spreads	Blended cream and vegetable oil, spreads easily	72–75
Reduced fat spreads	Mainly vegetable oils, may be some animal or dairy fat	60–70
Low-fat spreads	May contain dairy fat and vegetable oils; not suitable for cooking use	37–40
Very low-fat spreads	May contain dairy fat and vegetable oils; not suitable for cooking use	20–25
Extremely low-fat spreads	Made with fat substitutes (e.g. Simplesse, a modified protein) to replace almost all of the fat	5

Butter and margarine are legally defined, and hence low-fat substitutes cannot legally be called margarine. Low-fat spreads contain less fat, and hence more water, than margarine. They may also be whipped, so as to be lighter. They are intended for spreading, and are not suitable for cooking use.

The type of fat in the diet Not only should the total intake of fat be

19

30% of energy intake, but the type of fat that we eat is also important. The fatty acids which make up the fats of our diet can be chemically saturated or unsaturated. These chemically different types of fat have different actions in the body, so we have to have an understanding of the chemistry of the foods we eat. The chemistry of fats and fatty acids is discussed on p. 79. In saturated fatty acids there are only single bonds between the carbon atoms which make up the molecule, while in unsaturated fatty acids there may be one (mono-unsaturated) or more (polyunsaturated) double bonds between carbon atoms. In general, fats that contain mainly saturated fatty acids are hard at room temperature, while those that contain mainly unsaturated fatty acids are oils at room temperature. Table 2.6 shows the main sources of different types of fats in the average diet, and Table 2.7 shows the relative amounts of saturated, mono-unsaturated and polyunsaturated fatty acids in different types of cooking oil and fat.

Table 2.6 Sources of different types of fat in the average diet. The figures show the percentage of the total intake of different types of fat obtained from various foods in the average diet. It thus combines both the fat content of different foods and the amounts of various foods that people eat.

	Total	Saturated	Mono-unsat.	Poly-unsat.
Meat and meat products	24	23	31	17
Butter and margarine	16	17	11	20
Milk and cheese	15	23	12	2
Cakes, biscuits, etc.*	13	14	–	–
Vegetables (including cooking oil)*	11	6	12	24
Eggs	4	3	5	4
Fish	3	2	3	4

* Obviously, the relative amounts of different types of fat in baked and other cooked foods will depend on the fat or oil used in cooking.

The different types of fatty acid have different effects on the body's metabolism. Most studies of fat intake, heart disease and plasma cholesterol have shown that it is mainly saturated fats which pose hazards to health, and that unsaturated fatty acids have a beneficial effect, lowering LDL cholesterol, reducing the coagulability of blood platelets and reducing the risk of heart disease.

Therefore it is recommended that we should reduce our intake of saturated fats considerably more than just in proportion with the reduction in total fat intake. Total fat intake should be 30% of energy intake, with no more than 10% from saturated fats (compared with the present average of 17% of energy from saturated fat, see Table 2.3). The present average intakes of 6% of energy from polyunsaturated fats and 12% from mono-unsaturated fats match what is considered to be desirable, on the basis of epidemiological studies. (The missing 2% of energy intake in this calculation is accounted for by the *trans*-isomers of unsaturated fatty acids (see p. 58); it is considered that this should not increase.)

Table 2.7 The proportion of saturated and unsaturated fatty acids in different types of cooking oil and fat. The figures show the percentage of the total fatty acids present that are saturated, mono-unsaturated and polyunsaturated (see p. 79 for a discussion of saturated and unsaturated fatty acids).

	Saturated	Mono-unsaturated	Polyunsaturated
Butter	64	33	3
Hard margarine[*]	38	49	13
Soft margarine[*]	33	44	23
pufa margarine[*]	20	17	63
Lard	45	45	10
Coconut oil	91	7	2
Cottonseed oil	27	22	51
Corn oil	17	31	52
Olive oil	15	74	11
Palm oil	47	44	9
Peanut oil[†]	20	50	30
Soya bean oil	15	25	60
Sunflower oil	14	34	52

[*]   These are "typical" values; the precise composition of the mixture of vegetable oils used in making margarines will vary from one type to another. Similarly, "mixed vegetable oil" may well have a variable composition, containing different amounts of the various oils listed here.

[†]   Peanut oil is sometimes also called ground-nut or arachis oil.

Carbohydrates

If the total energy intake is to remain constant, but the proportion supplied by fat is to be reduced from the present average of about 39% to about 30%, and the proportion supplied by protein is to remain at about 15%, then, obviously, the proportion supplied by carbohydrates will increase. The guideline is that 55% of energy should come from carbohydrates.

We divide carbohydrates into two main groups: starches and sugars (this is a chemical term for a variety of carbohydrates, one of which is sucrose, cane or beet sugar, see p. 69). The guideline is that we should increase the proportion of energy that is derived from starches, and reduce that from sugars. Table 2.8 shows the average intakes of carbohydrate as a percentage of energy intake, and Table 2.9 shows those foods which are the main sources of carbohydrate in the diet.

Table 2.8 Average intakes of carbohydrates. The figures show the percentage of food energy intake (i.e. excluding that from alcohol) which is derived from different types of carbohydrates. The guideline is that 55% of energy intake should be from carbohydrate and 10% from non-milk extrinsic sugars).

	Average	Range
Total carbohydrate	42	30–55
Starch	25	21–27
Sugars	20	10–28

Table 2.9 Major sources of carbohydrate in the average diet. The figures show the percentage of total carbohydrate intake (column 2) or sugar (column 3) from various types of food.

	% total	% sugar
Cereal products	46	23
(bread)	22	–)
Fruit and vegetables	27	14[*]
Sugar, confectionery, jams	13	29
Soft drinks	7	17
Milk and milk products	6	13[†]

[*] This is mainly as intrinsic sugars within plant cell walls.

We can divide the sugars in the diet into two groups:
(a) **intrinsic sugars** in fruits, which are contained within plant cell walls; and
(b) **extrinsic sugars**, which are free in solution in the food and not contained within plant cell walls.

Extrinsic sugars consist of the sugars released into solution when fruit juice is prepared, sugar and honey added to foods and the lactose in milk. Milk is an excellent source of a variety of nutrients, most notably calcium (see p. 282) and riboflavin (see p. 257). Apart from people who are intolerant of lactose (the sugar of milk, see p. 133), there is no evidence that lactose is associated with any health hazards. It is the **non-milk extrinsic sugars** which give cause for concern, and for which we have guidelines.

Although there are many different sugars in the diet, the ones that cause most concern are sucrose (cane or beet sugar, a disaccharide of glucose and fructose, see p. 73) and honey (which is a mixture of glucose and fructose). There is some evidence that a high intake of sugar is a factor in the development of maturity-onset diabetes and atherosclerosis, although the evidence is less convincing than for the deleterious effects of a high intake of saturated fats. However, there is strong evidence for a harmful effect of sugar in the development of obesity and dental caries.

Sugar added to foods is a source of additional energy, but provides no nutrients. It makes many foods more palatable, and hence increases consumption. It may thus have a significant rôle in the development of obesity (see Ch. 7). This added sugar is mainly sucrose, although glucose syrups and mixtures of glucose and fructose are widely used in food manufacturing.

Extrinsic sugars have a major rôle in the development of dental caries. Sucrose especially (but also other sugars) encourages the growth of the bacteria which form dental plaque, and provides a metabolic substrate for the production by other bacteria of the acid that attacks dental enamel. Other factors are also important in the development of dental caries, including general oral hygiene and, perhaps most importantly, the intake of fluoride (see p. 281). The use of fluoride-containing toothpaste and the addition of fluoride to drinking water have led to a very dramatic decrease in dental decay over the past 20 years, despite a high intake of sucrose.

The guideline is that 10–11% of energy intake should be from non-milk extrinsic sugars. This can readily be achieved by reducing consumption of soft drinks, sweets, sugar added to foods, jams and honey, etc.

Non-starch polysaccharides (dietary fibre) The residue of plant cell walls is not digested by human enzymes, but provides bulk in the diet (and hence in the intestines). It is measured by weighing the fraction of foods which remains after treatment with a variety of digestive enzymes. This is what is known as dietary fibre. It is a misleading term, since not all the components of dietary fibre are fibrous; some are soluble and form viscous gels.

Several different compounds are grouped together under the heading of "dietary fibre". Chemically, the important compounds are polysaccharides (complex carbohydrates) other than starch, and a relatively recent development has been to distinguish between starch and non-starch polysaccharides by measuring the different polysaccharides in food specifically (see p. 75).

The two methods of analysis give different results. Measurement of non-starch polysaccharide in the diet gives average intakes in Britain of between 11 and 13g/day, compared with an intake of "dietary fibre" of about 20g/day, as measured by the less specific method. Non-starch polysaccharides are found only foods of vegetable origin, and **vegetarians** in Britain have a higher intake than omnivores (of the order of 21g/day).

Non-starch polysaccharides have little nutritional value in their own

23

right, since they are compounds that are not digested or absorbed to any significant extent. Nevertheless, they are a valuable component of the diet.

Diets low in non-starch polysaccharide are associated with the excretion of a small bulk of faeces, and frequently with constipation and straining while defecating. This has been linked with the development of haemorrhoids, varicose veins and diverticular disease of the colon. These diseases are more common in Western countries, where people generally have a relatively low intake of non-starch polysaccharide, than in parts of the world where the intake is higher.

Non-starch polysaccharides may bind potentially undesirable compounds in the intestinal lumen, and so reduce their absorption. This may be especially important with respect to colon cancer. Compounds which are believed to be involved in causing or promoting cancer of the colon occur in the contents of the intestinal tract, both because they are present in foods and as a result of bacterial metabolism in the colon. They are bound by non-starch polysaccharides, and so cannot interact with the cells of the gut wall, but are eliminated in the faeces. Epidemiological studies show that diets high in non-starch polysaccharides are associated with a low risk of colon cancer. However, diets rich in non-starch polysaccharides are those which contain a relatively large amount of fruit and vegetables, and therefore such diets are generally also rich in vitamins C and E and carotene, which also have some protective action against the development of cancer (see Ch. 11). Furthermore, since they contain more fruit and vegetables, and less meat, such diets are also generally relatively low in saturated fats, and there is some evidence that a high intake of saturated fats is a separate risk factor for colon cancer.

A diet rich in non-starch polysaccharide may help to lower blood cholesterol. This is because the bile salts, which are required for the absorption of fats (see p. 133) are formed in the liver from cholesterol and are secreted in the bile. Normally a considerable proportion of the bile salts is reabsorbed; when the diet is rich in non-starch polysaccharides, bile salts are bound, and so cannot be reabsorbed. This means that more bile salts have to be synthesized, so using up more cholesterol.

A total intake of about 18g of non-starch polysaccharides/day is recommended (equivalent to about 30g/day of "dietary fibre"). In general this should come from fibre-rich foods – whole-grain cereals and wholemeal cereal products, fruits and vegetables – rather than supplements. This is because as well as the fibre, these fibre-rich foods are valuable sources of a variety of nutrients. There is no evidence that intakes of more than about 30g/day of non-starch polysaccharide confer any benefit, other than in the treatment of bowel disease. Above this level of intake it is likely that you would reach satiety (or at least feel full, or even bloated) without eating enough food to satisfy energy needs. This may be a problem for children fed on a diet very high in non-starch polysaccharides; they may be physically full but still physiologically hungry.

Salt

There is a physiological requirement for the mineral sodium, and salt (chemically sodium chloride) is the major dietary source of sodium. One of the basic senses of taste is for saltiness – a pleasant sensation (see p. 6). However, average intakes of salt in Western countries are considerably higher than the physiological requirement for sodium. Most people are able to cope with this excessive intake with no problem; they just excrete the excess. However, people with a familial tendency to develop high blood pressure are sensitive to the amount of sodium in their diet. One of the ways of treating dangerously high blood pressure (hypertension) is by a severe restriction of salt intake. It is estimated that about 10% of the population have a genetic predisposition to develop hypertension in response to a high salt intake, and epidemiologically there is a relationship between sodium intake and the increase in blood pressure which occurs with increasing age.

The problem in terms of public health and general dietary advice (as opposed to specific advice to people known to be at risk of, or suffering from, hypertension) is one of extrapolating from clinical studies in people who have severe hypertension, and who benefit from a severe restriction in salt intake, to the population at large. We do not know whether a modest reduction in salt intake will benefit either the population at large, or those salt-sensitive individuals who might go on to develop severe hypertension. Nevertheless, it is prudent to recommend reducing the average intake of salt by about one-quarter, to a level that meets requirements for sodium without providing so great an excess over requirements as is seen in average diets at present. This can be achieved quite easily by reducing the amount of salt added in cooking, tasting food before adding salt at the table, and reducing the intake of salty snack foods. Low-sodium salt substitutes, containing mixtures of sodium and potassium chlorides (commonly called "light salt") are available. They can be used in place of ordinary salt to help reduce the intake of sodium.

Alcohol

A high intake of alcoholic drinks can be a factor in causing obesity, both as a result of the energy yield of the alcohol itself, and also because of the relatively high carbohydrate content of many alcoholic beverages. People who satisfy much of their energy requirement from alcohol frequently show vitamin deficiencies, because they are meeting their energy needs from drink, and therefore are not eating enough foods to provide adequate amounts of vitamins and minerals. Deficiency of vitamin B_1 is especially a problem among heavy drinkers (see p. 255).

In moderate amounts, alcohol has an appetite-stimulating effect, and may also help the social aspect of meals. However, in excess it has harmful effects, not only in the short term, when drunkenness may have undesirable consequences, but also in the longer term. Excess consumption of alcohol is associated with long-term health problems, including loss of mental capacity, liver damage and cancer of the oesophagus. Continued abuse can lead to physical and psychological addiction. The infants of mothers who drink more than a very small amount of alcohol during pregnancy are at risk of congenital abnormalities, and heavy alcohol consumption during pregnancy can result in the fetal alcohol syndrome: low birth weight and lasting impairment of intelligence, as well as congenital deformities.

The guidelines on alcohol intake are summarized in Table 2.10.

Table 2.10 The alcohol content of beverages.

	% alcohol by volume
Beer and cider	4–6
Table wine	9.5–12.5
Vermouth, aperitifs	15–18
Port and sherry	18–20
Spirits	35–45

We can calculate alcohol intake in "units of alcohol":
1 unit = 8g of alcohol
      = ½ pint beer
      = 1 glass of wine
      = 1 single measure of spirits
The limits of upper habitual intake recommended by the Royal College of Physicians are:
men: 21 units/week = 168g alcohol
women: 14 units/week = 112g alcohol

Food labelling

By law, food labels must contain a list of the ingredients of the food, in order of the quantities present. Food additives may be listed by either their chemical names or numbers in the list of permitted additives (the "E" numbers).

The weight or volume of the contents must also be shown on the label; where this is a size that has been registered with the appropriate authority of the European Community, the weight or volume is preceded by a small letter "e". The name of the manufacturer must also appear on the label.

Increasingly, food labels give more information: the energy yield, and the content of fat, protein and carbohydrate. This nutritional labelling is intended to give the consumer enough information to make sensible choices about what to eat in order to achieve the nutritional goals discussed in this chapter.

Many manufacturers provide additional information, listing the proportion or amount of saturated and unsaturated fats in the foods, and sometimes the proportion of the total carbohydrate which is present as starches and sugars. This more detailed nutritional labelling is not yet obligatory, but if the information is provided, it must be in a standard format. If *any* nutritional claims are made then full nutritional information must be given, in the prescribed form.

Claims for the vitamin and mineral content of foods must similarly be made in a standard format, and may only be made if the food in question provides a significant percentage of requirements. The content of vitamins and minerals must be shown as both the amount present and as the percentage of the reference intake (see p. 232).

Is there any need for nutritional supplements?

Average intakes of vitamins and minerals in developed countries are more than adequate to meet requirements, and deficiency diseases are rarely, if ever, due simply to an inadequate intake. The main nutritional problems in developed countries are associated with an excessive intake of food, and especially saturated fats and sugars, not with inadequate intakes of nutrients. There is no evidence that supplements of vitamins and minerals will increase a child's intelligence or ability to learn, although if the child was marginally deficient then supplements would, of course, be beneficial. Nevertheless, there is an ever-growing market for vitamin and mineral supplements, as well as a host of compounds of dubious nutritional value.

Apart from vitamin and mineral supplements which provide about the reference nutrient intake of the various nutrients (itself an amount greater than average requirements, see p. 232), preparations are available which provide very large amounts of individual vitamins, minerals or amino acids. Here we are not considering nutritional factors at all, but rather possible pharmacological or drug-like actions of compounds which also happen to be nutrients. Because they are nutrients, they are subject to food laws, and hence freely available, rather than the laws governing the sale of medicines, which would require clear evidence of efficacy and safety before a Medicines Licence could be issued. The possible pharmacological actions of some vitamins and minerals, and the dangers of excessive intakes, are discussed in Chapter 11.

Summary

We can summarize the nutritional guidelines and goals very simply:
(a) Eat as wide variety of foods as you can.
(b) Read the labels on foods. These will generally give you a great deal of information, but read the small print containing the nutrition information on the side of the package as well as the bold flash on the front which claims that the contents are "low in fat" or "low in sugar".
(c) Eat at least one meal of fish a week.
(d) Eat at least one portion of fruit or green vegetables each day.
(e) Try eating vegetarian dishes instead of meat now and again.
(f) Preferably eat wholemeal bread and whole-grain cereal products.
(g) Trim visible fat off meat, grill or roast meat rather than frying it.
(h) Buy low-fat mince, sausages, etc.
(i) Use vegetable oils and margarine rich in polyunsaturated fats in preference to saturated cooking fats and butter. Perhaps use low-fat spreads rather than butter or margarine.
(j) Try using semi-skimmed or skimmed milk instead of full-cream milk (but not for young children).
(k) Try using yoghurt rather than cream; but be warned that fruit-flavoured yoghurts contain a lot of sugar.
(l) Reduce your intake of sugar; if you must sweeten tea and coffee, use non-nutritive sweeteners; try "low calorie" lemonades made with non-nutritive sweeteners (see p. 176).
(m) Do not add salt to food unless you have tasted it and know you need to add it.
(n) Drink alcohol in moderation and try to have an "alcohol-free" day now and again.
Finally, remember that there is nothing "wrong" with white bread, cakes, whipped cream, hamburgers, etc., occasionally!

CHAPTER THREE

The chemical basis of life

If we are to understand the basis of the dietary guidelines discussed in Chapter 2, to interpret and evaluate new evidence of health risks and benefits from changes in our diet and appreciate the way in which nutrition is important for the maintenance of the normal integrity and functions of the body, we have to understand the chemistry and metabolism of the body. This chapter reviews the basic principles of chemistry which are important for an understanding of nutrition and metabolism, and Chapter 4 reviews the structures of biologically and metabolically important compounds.

Elements and atoms

The basic unit of chemical structure is the atom. There are 112 different chemical **elements** known, of which 96 occur naturally, the remainder being the products of nuclear reactions. Only a few of the elements are important in biological systems. Each element has a characteristic atomic composition, but the underlying structure of all atoms is similar.

An **atom** consists of a **nucleus**, which has a positive electric charge, surrounded by a cloud of **electrons**, which have a negative electric charge. The number of positively charged particles in the nucleus (protons) is equal to the number of electrons surrounding the nucleus, so that an atom has a no net electrical charge.

The simplest element is hydrogen, which consists of a single proton, accompanied by a single electron. We can classify the different elements by the number of protons in the nucleus (and hence the number of electrons surrounding the nucleus). This is the atomic number of that element. Each element has a unique atomic number.

As well as protons, the nuclei of most elements contain uncharged particles, the most important of which are the **neutrons**. The mass of a neutron is almost the same as that of a proton (which is 1.67×10^{-24} g; the mass of an electron is only 1/1840 of that of a proton, and we can consider it to be negligible). We assign a relative **atomic mass** or weight to each element, based on the number of protons and neutrons in the atomic nucleus, with 1 unit of mass for each proton or neutron. Table 3.1 lists some of the elements which are important in biological systems, together with their atomic numbers and relative atomic masses.

For convenience when we are writing chemical formulae, we use one- or two-letter abbreviations of the names of the elements. Some are obvious and simple, for example H for hydrogen, C for carbon, Ca for calcium. Others are less obvious. This is because two or more different elements could have the same abbreviation. Therefore, we use abbreviations based on the old Latin names. Thus copper is Cu, from *cuprum*, to avoid confusion with cobalt, which is Co; iron is Fe, from *ferrum*; sodium is Na, from *natrium* and potassium is K, from *kalium*. These abbreviations are also shown in Table 3.1.

Although the composition of the nucleus is unique for any element, the distribution of electrons around the nucleus determines the chemical reactivity of the atom, and hence the characteristic chemistry of that element.

Electrons are not randomly distributed around the nucleus, but occupy a series of concentric shells or orbitals. Those orbitals nearest to the nucleus are filled first. Elements with a higher atomic number will have a greater total number of electrons surrounding the nucleus, and hence their atoms will be larger than those of elements with lower atomic numbers. As an idea of the size of atoms, the diameter of the outermost orbital of electrons around the carbon atom (atomic number = 6) is 0.154 nm, about 10^4 times larger than the nucleus.

The outermost electrons participate in chemical reactions. This means that elements with a similar distribution of electrons in the outermost orbitals will have similar chemistry.

Isotopes

The chemistry of the elements is determined by their atomic number, and therefore the electron distribution around the nucleus. Some elements exist in multiple forms, called **isotopes**, with differing nuclear composition. As discussed below, isotopes are widely used in biochemical, nutritional and medical research.

Table 3.1 The biologically important elements.

	Symbol	Atomic number	Atomic mass
Carbon	C	6	12.01
Hydrogen	H	1	1.00
Oxygen	O	8	16.00
Nitrogen	N	7	14.00
Phosphorus	P	15	30.98
Aluminium	Al	13	26.97
Calcium	Ca	20	40.08
Chlorine	Cl	17	35.46
Chromium	Cr	24	52.01
Cobalt	Co	27	58.94
Copper	Cu	29	63.57
Fluorine	F	9	19.00
Iodine	I	53	126.91
Iron	Fe	26	55.85
Lead	Pb	82	207.21
Lithium	Li	3	6.94
Magnesium	Mg	12	24.32
Manganese	Mn	25	54.93
Mercury	Hg	80	200.61
Molybdenum	Mo	42	95.95
Nickel	Ni	28	58.69
Potassium	K	19	39.09
Selenium	Se	34	78.96
Sodium	Na	11	22.97
Sulphur	S	16	32.06
Tin	Sn	50	118.70
Zinc	Zn	30	65.38

The nuclei of the different isotopes of any element contain the same number of protons, and therefore they have the same number of electrons, and chemically they react in the same way. However, the nuclei of the different isotopes contain different numbers of neutrons, so that the isotopes differ from each other in their atomic mass, which is measurable.

Some of the isotopes of some elements are unstable, and their nuclei break down, emitting radiation. These are the radioactive isotopes, and we can detect and measure them by the radiation they emit. Other isotopes are stable; their nuclei do not decay, and they do not emit any radiation. We can detect and measure them only by their atomic mass.

If we wish to specify that we are considering a particular isotope, we do this by writing the atomic mass of that isotope as a superscript before the abbreviation for the element. Thus, the most commonly occurring form of carbon has atomic mass $= 12$, while the radioactive isotope has atomic mass $= 14$. We show this by writing ^{14}C when we need to specify that this is the isotope of carbon that we are considering.

Table 3.2 Isotopes commonly used in biochemical and nutritional research.

Hydrogen[*]	^{2}H stable
	^{3}H radioactive
Carbon	^{13}C stable
	^{14}C radioactive
Oxygen	^{18}O stable
Nitrogen	^{15}N stable
Sulphur	^{35}S radioactive
Phosphorus	^{32}P radioactive
Iron	^{57}Fe radioactive
	^{59}Fe radioactive
Iodine	^{125}I radioactive
	^{131}I radioactive
Sodium	^{23}Na radioactive
Calcium	^{45}Ca radioactive
Cobalt	^{65}Co radioactive

[*] The isotopes of hydrogen are sometimes called deuterium (^{2}H) and tritium (^{3}H).

Both stable and radioactive isotopes are widely used in biochemical and nutritional research; they are shown Table 3.2. A chemical compound containing one or more atoms of either a radioactive or stable isotope is **labelled** by that isotope. Although we can detect the presence of the isotope by measuring the radiation emitted as it decays, or its abnormal atomic mass, chemically the labelled compound behaves in exactly the same way as the unlabelled compound. We can use such labelled compounds to follow their metabolic fate. Many of the metabolic pathways discussed in later chapters of this book have been established in this way. We will see in Chapter 6 how the use of water labelled with ^{2}H and ^{18}O

enables us to measure peoples' average energy expenditure over a period of several weeks, and how such studies have enabled us to revise some of our estimates of energy requirements (see p. 159). In the same way, use of proteins containing the stable isotope of nitrogen, ^{15}N, allows us to follow changes in protein metabolism in the body, and so estimate protein requirements more precisely.

The radiation emitted when radioactive isotopes decay may penetrate solid matter for quite a distance before it interacts with an atom. Excessive exposure to such penetrating radiation is dangerous, because the radiation can interact with body constituents, producing highly reactive free radicals (see p. 67), causing genetic damage, or even killing cells. We frequently use controlled exposure to small amounts of such radiation, for example in X-rays to visualize internal organs, and in radiotherapy, where we rely on the damaging action of the radiation to kill the cancer cells it is focused on.

Other radioactive isotopes produce radiation with very much lower energy, which is absorbed by only a few centimetres of air, a thin layer of paper or plastic gloves. Such isotopes include ^{14}C and ^{3}H, which are commonly used in studies of metabolism. Although radioactive isotopes of carbon and hydrogen have been given to human beings in the past for experimental purposes, this is rarely done, because even though the radiation has very low energy, it can still cause tissue damage when taken internally. We do sometimes give radioactive isotopes to patients, for example when there is no other means of investigating a rare disease, or as a means of imaging specific glands and organs.

Compounds and molecules:
the formation of chemical bonds

The electrons surrounding the nucleus of an atom occupy **orbitals** in a series of defined shells. The innermost shell can contain two electrons. The next can contain eight, and the third 18. When these three sets of orbitals are filled, so a further set begins, consisting of shells capable of containing eight and 18 electrons. This is repeated as necessary to make up the characteristic pattern of electrons of the various elements.

Isolated atoms are unstable if they have unfilled "spaces" (empty orbitals) in their outer electron shells (see Fig. 3.1). The only elements whose atoms have stable, filled electron shells are the inert gases (helium, argon, neon, etc.). These gases exist stably as isolated atoms, and have very little chemical reactivity because of their stable outer electron configuration.

For all the other elements, isolated atoms are unstable, because they have unfilled orbitals. Isolated atoms of most elements only exist under extreme conditions, for example at very high temperatures, as in a flame.

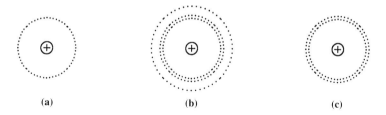

(a)   (b)   (c)

Figure 3.1 Atoms: the arrangement of electrons around the nucleus
(a) The hydrogen atom, a single positive charge in the nucleus and a single electron; (b) an unstable arrangement of electrons, a filled inner shell of two electrons, but only a single electron in the outer shell; (c) a stable arrangement of electrons, the outer shell has its full complement of electrons.

The empty orbitals can be filled, to create a stable configuration, in two ways: transfer of electrons from one atom to another to create charged particles (ions); or by the sharing of electrons between atoms, forming a covalent bond (see p. 36).

Ions and ionic bonds

The basis of ionic bonding is the transfer of electrons from one atom to another. The atoms of some elements can achieve a stable electron configuration by giving up one or more electrons to a suitable acceptor atom. Other elements achieve a stable electron configuration by accepting one or more electrons.

The result of donation or acceptance of electrons is the formation of a charged particle – an **ion**. Donation of electrons results in the formation of a positively charged ion, because there are now fewer electrons (which have a negative charge) surrounding the nucleus than there are protons (which have a positive charge) in the nucleus. Similarly, acceptance of electrons results in the formation of a negatively charged ion, since there are now more electrons surrounding the nucleus than protons within the nucleus.

Elements that can achieve a stable electron configuration by the donation of electrons, forming positive ions, are said to be **electropositive**, and are **metallic elements**. Elements that can achieve a stable electron configuration by the acceptance of electrons, forming negative ions, are said to be **electronegative**, and are **non-metallic** elements. Hydrogen occupies an interesting position; it has one electron, and can achieve stability by either donating that electron, resulting in the formation of a proton (H^+ ion) or, less commonly, accepting an electron from a donor, resulting in the formation of the H^- (hydride) ion.

The magnitude of the positive charge on a metal ion depends on the number of electrons it has donated.

A metal which has one "spare" electron can achieve a stable configuration by donating one electron to an acceptor, so forming an ion with a single positive charge. Biologically important metals which form ions with a single positive charge include sodium (Na^+) and potassium (K^+).

A metal which has two "spare" electrons can achieve a stable configuration by donating two electrons to an acceptor, so forming an ion with a double positive charge. Biologically important metals which form ions with a double positive charge include calcium (Ca^{2+}), magnesium (Mg^{2+}) and zinc (Zn^{2+}).

Some metals can achieve more than one stable configuration of electrons, and thus can form more than one positively charged ion. For example, copper can form ions with single or double positive charges (Cu^+ or Cu^{2+}) and iron can similarly form ions with two or three positive charges (Fe^{2+} or Fe^{3+}).

In the same way as different metals can achieve a stable electron configuration by donating different numbers of electrons, and hence forming ions with different positive charges, so different non-metals can form stable ions with different negative charges, by accepting different numbers of electrons.

An element which lacks one electron to achieve stability can accept one electron from a donor, forming an ion with a single negative charge. Biologically important elements in this group include chlorine, which forms the chloride ion (Cl^-), fluorine (forming the fluoride ion, F^-) and iodine (forming the iodide ion, I^-).

An element which lacks two electrons to achieve stability can accept two electrons from a donor, forming an ion with a double negative charge. Biologically important elements in this group include oxygen, which forms the oxide ion (O^{2-}) and sulphur, which forms the sulphide ion (S^{2-}).

Ions do not exist in isolation. The total number of positive and negative charges is always equal, with no net electric charge. Thus, ordinary salt is sodium chloride; we can write its formula as NaCl, although it consists of Na^+ and Cl^- ions. Calcium chloride is $CaCl_2$: $Ca^{2+} + 2 \times Cl^-$.

Covalent bonding – the sharing of electrons between atoms

In addition to achieving a stable electron configuration by an overall transfer of electrons between atoms, to form ions, atoms can achieve stability by sharing electrons. An electron which is shared between two atoms can be considered to spend part of its time in the empty orbitals of each atom, thus creating a stable configuration of partially occupied orbitals around the two nuclei. This sharing of electrons forms a **bond** between the atoms, and we now talk about a **molecule** rather than separate atoms or ions.

Each atom requires to share a characteristic number of electrons with other atoms to achieve a stable configuration. This means that each element forms a characteristic number of bonds to other atoms in a molecule. We call the number of bonds which must be formed by an element to achieve a stable electron configuration the **valency** of that element.

This type of chemical bond between atoms is called **covalent bonding**, because the individual atoms making up the molecule share electrons in such a way that each achieves a share in the number of electrons required to meet its valency requirement and so complete a stable outer shell of electrons.

Hydrogen has one electron per atom, and therefore requires to share one more to achieve a stable electron configuration. Hydrogen thus forms one bond to another atom and has a valency of 1.

Oxygen has six electrons in its outermost electron shell, and requires to share two more to achieve a stable electron configuration. Oxygen thus forms two bonds to other atoms and has a valency of 2.

Nitrogen has five electrons in its outermost electron shell, and requires to share three more to achieve a stable electron configuration. Nitrogen thus forms three bonds to other atoms and has a valency of 3.

Carbon has four electrons in its outermost electron shell, and requires to share four more to achieve a stable electron configuration. Carbon thus forms four bonds to other atoms and has a valency of 4.

The simplest molecules consist of two atoms of the same kind, as occurs in the gases hydrogen, oxygen and nitrogen, forming molecules written as H_2, O_2 or N_2 (see Fig. 3.2). The two atoms each share electrons so as to achieve a stable electron configuration as follows: two atoms of hydrogen share two electrons, forming one bond, H–H. Two atoms of oxygen share four electrons, forming two bonds, O=O. Two atoms of nitrogen share six electrons, forming three bonds, N≡N.

Covalent bonding also occurs between atoms of different elements (see Fig. 3.3). The number of bonds formed is determined by the number of empty orbitals in each atom, i.e. the valency of each element.

In water, two atoms of hydrogen each share two electrons with one atom of oxygen. The result is H–O–H (H_2O). Each hydrogen now has a

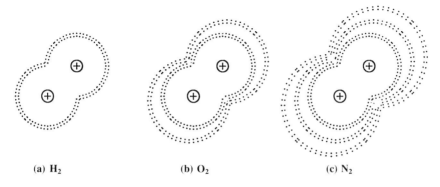

(a) H_2 (b) O_2 (c) N_2

Figure 3.2 Covalent bonding
The sharing of electrons between atoms to achieve a stable arrangement in the molecule.
(a) **Hydrogen** (H_2). Each atom of hydrogen has one electron, and requires to gain a share
in one more to achieve a stable arrangement. In the molecule of hydrogen (H_2) each atom
has a share in two electrons, and there is a single bond between the two hydrogen atoms
(H–H). (b) **Oxygen** (O_2). Each atom of oxygen requires four electrons in the outermost
shell to achieve a stable configuration. In the molecule of oxygen (O_2) four electrons are
shared between the two atoms, forming a double bond (O=O). (c) **Nitrogen** (N_2). Each
atom of nitrogen requires six electrons in the outermost shell to achieve a stable
configuration. In the molecule of nitrogen (N_2) six electrons are shared between the two
atoms, forming a triple bond (N≡N).

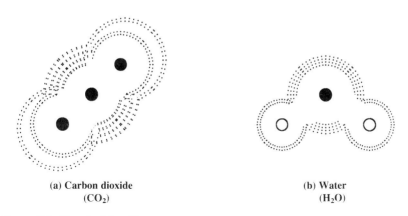

(a) **Carbon dioxide**   (b) **Water**
(CO_2)   (H_2O)

Figure 3.3 Covalent bonding
The sharing of electrons between different atoms to achieve a stable arrangement in the
molecule. (a) **Carbon dioxide**: two atoms of oxygen each share four electrons with an
atom of carbon. As a result, each oxygen atom now has a share in four electrons, and
so has a stable configuration. Similarly, the carbon atom has a share in eight electrons
in its outermost shell, and it too has a stable electron configuration. We show the
resultant molecule, consisting of one atom of carbon and two of oxygen, as CO_2. Each
oxygen has formed a double bond to the carbon atom (O=C=O). (b) **Water**: two atoms
of hydrogen each share two electrons with one atom of oxygen. As a result, each
hydrogen atom now has a share in two electrons, and so has a stable configuration.
Similarly, the oxygen atom has a share in four electrons in its outermost shell, and it too
has a stable configuration. We show the resultant molecule, consisting of two atoms of
hydrogen and one of oxygen as H_2O. Each atom of hydrogen has formed a single bond
to the oxygen atom (H–O–H).

37

share in two electrons, and forms one bond; the oxygen atom has a share in four electrons, and thus forms two bonds, one to each hydrogen.

In carbon dioxide, two atoms of oxygen each share four electrons with an atom of carbon. The result is O=C=O (CO_2). Each oxygen now has a share in four electrons, and the carbon has a share in eight.

If we consider simple compounds of carbon and hydrogen, we can see how valency can be satisfied by a mixture of single and double bonds.

The simplest such compound is the gas methane (CH_4). Here four atoms of hydrogen each share electrons with carbon, so completing the valency of hydrogen (1) and that of carbon (4).

The same occurs with the gas ethane (C_2H_6). Here there is one bond formed between the two carbon atoms, and the remaining three valencies of each carbon are completed by sharing electrons with hydrogen atoms: $H_3C–CH_3$.

In the gas ethene (sometimes also called ethylene, C_2H_4) a **double bond** is formed between the two carbon atoms, so that two of the four valencies of each carbon have been satisfied. Therefore each carbon only needs to share electrons with two hydrogens to complete its valency of four: $H_2C=CH_2$.

In the gas ethyne (sometimes also called acetylene, C_2H_2) a triple bond is formed between the two carbon atoms, so that three of the four valencies of each carbon have been satisfied. Therefore each carbon only needs to share electrons with one hydrogen to complete its valency: $HC{\equiv}CH$.

Such compounds, with carbon–carbon double or triple bonds, are called **unsaturated compounds**. Although they form stable molecules, in which all the valencies of carbon are occupied, they can react with more hydrogen, until they form what is called a **saturated** compound, i.e. one in which there is only a single bond between the carbon atoms, and all the remaining valencies of the carbon are occupied by sharing electrons with hydrogen. Ethyne can be partially saturated with hydrogen, to form ethene:

$$HC{\equiv}CH + H_2 \rightarrow H_2C=CH_2.$$

In turn, ethene can react with more hydrogen, becoming the fully saturated compound ethane:

$$H_2C=CH_2 + H_2 \rightarrow H_3C–CH_3.$$

Here, for clarity, we have shown the double and triple bonds between the separate carbon atoms. However, we could also write these reactions without showing the double and triple bonds, as:

$$C_2H_2 + H_2 \rightarrow C_2H_4$$
$$C_2H_4 + H_2 \rightarrow C_2H_6.$$

Triple bonds between carbon atoms are rare in biologically important molecules. However, you will see later on that carbon–carbon double bonds are extremely important in a variety of biochemical systems. We have already seen that saturated and unsaturated fatty acids have different effects in the body, and that we have guidelines not only about the total amount of fat in the diet, but also the proportion of saturated and unsaturated fat (see p. 19).

Molecular mass and moles

If we wish to talk about equivalent amounts of compounds, we need to know how many molecules of each compound we are considering, rather than the mass or weight of the compounds. We calculate the **relative molecular mass** (M_r, sometimes called the **molecular weight**) of any compound if we know its chemical formula, from the relative atomic masses of its constituent atoms (see Table 3.1). For example:

$$\text{methane} = CH_4 = 1 \times C\,(= 12) + 4 \times H\,(= 4 \times 1 = 4)$$
$$\text{therefore its molecular mass } (M_r) = 16$$
$$\text{water} = H_2O = 2 \times H\,(= 2 \times 1) + 1 \times O\,(= 16)$$
$$\text{therefore its molecular mass } (M_r) = 18$$
$$\text{carbon dioxide} = CO_2 = 1 \times C\,(= 12) + 2 \times O\,(= 2 \times 16 = 32)$$
$$\text{therefore its molecular mass } (M_r) = 44.$$

Since the molecules of methane, water and carbon dioxide have different masses, it is obvious that 1g of each will contain a different number of molecules; in other words, different amounts of each compound, although there will be the same mass of each compound present. There are more molecules of water ($M_r = 18$) in 1g of water than there are molecules of carbon dioxide in 1 g of carbon dioxide ($M_r = 44$). When we describe chemical or biochemical reactions, we have to consider the number of molecules that are present to react with each other, not the mass of material present.

When we want to talk about numbers of molecules of different compounds, rather than grams of those compounds, we use the term **mole** (abbreviated to mol, and derived from molecule). The mol is defined as the relative molecular mass of a compound, expressed in grams, and is the SI unit for the amount of substance present.

Thus we can say that for the reaction:

$$A + B \rightarrow C$$

one mol of compound A reacts with one mol of compound B to form one mol of the product C.

One mol of a compound has a mass equal to the relative molecular mass in grams; thus 1 mol of methane weighs 16 g, 1 mol of water 18 g and 1 mol of carbon dioxide 44 g. We can calculate the number of mol of a compound in a given mass from the same information; for example, 1g of methane contains $1/16$ mol $= 0.0625$ mol $= 62.5$ mmol.

The states of matter: solids, liquids and gases

Molecules move continuously. Indeed, the whole of chemistry depends on the fact that molecules do move around, and hence different molecules can come together to undergo chemical reactions. The extent of their movement depends mainly on the size of the molecules (and hence on their relative molecular mass), and the temperature. At higher temperatures, molecules move faster, and farther from each other.

In a **solid**, the molecules move only relatively slowly, and do not move far from each other. Because of this, a solid has a defined shape. It expands as the temperature increases, because the molecules can move slightly farther from each other.

As the temperature of a solid increases, so the molecules move faster, and farther from each other. Eventually they reach such a speed of movement that the defined shape of the solid is lost; the solid has melted to a **liquid**. The temperature at which each compound melts is a characteristic of that particular compound, and depends on two main factors:

(a) The size of the molecules (i.e. the relative molecular mass). Larger, heavier, molecules will remain closely associated, as solids, at higher temperatures than smaller molecules.

(b) The shape of the molecules. Some molecules have a regular shape, and can interact very closely with each other. Such molecules require a greater input of energy (in the form of heat) to break away from each other and melt, than do molecules which cannot fit so closely to each other. The different shapes of saturated and unsaturated fatty acids (see p. 79) mean that unsaturated fats melt at a lower temperature than saturated fats. Indeed, unsaturated fats are liquids (oils) at ordinary temperatures, while saturated fats are solids.

As the temperature of a liquid increases, so the molecules move faster and farther from each other. We can see this by the increase in volume as a liquid is heated; for example, the thermometer we use to measure temperature depends on the fact that the mercury or alcohol inside expands, and so takes up more room, as its temperature increases.

As a liquid is heated further, so it reaches the point where the molecules break away from each other altogether, and form a gas. We say that the liquid has boiled. Like the temperature at which a compound melts, the temperature at which it boils is a characteristic, and it depends on three main factors:

(a) The size of the molecule, and hence its relative molecular mass. As with melting, larger, heavier molecules require a greater input of energy in order to break away from the liquid.

(b) Interactions between the molecules. These may depend on the shape of the molecules, as described above for melting, or may be more complex interactions, as discussed below.

(c) The pressure. Boiling requires the molecules to break away from the liquid and join other molecules in the gas phase. At higher pressure, the molecules have to move faster to join the gas phase, and therefore have to be heated to a higher temperature. We can see this, for example, in a pressure cooker or autoclave. At a pressure of 15 lb above atmospheric pressure, water reaches a temperature of 121 °C without boiling. Not only does this cook food faster, it is also a high enough temperature to kill more or less all micro-organisms within about 15 min. This is the basis of the autoclave which is used to sterilize surgical instruments, dressings, etc.

Interactions between molecules – why water is a liquid

Both methane ($M_r = 16$) and carbon dioxide ($M_r = 44$) are gases at ordinary temperature and pressure, yet water ($M_r = 18$) is a liquid. This is because water molecules can interact with each other in a way which carbon dioxide and methane molecules cannot.

Although we show the formation of a covalent bond as the sharing of one or more electrons between the atoms making up the molecule, this is not always completely even sharing. Some atoms exert a greater attraction for the shared electrons than do their partners (see Fig. 3.4). This means that often one atom has a greater share of the electrons forming a covalent bond than does the other. The atom which attracts the shared electrons more strongly is said to be more **electronegative** than the other atom.

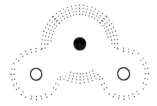

Figure 3.4 Unequal sharing of electrons in covalent bonding
The oxygen atom of the water molecule exerts a slightly greater attraction for the shared electrons than do the hydrogen atoms. Oxygen is more electronegative than hydrogen. As a result, the electrons spend more of their time associated with the oxygen than with either of the hydrogens. Overall, the oxygen has a small (partial) negative charge (shown as δ^-) and the hydrogen atoms have a small (partial) positive charge (shown as δ^+).

Oxygen is more electronegative than hydrogen. This means that in water the oxygen atom tends to attract the shared electrons more strongly than the hydrogen atoms. The result is that the oxygen atom has a slight excess of negative charge, and the hydrogen atoms have a slight excess of positive charge. As shown in Figure 3.5, we show this as δ^- associated with the oxygen and δ^+ associated with the hydrogen, where the δ^- or δ^+ indicates a partial charge, not the full charge associated with the transfer of an electron from one atom to the other. Therefore water has (small) positive and negative charges in the same molecule. Opposite charges attract each other, so we can see that water can form weak bonds from the δ^- of its oxygen to the δ^+ charge of a hydrogen on another molecule. These intermolecular bonds are called **hydrogen bonds**.

Because of this hydrogen bonding, water molecules require a greater input of heat in order to break away from each other and boil than would be expected from the M_r of water. Therefore, at temperatures between 0° and 100°C water is a liquid, while carbon dioxide and methane are both gases. There is equal sharing of the electrons in the covalent bonds in carbon dioxide and methane, and therefore no development of partial charges to form hydrogen bonds.

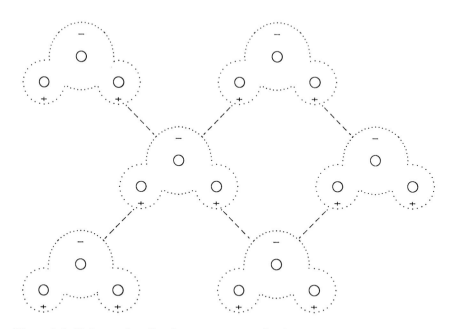

Figure 3.5 Hydrogen bonding between water molecules
The partial negative charges (δ^-) on the oxygen atoms of individual water molecules attract the partial positive (δ^+) charges on the hydrogen atoms of different molecules. As a result there is a some electrical bonding between adjacent water molecules. This is hydrogen bonding.

Solution in water – ions and electrolytes When compounds which are formed by ionic bonding are dissolved in water, the ions separate from each other and interact with the water molecules. Since opposite charges attract each other, positively charged ions interact with the δ^- charges on the oxygen atoms of the water molecule, while negatively charged ions interact with the δ^+ charges on the hydrogen atoms of the water molecule. We say that such compounds **ionize** when they are dissolved in water.

Compounds which ionize on solution in water are called **electrolytes**, because they will carry an electric current. The ions move to the oppositely charged electric pole:

(a) Positively charged ions move to the negative pole. This pole is called the cathode, and ions that move to the cathode are called **cations**.

(b) Negatively charged ions move to the positive pole, which is called the anode. Such ions are called **anions**.

Solution of non-ionic compounds in water Any compound that contains atoms which are relatively electropositive or electronegative, so that there is uneven sharing of electrons in covalent bonds, and the development of δ^- and δ^+ partial charges on the surface of the molecule, can interact with the partial charges on the water molecules, and so dissolve.

If a compound is dissolved in water, it appears to disappear. This is because the many molecules of the compound which made up the crystal of the solid separate from each other and become dispersed in the water, because the molecules can interact with water molecules rather than each other. The result is a **solution**. We can call water the **solvent**, and the compound which has dissolved in the water to form the solution is the **solute**.

Although the individual molecules of the solute have been separated from each other, and dispersed throughout the solution, they are still present as molecules. Dissolving a compound does not break covalent bonds which make up the molecules; it simply disperses the individual molecules uniformly throughout the solution.

More complex ions

Not all ions are formed by single atoms of elements donating or accepting electrons. Atoms can achieve a stable electron configuration by covalent bonding, ion formation or a mixture of the two.

Many of the biologically important ions are of this type: a covalent molecule which also donates or accepts electrons to achieve a stable configuration. Examples of such ions are shown in Table 3.3.

The ammonium ion, NH_4^+, arises when ammonia gas (NH_3) dissolves in water, as a result of interaction between ammonia and water:

$$NH_3 + H_2O \rightleftharpoons NH_4^+ + OH^-.$$

Note here that the ammonia has attracted a hydrogen ion (H^+) from the water, to form the positively charged **ammonium ion** (NH_4^+), and a negative **hydroxyl ion** (OH^-) from the rest of the water molecule. Note also that we write this reaction with arrows in both directions. It is a readily reversible process. The solution will contain both unionized ammonia (NH_3) and ammonium ions (NH_4^+).

Table 3.3 Some biologically important complex ions.

Ion	Formula	M_r
Ammonium	NH_4^+	18
Carbonate	CO_3^{2-}	60
Bicarbonate	HCO_3^-	61
Phosphate	PO_4^{3-}	95
Sulphate	SO_4^{2-}	96
Nitrate	NO_3^-	62
Acetate	CH_3COO^-	59

We see a similar process, but this time with a different effect on the water molecule, when carbon dioxide dissolves in water:

$$CO_2 + H_2O \rightleftharpoons H^+ + HCO_3^-.$$

In this case the carbon dioxide has interacted with a hydroxyl ion (OH^-) derived from water, to form the **bicarbonate ion**, leaving a hydrogen ion (H^+) to balance the charge in the solution. Again, the process is reversible and the solution will contain both bicarbonate ions and unionized carbon dioxide.

Acids and bases: pH and buffers

We saw above how when carbon dioxide dissolves in water it interacts with water to form a bicarbonate ion (HCO_3^-) and a hydrogen ion (H^+). Compounds of this type, which **dissociate** when dissolved in water to give rise to hydrogen ions and an anion are called **acids**. Indeed, carbon dioxide is sometimes still called by its old name of "carbonic acid".

Other examples of acids include hydrochloric acid (HCl) and acetic acid (CH_3COOH). Both of these dissociate in the same way when they dissolve in water: hydrochloric acid gives the chloride ion (Cl^-) and a hydrogen ion, while acetic acid yields the acetate ion (CH_3COO^-) and a hydrogen ion. (You may sometimes see acetic acid referred to by its formal systematic chemical name, ethanoic acid.)

Acids do not always dissociate completely into ions when they are dissolved in water. We can classify the strength of acids by the extent to which they do dissociate; in other words, by how much is present in a solution as the undissociated acid, and how much as ions. The acidity of a solution will depend on both the strength of the acid and its concentration, i.e. how much is present in the solution.

Hydrochloric acid a strong acid; it is more or less completely dissociated in water. Acetic acid and carbon dioxide are a relatively weak acids; they are only partially dissociated in water.

The opposite of acids are the **alkalis** or **bases**. These are compounds which dissolve in water to give positively charged ions (cations) and a negatively charged hydroxide ion (OH^-). An example of a strong base is sodium hydroxide (NaOH, caustic soda):

$$NaOH + H_2O \rightarrow Na^+ + OH^- + H_2O.$$

Like a strong acid, it is more or less completely dissociated in solution.

An example of a relatively weak base is ammonia (NH_3):

$$NH_3 + H_2O \rightleftharpoons NH_4^+ + OH^-.$$

In this case we can see that some ammonia (NH_3) remains in the solution, although some has gained a hydrogen ion from water to form the ammonium ion (NH_4^+).

If we mix equal amounts of solutions of an acid and a base, the hydrogen ions of the acid solution react with the hydroxyl ions of the base, forming water:

$$H^+ + OH^- \rightarrow H_2O.$$

The result is a mixture of the positively charged ion of the base and the negatively charged ion of the acid. This is a **salt**. For example, if we mix hydrochloric acid and sodium hydroxide together, the result is sodium chloride (a mixture of Na^+ and Cl^- ions) – sodium chloride is what we call ordinary table salt.

$$Na^+ + OH^- + H^+ + Cl^- \rightarrow Na^+ + Cl^- + H_2O.$$

The reaction between hydrogen ions and hydroxide ions to form water proceeds with the production of a great deal of heat; if you mix an acid and an alkali the solution becomes hot, and indeed may even boil explosively in a concentrated solution. This is because, all other things being equal, H_2O is very much more stable than a mixture of H^+ and OH^- ions. In other words, the equilibrium

$$H^+ + OH^- \rightleftharpoons H_2O$$

lies well over to the right-hand side.

If we take pure water, we find that only a minute proportion is present as hydrogen and hydroxyl ions. The concentration of H^+ ions is only 10^{-7} mol/litre, while there are 55mol/litre of H_2O. In pure water the concentration of OH^- ions equals that of H^+ ions, i.e. we have **neutrality**.

Since an acid is a compound which dissociates in solution to give hydrogen ions and negatively charged ions, we can measure the acidity of a solution by measuring the concentration of H^+ ions present. The higher the concentration of H^+ ions, the more acid it is. Conversely, an alkaline solution is one in which the concentration of H^+ ions is lower than 10^{-7} mol/litre (and the concentration of OH^- ions is higher).

We could express acidity and alkalinity as simple concentrations of hydrogen ions, but this becomes rather cumbersome, and what is normally done is to take the logarithm of the concentration of hydrogen ions:

At neutrality the concentration of hydrogen ions $= 10^{-7}$ mol/l
$$\log(10^{-7}) = -7.$$
For convenience, to avoid negative numbers, we use the negative logarithm of the concentration of hydrogen ions:
$$-\log(10^{-7}) = 7.$$
We call this negative logarithm of the concentration of hydrogen ions the **pH** (for potential hydrogen). A neutral solution, in which the concentration of both H^+ and OH^- ions is 10^{-7} mol/l has a pH of 7.0. An acid solution has a pH lower than 7, because there are more than 10^{-7} mol of H^+ ions per litre. Similarly, an alkaline solution has a pH higher than 7, because there are fewer than 10^{-7} mol of H^+ ions per litre.

The complete range of the pH scale is from 1 (which is very strongly acid) to 14 (which is very strongly alkaline). In biological systems we are generally concerned with a narrow range of pH around neutrality, from about 5 to 9, although it is noteworthy that the gastric juice is strongly acid, with a pH of about 1.5–2.

Using a logarithmic scale for pH disguises the fact that an apparently small change in pH is a very large change in the concentration of H^+ ions, and hence a large change in acidity or alkalinity. A change of one pH unit represents a ten-fold change in the concentration of H^+ ions.

We can see how important this is by considering the pH of blood plasma. Normally plasma is at pH 7.4; if the pH falls to 7.2, the patient is seriously ill (we call the condition acidosis), and a fall to as low as pH 7.2 is life-threatening.

Buffers Since it is important to maintain the pH of tissue fluids as nearly constant as possible, we have to consider how this can be achieved. What we need is some kind of a system which can "mop up" spare H^+ ions when the pH begins to fall, and release H^+ ions as the pH begins to rise again. Consider the reaction between carbon dioxide and water:
$$CO_2 + H_2O \rightleftharpoons H^+ + HCO_3^-.$$
We saw above that carbon dioxide is a weak acid. The position of the equilibrium (i.e. how much is present in the solution as CO_2, compared

with how much is present as HCO_3^- and H^+ ions) depends on the relative concentrations of carbon dioxide and hydrogen ions. If the concentration of hydrogen ions rises, the equilibrium will shift to the left. Bicarbonate ions will break down to carbon dioxide and hydroxyl ions (OH^-), which then react with the hydrogen ions to form water. Conversely, if the concentration of hydrogen ions begins to fall, so more of the carbon dioxide will react to form bicarbonate and hydrogen ions.

This equilibrium between carbon dioxide and bicarbonate thus acts to stabilize the concentration of hydrogen ions in a solution. We call such a system a **buffer** – it acts to absorb changes in hydrogen ion concentration and reduce their impact. It is only when the change in hydrogen ion concentration is greater than the capacity of the buffer system that we see a detectable change in pH.

The carbon dioxide/bicarbonate system is only one of many different buffer systems in the body, although it is one of the most important in terms of maintaining the pH of plasma.

Any weak acid or base can act as a buffer around the pH at which it undergoes ionization, stabilizing the pH as the concentration of H^+ ions changes, by changing between its ionized and unionized forms. Figure 3.6

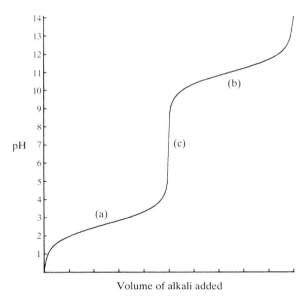

Volume of alkali added

Figure 3.6 The rôle of weak acids and weak bases as buffers
The curve shows the effect on the pH of a solution containing a weak acid (a) and a weak base (b) of adding increasing amounts of alkali. It is based on experiments with the amino acid glycine, which has both a weakly acidic group (–COOH) and a weakly basic group (–NH$_2$) in the same molecule. The formula of glycine is $H_2N–CH_2–COOH$. Both reactive groups can ionize: the –NH$_2$ group can accept a hydrogen ion (H^+), to form –NH$_3^+$; the –COOH group can lose a hydrogen ion (H^+) to form –COO$^-$.

shows the effect on pH of adding increasing amounts of alkali to a solution of the amino acid glycine ($H_2N–CH_2–COOH$). Glycine has both a weak acid group (–COOH, which can donate a hydrogen ion to form COO^-) and a weak basic group (–NH_2, which can accept a hydrogen ion to form –NH_3^+). At pH 2.4 the –COOH group is half-ionized, and it can therefore act as a buffer. At pH 9.8 the –NH_2 group is half-ionized, and it can act as a buffer around this pH.

Chemical reactions: breaking and making covalent bonds

We have seen that covalent bonds are the result of the sharing of electrons between atoms, with the result that each has a stable configuration of electrons. Elements can react with each other in different ways, to form a very wide variety of different compounds, each of which has a stable configuration of electrons. Compounds can also react with each other, by breaking some covalent bonds, and forming others.

Breaking covalent bonds requires an input of energy in some form, normally as heat, but in some cases also light or other radiation. This is the **activation energy** of the reaction. The process of breaking a bond requires activation of the electrons forming the bond – a temporary shift of one or more electrons from orbitals in which they have a stable configuration to other orbitals, farther from the nucleus. Electrons which have been activated in this way now have unstable configurations, and the covalent bonds they had contributed to are broken. Electrons cannot remain in this unstable activated state for more than a fraction of a second. They may undergo one of two fates:

(a) They may return to the configuration they had before. In other words they may re-form the same covalent bonds as existed before the compound was heated or exposed to radiation. In this case there is an output of energy equal to the activation energy of the reaction which was required to excite the electrons. Overall there is no change.

(b) They may adopt a different stable configuration, by interacting with electrons associated with different atoms and molecules. The result is the formation of new covalent bonds, and hence the formation of new compounds. In this case, there are three possibilities (as shown in Fig. 3.7):

   (i) There may be an output of energy equal to the activation energy of the reaction. Such a reaction is **energetically neutral**.

   (ii) There may be an output of energy greater than the activation of the reaction. This is called an **exergonic reaction**; it proceeds with the output of energy, frequently as heat. As the reaction proceeds, so the solution gets hotter. An exergonic reaction will proceed spontaneously once the initial activation energy has been provided.

(iii) There may be an output of energy less than the activation energy, or even a requirement for additional energy, i.e. the solution will take up heat from its surroundings, and therefore we will have to heat it for the reaction to proceed. This is called an **endergonic reaction**. An endergonic reaction will not proceed unless there is a continuing input of energy to allow for the difference in energy level between the starting materials and the products.

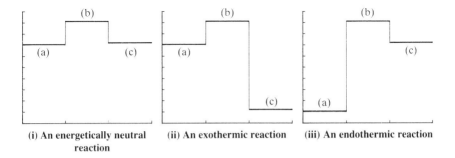

(i) An energetically neutral reaction

(ii) An exothermic reaction

(iii) An endothermic reaction

Figure 3.7 The activation energy of chemical reactions
(a) The initial energy level of the electrons in the substrate for the reaction. (b) The excited energy level of the electrons; when the electrons are excited to this energy level the bonds in the substrates can be broken, and there is the chance of forming new bonds between different atoms. (c) The final energy level of the electrons in the product of the reaction: (i) The final energy level of the electrons in the product is the same as in the substrate. Overall there is no change in the energy level of the electrons; such a reaction is energetically neutral. (ii) The final energy level of the electrons in the product is lower than the energy level of the electrons in the substrate. This is an exergonic reaction. (iii) The final energy level of the electrons in the product is higher than the energy level of the electrons in the substrate. This is an endergonic reaction.

As a rule, reactions in which relatively large complex molecules are broken down to smaller molecules are generally exergonic and proceed with the output of energy. We see this, for example, when we burn something in air. Although we have to apply a small amount of heat to start the reaction, once the reaction has started, it proceeds with the output of heat and light. Reactions in which relatively large complex molecules are synthesized from smaller molecules are generally endergonic, and require the input of energy to proceed – we generally have to heat the solution for the reaction to proceed.

Equilibrium

Some reactions, such as the burning of a hydrocarbon in air to form carbon dioxide and water, are highly exergonic, and the products of the reaction are widely dispersed. Such reactions proceed essentially in one direction only. However, most reactions do not proceed in only one direction. If we consider the reaction between two compounds, A and B, to form the products X and Y, we must also consider the reverse reaction between X and Y to form A and B:

$$\text{(i)} \quad A + B \rightarrow X + Y$$
$$\text{(ii)} \quad A + B \leftarrow X + Y.$$

If we start with only A and B in the solution, then at first there will only be reaction (i) to form X and Y. However, as X and Y accumulate, so they will be available to undergo the reverse reaction (ii), forming A and B.

Similarly, if we start with only X and Y in the solution, then at first there will only be reaction (ii), to form A and B. However, as A and B accumulate, so they will be available to undergo reaction (i) to form X and Y.

In both cases, the final result will be a solution containing A, B, X and Y. The relative amounts of [A + B] and [X + Y] will be the same whether we have started with A + B or X + Y. At this stage, the rate of reaction (i), forming X + Y from A + B is equal to the rate of reaction (ii), which forms A + B from X + Y. We call this **equilibrium**, and we can write the reaction as:

$$A + B \rightleftharpoons X + Y.$$

If there is a large uptake or output of energy (i.e. in endergonic or exergonic reactions) the equilibrium is such that the rate of reaction in one direction is very much greater than that in the other. This means that, if the reaction of $A + B \rightarrow X + Y$ is exergonic, at equilibrium there will be very little of A and B remaining, most will have gone to form X + Y.

If the reaction $A + B \rightarrow X + Y$ is endergonic, then at equilibrium there will still be a relatively large amount of A and B remaining, and relatively little X and Y will have been formed. If we heat the solution, to provide the energy which is taken up in the formation of X and Y from A and B, we can shift the equilibrium towards increased formation of X and Y.

The effect of concentration Chemical reactions depend on molecules colliding with each other, under appropriate conditions. This means that the more molecules that are present in our reaction mixture, the greater the chance of such a collision, and hence the greater the rate of reaction. Therefore equilibrium will be reached sooner in a more concentrated solution.

We can use changes in concentrations to force a change in the apparent position of the equilibrium. If we have a constant addition of A and B in the reaction shown above, then we will continue to disturb the equilibrium, and what we will observe is a net formation of the products X and Y. In the same way, if we remove one of the products from the reaction mixture in some way, then again we will disturb the equilibrium, and we will observe continuing formation of the products.

The rôle of catalysts A **catalyst** is something which speeds up a chemical reaction, or, more correctly, speeds the rate at which equilibrium is attained, without itself being altered by the reaction. The whole of metabolism depends on the enzymes that catalyse biochemical reactions (see p. 105).

Commonly, catalysts act to provide a surface on which the reactants can be brought together in higher concentration than would otherwise be possible in free solution. Because of this local increase in concentration, the chances of molecules colliding in the correct orientation for reaction to occur are increased, and so the reaction reaches equilibrium faster.

Catalysts may also act either to withdraw electrons from covalent bonds or donate a share in additional electrons. In this way they participate in the reaction by easing the breaking and formation of bonds.

Forces between molecules

We have seen that there are two types of interaction between atoms to form molecules: the formation of covalent bonds by sharing electrons; and the transfer of electrons to form ions. Obviously, ionic (i.e. charged) compounds can interact with each other. Compounds with opposite charges will attract each other, in the same way as we can say that a mixture of Na^+ ions and Cl^- ions forms the compound sodium chloride.

Covalently bonded molecules also interact with each other, in three main ways: the formation of hydrogen bonds between molecules; van der Waals forces between molecules; and hydrophobic interactions. These interactions are responsible for the maintenance of the structures of proteins and nucleic acids which are essential for their functions in the body (see Ch. 4).

Hydrogen bonding

Any compound in which one of the atoms sharing electrons in a bond exerts a greater attraction for the shared electrons than the other will show δ^- and δ^+ charges, as discussed for water on p. 42. The atoms that exert a relatively strong attraction for shared electrons, and hence tend to accumulate a δ^- charge, are called electronegative atoms. Those atoms that exert a smaller attraction for the shared electrons, and hence tend to develop a δ^+ charge, are called electropositive atoms.

When an electronegative atom or group faces outwards from the overall molecule, there will be an exposed δ^- at the surface of the molecule. Similarly, if an electropositive atom or group faces outwards from the surface of the molecule, there will be an exposed δ^+ charge at the surface of the molecule.

These δ^+ and δ^- partial charges at the surface of molecules are capable of interacting with the oppositely charged poles of water molecules. As discussed above, this is the basis for the solubility of non-ionic compounds in water. Although there is no overall charge on the molecule, the partial charges allow considerable interaction with water molecules, and thus the molecules of the compound can readily be distributed through the water. For obvious reasons, we generally call such compounds **water-soluble**. They are also sometimes called **hydrophilic** (from the Greek for water-loving) compounds.

Compounds which do not form such δ^+ and δ^- partial charges cannot interact with water, and are generally insoluble in water. They are sometimes called **hydrophobic** (from the Greek for water-hating) compounds.

If we are considering relatively large molecules, we may find that they have some regions which develop partial δ^+ and δ^- charges, and therefore can interact with water (i.e. hydrophilic regions) and other regions which do not develop partial charges, and do not interact with water (hydrophobic regions). Compounds with both hydrophilic and hydrophobic regions in the molecule are sparingly soluble in water; the extent to which they dissolve depends on the relative sizes of the hydrophilic and hydrophobic regions.

Hydrophilic compounds in which δ^+ or δ^- partial charges can develop do not only interact with water molecules. They can also interact with other hydrophilic molecules, forming partial bonds between partial charges of opposite polarity, known as **hydrogen bonds**. Hydrogen bonds between molecules are of critical importance in the structure and functions of proteins (see p. 88) and nucleic acids (see pp. 95 and 98). Although individual hydrogen bonds are weak, in large molecules the sum of a large number of such weak bonds can result in very great structural stability.

van der Waals forces

Even when the different atoms in a chemical bond exert the same overall attraction on the shared electrons, so that there is no development of δ^+ and δ^- partial charges, there can be transient partial charges. This is because the electrons surrounding a nucleus are not static, but move around the nucleus in their orbitals. In a covalent bond, the shared electrons are oscillating around both nuclei. At any instant, one atom will have a greater share in the electron than the other. This means that one atom will develop a minute negative charge, and the other an equally minute positive charge. This is only a transient separation of charge, and at another instant there may be either the opposite separation of charges, or an equal distribution of charge associated with both atoms. Nevertheless, for as long as a charge separation of this type exists, it provides the possibility of attraction to an opposite transient charge in a nearby molecule (or a nearby region of the same molecule in a large compound such as a protein).

Attractions between molecules based on transient minute inequality of the sharing of electrons of this type, are called **van der Waals forces**, after their original discoverer. Individually, van der Waals forces are very much weaker than hydrogen bonds, and only last for an infinitesimally short time. Nevertheless, at any time there are a great many such temporary charge separations in any molecule, and the sum of the van der Waals forces makes a considerable contribution to the structure of large molecules.

Hydrophobic interactions

We have already seen how compounds with electronegative or electropositive atoms or groups at the surface can form hydrogen bonds to water, and so are water-soluble. Compounds which cannot interact with water in this way are insoluble in water. They are actually repelled by the slightly charged water molecules.

We can see this easily if we shake an oil in water. Oils are hydrophobic molecules, and do not dissolve in water. If we shake hard enough, the oil will be dispersed in the water. However, it has not been dissolved. It has just been broken up into a large number of very small droplets. The result is a milky-looking suspension of those droplets in water – an **emulsion**. Under a microscope, we would be able to see that the droplets take up a spherical shape. This is the shape in which they have least need to interact with water.

As we watch our mixture of oil and water, it begins to clear, and the

53

oil forms larger and larger droplets. Eventually it separates from the water completely. This separation is again the result of repulsion between the slightly charged water molecules and the hydrophobic molecules. In order to minimize contact with water, the hydrophobic molecules associate with each other as much as possible.

If we consider molecules which have both hydrophobic and hydrophilic regions, we find that the different regions of the molecule behave as we would predict. The hydrophilic regions of the molecule interact with water, while the hydrophobic regions are repelled by the water, and interact with each other. This is illustrated by fatty acids (see p. 79).

Fatty acids are compounds with both hydrophobic and hydrophilic regions: they have a charged (and hence hydrophilic) group at one end of the molecule, and a chain of $-CH_2-$ groups, which is hydrophobic. Thus the sodium salt of palmitic acid is:

$$CH_3-(CH_2)_{16}-COO^- + Na^+.$$

As shown in Figure 3.8, we can dissolve a fatty acid in water, but as we do so, the hydrophobic "tail" regions group together, and the end result is a spherical globule called a **micelle**. The hydrophobic tails are inside and the hydrophilic groups face outwards, interacting with water. The sodium ions will interact with water, and will be freely dispersed in the solution.

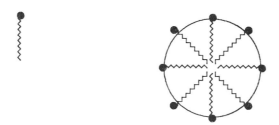

Figure 3.8 The formation of micelles by fatty acids
Fatty acids have a hydrophilic carboxylic acid (–COOH) group, and a hydrophobic tail composed of multiple –CH$_2$– units. This is shown diagrammatically on the left, where the round blob represents the hydrophilic –COOH group, and the zigzag the hydrophobic tail. In water, fatty acids will align themselves in such as way as to maximize the interaction of the hydrophilic –COOH group, and minimize the interaction of the hydrophobic tail, with water. This means that they will form spherical globules (micelles), as shown on the right, with the hydrophobic tails inside, in a lipid environment.

If we now repeat our experiment of shaking oil and water together, but this time add some sodium palmitate (or the salt of another fatty acid), we find that the emulsion does not separate into larger droplets of oil. Both the oil and the hydrophobic tails of the fatty acid molecules have been repelled by the water, and have formed mixed micelles. The hydrophilic charged groups of the fatty acid molecules stick out from the micelles and interact with water. Now the micelles do not come together to form larger droplets, because each one has an outer "coat" of hydrophilic groups which interact with water. We now have a stable emulsion of oil in water.

This is the basis of the action of soaps and detergents; soap is a mixture of salts of fatty acids such as palmitate. Emulsification of dietary fats in the aqueous medium of the gut contents is essential for the digestion and absorption of fats (see p. 133). Both the bile salts, secreted into the gut by the gallbladder, and the fatty acids formed from the digestion of fats, act to stabilize the emulsion. As discussed on p. 83, molecules which have both hydrophobic and hydrophilic regions are important in forming cell membranes.

Oxidation and reduction

In its simplest form, oxidation is the combination of a molecule with oxygen. Thus, if we burn carbon in air, we oxidize it to carbon dioxide:

$$C + O_2 \rightarrow CO_2.$$

Similarly, if we burn a simple carbohydrate, such as glucose ($C_6H_{12}O_6$) in air, we oxidize it to carbon dioxide and water:

$$C_6H_{12}O_6 + 6 \times O_2 \rightarrow 6 \times CO_2 + 6 \times H_2O.$$

Oxidation reactions need not always involve the addition of oxygen to the compound being oxidized. Oxidation can also be considered as a process of removing electrons from a molecule. Thus, the conversion of the iron Fe^{2+} ion to Fe^{3+} is also an oxidation, although in this case there is no direct involvement of oxygen.

In some chemical reactions, the removal of electrons in an oxidation reaction does not result in the formation of a positive ion; hydrogen ions (H^+) are removed together with the electrons. This means that the removal of hydrogen from a compound is also oxidation. For example, we can oxidize a simple hydrocarbon such as ethane (C_2H_6) to ethene (C_2H_4) by removing two hydrogen atoms onto a suitable carrier:

$$CH_3\text{-}CH_3 + carrier \rightleftharpoons CH_2{=}CH_2 + carrier\text{-}H_2.$$

Having removed one hydrogen atom from each carbon, the carbon atoms have "spare" bonds, and form a carbon–carbon double bond. We will see in later chapters how this type of oxidation reaction to form double bonds between carbon atoms is a common reaction in the oxidation of metabolic fuels.

Reduction is the reverse of oxidation – the addition of hydrogen, or electrons, or the removal of oxygen, are all reduction reactions.

In the reaction sequence above, ethane was oxidized to ethene at the expense of a carrier, which was reduced in the process. The addition of hydrogen to the carrier is a reduction reaction. Similarly, the addition of electrons to a molecule is a reduction, so just as the conversion of Fe^{2+} to Fe^{3+} is an oxidation reaction, the reverse reaction, the conversion of Fe^{3+} to Fe^{2+}, is a reduction. In the oxidation of glucose, while we can say that the glucose has been oxidized to carbon dioxide and water, it is equally true to say the oxygen has been reduced to water by its reaction with glucose.

As a broad generalization, we can say that in biological systems most of the reactions involved in the generation of metabolically useful energy involve oxidation, while many of the biosynthetic reactions involved in the formation of metabolic fuel reserves and the synthesis of body components are reductions.

Biologically important molecules

Although there are 96 naturally occurring chemical elements, relatively few of them are important in biological systems. Indeed most of the important compounds in biochemistry are composed of carbon, hydrogen, oxygen and nitrogen; sulphur and phosphorus also have important rôles. Some other elements (Table 3.1) are also important in biochemistry, and a few elements may be important because we are exposed to them, and they may be poisonous (for example cadmium, lead and mercury), but for the most part we do not need to concern ourselves with the remainder.

The chemistry of biological systems is essentially the chemistry of carbon compounds; these are generally known as **organic** compounds, because they were originally discovered in living (organic) matter. Simple carbonates and bicarbonates, and the whole host of compounds not involving carbon are known as inorganic compounds. Note that this chemical use of the word "organic" is quite different from that used to describe foods grown without the use of pesticides, fertilizers, etc., which are sometimes known as "organic" foods. Chemically, they are exactly the same as "conventional" foods.

We frequently refer to the **inorganic compounds** which are nutritionally important as **minerals**, because they are compounds which are (or can be) obtained by mining.

We have already seen how we can simplify the writing of chemical formulae by using abbreviations for the names of the elements. When we are considering organic compounds, we can simplify things further, by omitting many of the carbon atoms, and just drawing a skeleton of the structure of the molecule we are discussing. Indeed, we do not even draw

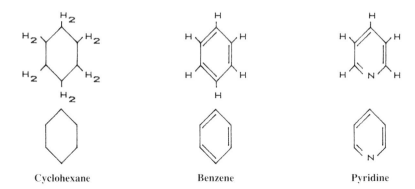

Figure 3.9 Three types of cyclic compound: cyclohexane, benzene and pyridine
Note that each point in the hexagon drawn for cyclohexane and benzene is a carbon atom; in pyridine, where one of the six atoms of the ring is nitrogen rather than carbon, we show this with N for nitrogen. In the upper row we show all of the hydrogen atoms involved in forming the molecule. Normally, we do not do this, but draw the molecules as shown in the lower line, omitting the hydrogen atoms as well as the carbon atoms.

in hydrogen atoms unless there is some reason to do so. Figure 3.9 shows how we can draw the structure of two related compounds, cyclohexane (a cyclic compound containing six carbon atoms in a ring, C_6H_{12}) and benzene (C_6H_6), which can be regarded as an oxidized form of cyclohexane in which six hydrogens have been removed, and replaced with three carbon–carbon double bonds.

When there is an atom other than carbon in the molecule, of course it has to be shown, since otherwise we would assume that there was a carbon atom there. For example, the third compound shown in Figure 3.9 is pyridine. It has a nitrogen atom incorporated into the ring, the other five positions of the ring are all carbon atoms.

Important groups in organic compounds

The chemistry of organic compounds is determined by the chemically reactive groups in the molecule. While the rest of the molecule is obviously important, we find, for example, that the different fatty acids, shown in Figure 3.12, have more in common with each other than any one fatty acid does with the corresponding alkane, alcohol or aldehyde.

Hydrocarbons Hydrocarbons are compounds consisting of carbon and hydrogen only. They may consist of straight or branched chains of carbon atoms, or may form cyclic structures (rings), commonly of five or six carbon atoms in biologically important compounds. Hydrocarbons do not have to be saturated with hydrogen; they may contain one or more carbon–carbon double bonds.

Simple hydrocarbons are not important in nutrition or biochemistry. However, many compounds contain relatively large regions which are hydrocarbon chains or rings. These cannot interact with water, because they do not show charge separation in their covalent bonds, and so cannot form hydrogen bonds (see p. 51). Hydrocarbon regions of molecules are therefore hydrophobic.

Double bonds and cis-trans isomerism   Single bonds between carbon atoms permit free rotation of the various parts of the molecule. However, carbon–carbon double bonds do not. They impose rigidity on that part of the molecule. This means that we can consider two different arrangements around a carbon–carbon double bond, as shown in Figure 3.10:

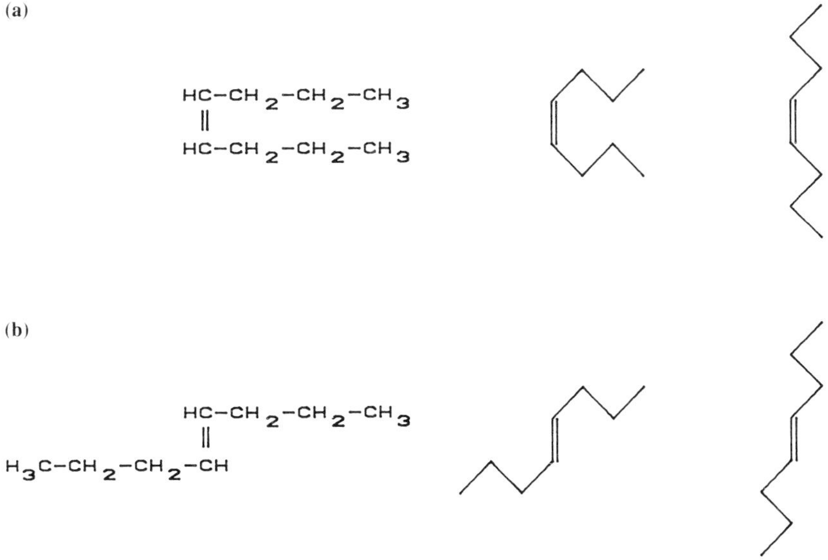

(a)

HC–CH$_2$–CH$_2$–CH$_3$
||
HC–CH$_2$–CH$_2$–CH$_3$

(b)

HC–CH$_2$–CH$_2$–CH$_3$
||
H$_3$C–CH$_2$–CH$_2$–CH

Figure 3.10 *Cis-* and *trans*-isomerism
Single bonds between carbon atoms (–CH$_2$–CH$_2$–) allow free rotation. However, double bonds (–CH=CH–) impose rigidity on the molecule. This means that the configuration of the carbon chain may be such that: (a) both parts of the molecule lie on the same side of the carbon–carbon double bond (the *cis*-isomer); (b) the two parts of the molecule lie on opposite sides of the carbon–carbon double bond (the *trans*-isomer). We can draw *cis-trans* isomers in three different ways: on the left we show all of the carbon and hydrogen atoms, while on the right we can see two different ways of showing the arrangement of the bonds, omitting the carbon and hydrogen atoms.

(a) Both parts of the chain may be on the same side of the double bond. This is the *cis*-**configuration**.

(b) The chain on one side of the double bond may be on the opposite side from the other. This is the *trans*-**configuration**.

Compounds that can exist in two or more different forms, with the same chemical composition, are called **isomers** of each other, and the phenomenon is isomerism. This type of isomerism, where groups may be on the same side of a double bond (*cis*-) or opposite sides (*trans*-) is called *cis–trans* isomerism.

Cis–trans isomerism is extremely important in biochemistry, since the two isomers have very different shapes, and the overall shape of molecules is important in enzyme-catalysed reactions (see p. 105). For example, interconversion between the *cis*- and *trans*-isomers of retinol (vitamin A) is crucially important for its function in vision (see p. 239).

Aromatic compounds An important group of unsaturated hydrocarbons have a cyclic structure, with multiple double bonds in the ring. The simplest such compound is benzene. As shown in Figure 3.11, benzene is C_6H_6, and has three carbon–carbon double bonds in the six-carbon ring. Although we can draw separate double bonds, these could be in either of the arrangements shown in Figure 3.11. In fact, we can consider that they alternate rapidly between both of these arrangements. It is more correct to draw the molecule with a circle in the middle of the ring, to show the alternation of double and single bonds, and the fact that we cannot localize the single and double bonds to individual carbon atoms.

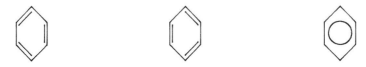

Figure 3.11 The benzene ring
Aromatic compounds have alternating double and single bonds between carbon atoms. We could draw benzene (C_6H_6) equally correctly with the double bonds in either of the arrangements shown in the two figures on the left. In fact, the electrons are shared around the ring in such a way that all of the bonds between the carbon atoms have some characteristics of carbon–carbon single bonds and some of the characteristics of carbon–carbon double bonds. You will sometimes see aromatic compounds represented as shown on the right, with a circle in the middle of the ring, to show that the electrons are equally shared between the atoms of the ring, and all the bonds are equivalent to 1½ bonds.

In compounds of this type, the electrons forming the covalent bonds are evenly shared between all the atoms in the ring, so that all the bonds are intermediate between single and double bonds. Compounds of this type are called **aromatic**. This is a chemical term, and does not mean that all aromatic compounds have a smell or aroma, although the term was originally used because many of the aromatic oils from natural sources have this type of ring structure in their molecules.

In linear molecules which have alternating single and double bonds in the carbon chain, the electrons shared to form the covalent bonds are delocalized and shared between more than just two carbon atoms in almost the same way as occurs in aromatic compounds. Such compounds are not aromatic, but they share some chemical properties with aromatic compounds. A compound having alternating single and double bonds is said to have **conjugated double bonds**. They are important in the structure and function of compounds such as vitamin A and carotene (see p. 237).

Heterocyclic compounds Carbon is not the only element which can be incorporated into ring structures. We frequently find an oxygen or nitrogen atom, and sometimes also sulphur and other elements, incorporated into carbon ring structures. Such compounds are called **heterocyclic**, from the Greek *heteros*, meaning different, because they contain an atom other than carbon in the ring.

Heterocyclic compounds may be saturated or unsaturated, and indeed some are also aromatic. Nitrogen-containing heterocyclic rings are especially important in the purines and pyrimidines (see p. 93), as well as a variety of other important compounds.

Functional groups

Groups containing oxygen, nitrogen or sulphur, in addition to carbon, are attached to the hydrocarbon carbon "skeleton" of biologically important molecules. It is these groups which provide the chemical reactivity of the compounds. They are hydrophilic groups, and interact with water.

Hydroxyl groups A simple hydroxyl (–OH) group attached to a hydrocarbon chain forms an **alcohol** (see Fig. 3.12). Alcohols are important in nutrition and biochemistry, quite apart from ethanol (ethyl alcohol) which is what we consume in alcoholic beverages.

Hydroxyl groups are important in carbohydrates (see p. 69) and in the glycerol which forms fats and oils by reaction with the fatty acids (see p. 78), as well as in other compounds.

A hydroxyl group attached to an aromatic ring can ionize relatively readily, giving up H^+ to form $-O^-$. Such aromatic hydroxyl compounds are called **phenols**. Again, phenolic compounds are important in several compounds, including the amino acid tyrosine (see p. 87) and some of the steroid hormones (see p. 85).

Sulphydryl groups In some ways, the sulphydryl group (–SH) is similar to the hydroxyl group. Compounds bearing a sulphydryl group are sometimes called **thiols**.

Biologically, the most important feature of sulphydryl groups is that they readily undergo oxidation. For example, the -SH groups in two molecules of the amino acid cysteine can undergo oxidation, resulting in the formation of a new bond, between the two sulphur atoms, and joining the two cysteine molecules together to form the amino acid cystine. Oxidation of the sulphydryl groups of cysteine molecules in proteins, with the formation of cystine, plays an important rôle in the structure of proteins (see Fig. 4.15 on p. 92).

Carbonyl groups: aldehydes and ketones As shown in Figure 3.12, the carbonyl group (–C=O) is important in two main groups of compounds:

(a) **aldehydes**, in which one valency of the carbon of the carbonyl group is occupied by an aliphatic group (or sometimes an aromatic group), while the other is occupied by hydrogen; and

(b) **ketones**, in which two aliphatic groups are attached to the carbon which bears the carbonyl group.

Aldehydes and ketones arise from the oxidation of alcohols. For example, oxidation of ethyl alcohol (ethanol) results in the formation of acetaldehyde:

$$CH_3\text{--}CH_2\text{--}OH + \text{carrier} \rightleftharpoons CH_3\text{--}HC=O + \text{carrier-}H_2.$$

The reaction is reversible, and reduction of an aldehyde results in the formation of the corresponding alcohol.

Carbonyl groups also occur in a variety of compounds which are not strictly either aldehydes or ketones. Such a C=O group occurring in a molecule is sometimes called a **keto-group**, although it is more correct to call it an **oxo-group**. Oxo-acids are important intermediates in the metabolism of amino acids (see p. 198), and in other metabolic pathways.

Carboxylic acids The carbonyl group is also important in a further class of compounds, the carboxylic acids. The acid group arises from the further oxidation of an aldehyde. Thus, oxidation of acetaldehyde results in the formation of acetic acid (ethanoic acid):

$$CH_3\text{--}HC=O + \text{acceptor} + H_2O \rightleftharpoons CH_3\text{--}COOH + \text{acceptor-}H_2$$

Acetic acid is the acid of vinegar. Although it can be synthesized chemically, much of the vinegar we use is produced by fermentation of carbohydrates to form ethanol (see p. 139), followed by a further fermentation process to convert the alcohol to acetic acid.

In the reaction written above, we have shown the acid as $CH_3\text{--}COOH$. This is a chemical shorthand way of writing the structure on a single line. As shown in Figure 3.12, the four valencies of the carbon atoms are occu-

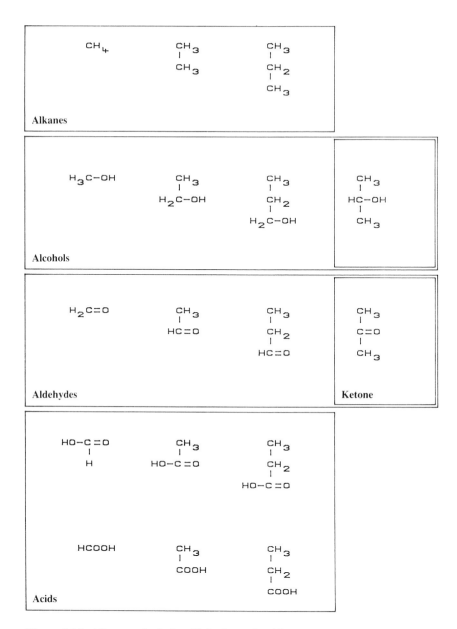

Figure 3.12 Alkanes, alcohols, aldehydes and acids

The first row shows three saturated hydrocarbons (alkanes): methane (CH_4), ethane (C_2H_6) and propane (C_3H_8). The second row shows the alcohols that can be formed by oxidation of these alkanes: methanol (methyl alcohol), ethanol (ethyl alcohol) and propanol (propyl alcohol). There are two possible isomers of propanol, since the hydroxyl group may be attached to either carbon-1 or carbon-2. The third row shows the result of further oxidation of the alcohol ($-CH_2OH$) group, to an oxo ($-C=O$) group. A compound with an $HC=O$ group is an aldehyde. The product of oxidizing *iso*-propanol to the oxo-compound is a ketone; this is dimethyl ketone, commonly known as acetone. The fourth row shows the result of further oxidation of the aldehydes to carboxylic acids.

pied as follows: one carbon atom has three valencies occupied by hydrogen, forming a methyl group (CH_3–) and the fourth by bonding to carbon; the other carbon atom has one valency occupied by binding to the carbon of the methyl group, one to the oxygen of the hydroxyl group (–OH) and the other two to oxygen (a carbonyl group, C=O).

The hydrogen of the hydroxyl group of carboxylic acids can readily be lost. We have already seen (see p. 44) that acetic acid is a (relatively weak) acid; it can dissociate in solution to form the acetate ion (CH_3–COO^-) and a hydrogen ion (H^+).

Almost all of the biologically important acids are carboxylic acids, including the fatty acids (see p. 79), the amino acids (see p. 87) and compounds which are formed as intermediates in the metabolism of fats, carbohydrates and proteins.

Esters   Under appropriate conditions, an alcohol and an acid can react together, with the elimination of water, forming an **ester**, as shown in Figure 3.13. The reaction is reversible, and esters can be cleaved to yield the acid and alcohol by the addition of water. The elimination of water to form an ester is a **condensation** reaction, while the reverse reaction, the cleavage of a bond by the addition of water, is **hydrolysis**.

Esters are important in biochemistry, especially in the formation of fats from fatty acids and the alcohol glycerol (which has three hydroxyl groups, and can therefore form esters to three fatty acid molecules at the same time (see p. 78).

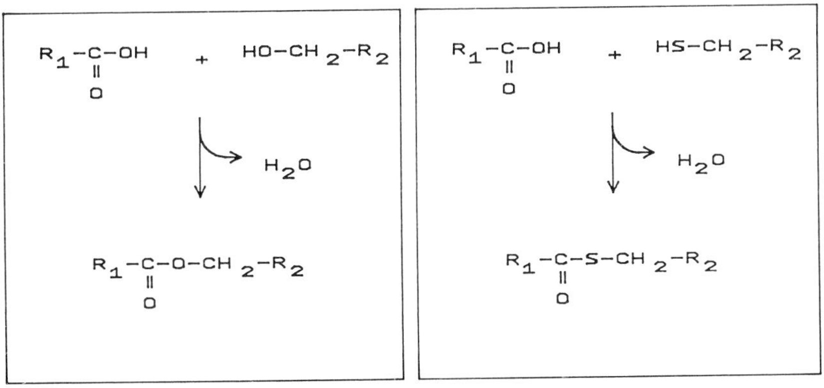

Figure 3.13 The formation of esters
An acid and an alcohol can undergo a reaction with the elimination of water, to form a new compound, an ester. This is shown in the left-hand box of this figure. Such a reaction, which involves the elimination of water, is known as a condensation reaction. The reverse, the cleavage of the bond by introducing the elements of water, is known as hydrolysis. Sulphydryl compounds (those with an –SH group rather than the –OH group of an alcohol) can undergo a similar reaction, to form a thio-ester. This is shown in the right-hand box of this figure.

Amides Carboxylic acids can react with ammonia to form amides. For example, acetic acid forms acetamide. Like ester formation, the formation of an amide is a condensation reaction, and the reverse reaction is a hydrolysis:

$$CH_3\text{–}COOH + NH_3 \rightleftharpoons CH_3\text{–}CO\text{–}NH_2 + H_2O.$$

Amides formed from carboxylic acids are found in the amino acids glutamine and asparagine (see p. 87) and the coenzymes NAD and NADP (see p. 117).

Amino groups and peptide bonds The commonest nitrogen-containing group in metabolically important compounds is the amino group, $-NH_2$. Amino groups are found in the amino acids of proteins (see p. 87), and in the purines and pyrimidines of nucleic acids (see p. 93).

Amino groups can undergo a condensation reaction with a carboxylic acid similar to the formation of esters (see above). The elimination of water between an amino group and carboxylic acid results in the formation of a **peptide bond**:

$$R\text{–}CH_2\text{–}COOH + H_2N\text{–}CH_2\text{–}R' \rightleftharpoons R\text{–}CH_2\text{–}CO\text{–}NH\text{–}CH_2\text{–}R' + H_2O.$$

(Note how we use the symbol $-R$ or $-R'$ to represent the rest of the molecule when it is not relevant to the reactive groups we are discussing.)

Again the reaction is reversible, and peptide bonds can be hydrolysed under appropriate conditions. The formation of peptide bonds is the basis of the formation of proteins from amino acids (see p. 88), and the hydrolysis of peptide bonds to release amino acids is the basis of the digestion of proteins (see p. 134).

The naming of organic compounds

There are systematic chemical rules for the naming of organic compounds, based on the functional groups and the size and type of hydrocarbon structure of the compound. Such systematic names uniquely identify any given compound, in the same way as the structural formula does. However, they tend to be cumbersome, and many metabolically important compounds have more convenient, officially accepted, trivial names. In general, we will use these trivial names in this book, and not the formal systematic names.

It is often necessary to be able to say which carbon atom of a compound has a reactive group attached. Here there is a simple rule. The carbon atoms are numbered from one end of the molecule. Carbon-1 is the one that carries the reactive group for which the compound is named. If the reactive group is an aldehyde or a carboxylic acid, then carbon-1 is the carbon of the carbonyl group.

There is also a slightly different system for numbering carbon atoms. Here we use the letters of the Greek alphabet. The α-carbon is the one to which to the functional group for which the compound is named is attached. The next carbon is the ß-carbon, etc. Thus in a fatty acid or aldehyde, the α-carbon is actually carbon-2, since the carbonyl group as a whole is the functional group. We sometimes call the carbon atom which is furthest from the α-carbon the ω-carbon; ω is the last letter of the Greek alphabet. (See, for example, Table 4.1 on p. 80, where this system is used in the naming of unsaturated fatty acids).

In cyclic compounds, the positions of the ring are numbered in such a way that the position to which the functional group for which the compound is named is attached has the lowest number. In heterocyclic compounds, the atom which is not carbon is given the number 1, and the carbon atoms are numbered from that position.

Asymmetry and the shape of molecules

We have already see that the position of groups around a carbon–carbon double bond can be such as to give two possible different arrangements, *cis–trans* isomers (see p. 58), which have very different shapes. We can also consider a further factor which affects the shape of a molecule, and is especially important in biochemistry. If four different groups are attached to a single carbon atom, we have to consider their arrangement. As shown in Figure 3.14, there are two possible arrangements of four groups. These two arrangements are mirror images of each other, and cannot be superimposed on each other – in the same way as right and left hands or feet are mirror images of each other. In other words, the compounds are **asymmetric**. The carbon atom to which the four different groups are attached is a **centre of asymmetry**.

The two forms of such compounds are **conformational isomers**. Chemically they react in the same way, but they have a different conformation or spatial arrangement of reactive groups in the molecule. This is important in biological systems, since, as discussed on p. 105, enzyme-catalysed reactions depend on binding of compounds to enzyme surfaces. The two isomers cannot bind to the same surface in the same way, and thus have different activity in enzyme-catalysed reactions.

The two conformational isomers of the sugar glyceraldehyde are shown in Figure 3.14. They are distinguished from each other by using the letters D (from the Greek *dextro* = right) and L (from the Greek *laevo* = left). The assignment of conformation to other compounds is based on their relationship to D- or L-glyceraldehyde.

This system for assigning conformation has a significant advantage in

```
        HC=O                          HC=O
         |                             |
      HO-CH                         HC-OH
         |                             |
       CH 2 OH                       CH 2 OH

    L-Glyceraldehyde              D-Glyceraldehyde


        COOH                          COOH
         |                             |
   H 2 N-CH                        HC-NH 2
         |                             |
        CH 3                          CH 3

      L-Alanine                     D-Alanine
```

Figure 3.14 D- and L-isomerism
The assignment of D- or L-configuration to an asymmetric compound is by reference to the spatial arrangement of the atoms around the asymmetric carbon in glyceraldehyde (shown in the upper row of the figure). The conformation of the amino acids is related to that of glyceraldehyde by comparison with alanine, shown in the lower row of the figure.

biochemistry. Almost all of the metabolically important sugars have the D-conformation. Thus, if we need to specify that we are talking about the (naturally occurring) D-isomer of glucose, we call it D-glucose. (You will sometimes see this referred to as dextrose.)

Similarly, almost all of the naturally occurring amino acids have the L-conformation. (Small amounts of D-amino acids occur in some bacteria, but these are not generally important in human biochemistry and nutrition.)

The opposite conformational isomer from the one that occurs naturally can have very different effects in the body. This is because it cannot bind to enzymes or receptors in the same way. We see this, for example, with the amino acid tryptophan. The metabolically important compound is L-tryptophan. Pure L-tryptophan has a very strong and unpleasant bitter flavour. However, D-tryptophan has a pleasant sweet taste. Indeed, it is some 40 times sweeter than sugar.

Chemical synthesis of compounds which have centres of asymmetry results in a mixture of equal amounts of the D- and L-isomers. This is called the **racemic mixture**, and is shown by using the prefix DL- before the name of the compound. Frequently we have to separate the D- and L-isomers of such synthesized compounds before they can be used, because the opposite isomer has undesirable effects. Increasingly, complex drugs are being synthesized by a mixture of chemical and biochemical (generally microbiological) techniques, in order to achieve the synthesis of only one isomer.

Although the system of naming asymmetric compounds by their relationship to the spatial arrangement of groups in glyceraldehyde has advantages for biochemistry, it does not follow the rigorous rules of chemistry. There is an alternative system, based on assignment of a strict hierarchy of chemically reactive groups around the asymmetric centre, which is the basis of systematic chemical nomenclature. Here the two possible stereo-isomers are called R (for right) and S (from the Latin *sinistra* = left; it would cause confusion with the D- and L- system of naming to use L for left as well!).

This system of nomenclature does not give the same conformation for all of the amino acids, and is relatively little used in biochemistry and nutrition. However, it is sometimes used, especially when considering complex molecules. For example, there are three asymmetric centres in the molecule of vitamin E (see p. 247). To distinguish between the possibilities, the conformation at each of these positions is given as R or S. The naturally occurring form of vitamin E is chemically RRR-α-tocopherol (sometimes also called all-R-α-tocopherol).

Free radicals

The formation of molecules involves the sharing of electrons in order to achieve a stable configuration of electrons in the outer shells of the individual atoms which make up the compound. A compound which loses or gains a single electron, and thus has an unpaired electron in its outermost shell, is extremely unstable, and very highly reactive. Such compounds are known as **free radicals**.

Free radicals usually exist for only extremely short periods of time, of the order of nanoseconds (10^{-9}s) or less, before they react with another molecule. However, this reaction in turn generates another molecule with an unpaired electron. Each time a radical reacts with a molecule, while it loses its unpaired electron and achieves stability, in turn it generates another radical, which is again short-lived and highly reactive. This is a **chain reaction**.

To show that a compound is a free radical, we sometimes show its chemical formula with a dot (·) to represent the unpaired electron.

If two radicals react together, each contributes its unpaired electron to the formation of a new, stable bond. This means that the chain reaction, in which reaction of radicals with other molecules generates new radicals, is stopped. We can call this **quenching** of the chain reaction, or quenching of the radicals. Since radicals are generally so short-lived, it is rare for two radicals to come together to quench each other in this way.

Some radicals are relatively stable. This applies especially to those which are formed from molecules with aromatic rings or conjugated double-bond systems. A single unpaired electron can be distributed or delocalized through such a system of double bonds, and the resultant radical is less reactive and longer lived. Compounds which are capable of forming relatively stable radicals are important in quenching radical chain reactions. They frequently have a long-enough life-time to permit two such stable radicals to come together, react with each other, and so terminate the chain. Vitamin E (see p. 247) and carotene (see p. 237) are especially important in quenching radical reactions in biological systems.

Chain reactions of free radicals can cause significant damage to the DNA in cells (see p. 98), possibly resulting in mutations or the induction of cancer. Radicals can also cause cell death, by interacting with membrane lipids, resulting in the lysis of cell membranes. We are exposed to a considerable burden of free radical attack, both as a result of environmental chemicals, and also as a result of normal oxidative metabolism; the oxidation of the reduced forms of riboflavin coenzymes (see p. 119) involves the generation of reactive oxygen radicals. Some nutrients, especially carotene (see p. 237), vitamin E (see p. 247) and vitamin C (see p. 273) and the mineral selenium (see p. 278), are important in protection against radical-induced tissue damage.

CHAPTER FOUR

Biologically important compounds: carbohydrates, lipids, proteins and nucleic acids

We can divide the biologically important types of compound into four main groups:

(a) **carbohydrates** – compounds containing carbon, hydrogen and oxygen, normally in the ratio $C_n:H_{2n}:O_n$;

(b) **lipids** – compounds mainly composed of carbon and hydrogen, for the most part in the ratio of $C_n:H_{2n}$, but with small amounts of oxygen, and in some lipids also phosphorus and nitrogen;

(c) **amino acids**, and the **proteins** formed from them, which contain carbon, hydrogen, oxygen, nitrogen and small amounts of sulphur; and

(d) **nucleotides**, and the **nucleic acids** formed from them, which contain carbon, hydrogen, oxygen, nitrogen and phosphorus.

Obviously, there are many other biologically important compounds which do not fall into these four main groups. These will be discussed as they become relevant, in later chapters.

Carbohydrates: sugars and starch

Carbohydrates are compounds of carbon, hydrogen and oxygen in the ratio $C_n:H_{2n}:O_n$. The basic unit of the carbohydrates is the sugar molecule or **monosaccharide**. Note that **sugar** is used here in a chemical sense, and includes a variety of simple carbohydrates, which are collectively known as sugars. Ordinary table sugar (cane sugar or beet sugar) is correctly known as sucrose; as discussed below, it is a disaccharide. It is just one of many different sugars.

The simplest type of sugar is a monosaccharide – a single sugar unit. **Monosaccharides** normally consist of between three and seven carbon atoms (and the corresponding number of hydrogen and oxygen atoms). A few larger monosaccharides also occur, although they are not generally important in nutrition and metabolism.

Two monosaccharides may be joined together, to form a **disaccharide**. This is a condensation reaction, i.e. it occurs by the elimination of water, to form a **glycoside bond** between the two monosaccharide units. The reverse reaction, cleavage of the glycoside bond to release the individual monosaccharides, is a hydrolysis.

Occasionally we come across sugars made up from three or four monosaccharide units (**trisaccharides** and **tetrasaccharides**). Nutritionally these are not particularly important, and indeed they are often not digested, although they may be fermented by intestinal bacteria and make a significant contribution to the production of intestinal gas.

We also find chains (polymers) of large numbers of monosaccharide units. These are known as **polysaccharides**. The most important are starch and glycogen (see below), both of which are polymers of the monosaccharide glucose. Other polysaccharides, composed of other monosaccharides, or of glucose linked in different ways from those found in starch and glycogen, also exist. Collectively these are known as **non-starch polysaccharides**. They are generally not digested, but have important rôles in nutrition (see p. 75).

Monosaccharides

The classes of monosaccharides are named by the number of carbon atoms in the ring, using the Greek names for the numbers, ending with "ose" to show that they are sugars. The names of all sugars end in "-ose": three-carbon monosaccharides are trioses; four-carbon monosaccharides are tetroses; five-carbon monosaccharides are pentoses; six-carbon monosaccharides are hexoses; seven-carbon monosaccharides are heptoses.

In general, trioses, tetroses and heptoses are important as intermediate compounds in the metabolism of pentoses and hexoses, which are the nutritionally important sugars.

The pentoses and hexoses can exist as either straight-chain compounds or can form heterocyclic rings. The two forms are shown in Figures 4.1

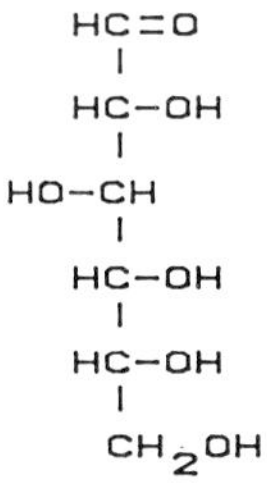

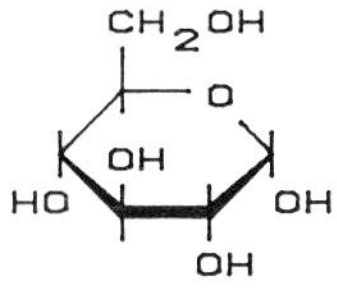

```
HC=O
 |
HC-OH
 |
HO-CH
 |
HC-OH
 |
HC-OH
 |
CH₂OH
```

Glucose

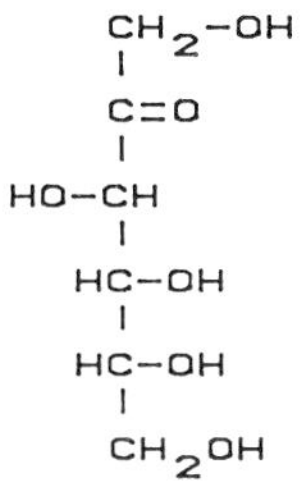

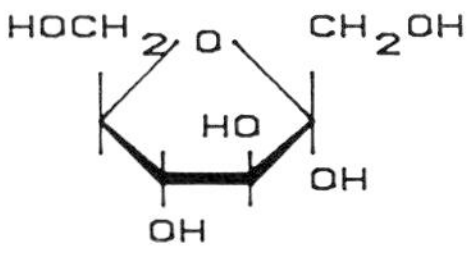

```
CH₂-OH
 |
C=O
 |
HO-CH
 |
HC-OH
 |
HC-OH
 |
CH₂OH
```

Fructose

```
HC=O
 |
HC-OH
 |
HO-CH
 |
HO-CH
 |
HC-OH
 |
CH₂OH
```

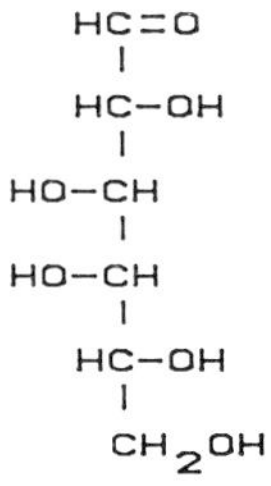

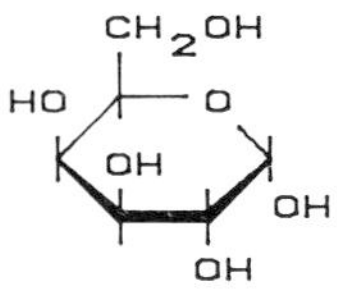

Galactose

Figure 4.1 The common six-carbon sugars (hexoses): glucose, fructose and galactose
We can draw the structures of the sugars in two ways: as a straight chain of carbon atoms, shown on the left, or as rings, shown on the right. You will find both straight-chain and ring forms used in various diagrams in this book, since in some cases it is clearer or more convenient to use one way of representing the structure rather than the other. In some diagrams you will also find the ring of a sugar drawn the other way up, because this is the most convenient way of representing it in a complex structure.

71

and 4.2. By convention, the ring of sugars is drawn with the bonds of one side thicker than the other. This is to show that the rings are planar, and can be considered to lie at right angles to the plane of the paper. The boldly drawn part of the molecule is then coming out of the paper towards you, while the lightly drawn part is going behind the paper. The hydroxyl groups lie above or below the plane of the ring, in the plane of the paper. Each carbon has a hydrogen atom attached as well as a hydroxyl group. For convenience in drawing the structures of sugars, we generally omit this hydrogen when we draw them as rings, although we show them when we draw the straight-chain forms of the molecules.

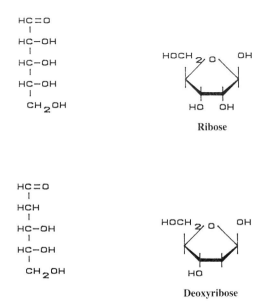

Figure 4.2 The common five-carbon sugars (pentoses): ribose and deoxyribose

The nutritionally important hexoses are shown in Figure 4.1. **Glucose** and **galactose** differ from each other only in the arrangement of the hydroxyl groups above and below the plane of the ring. **Fructose** differs from glucose and galactose in that it has a C=O (keto) group at carbon-2, while the other two sugars have an H–C=O (aldehyde) group at carbon-1.

There are two important pentose sugars, ribose and deoxyribose. As can be seen from Figure 4.2, deoxyribose is an unusual sugar, in that it has "lost" one of its hydroxyl groups. The main rôle of ribose and deoxyribose is in the nucleic acids, RNA and DNA (see p. 93). Xylose (not shown in Fig. 4.2) is an isomer of ribose.

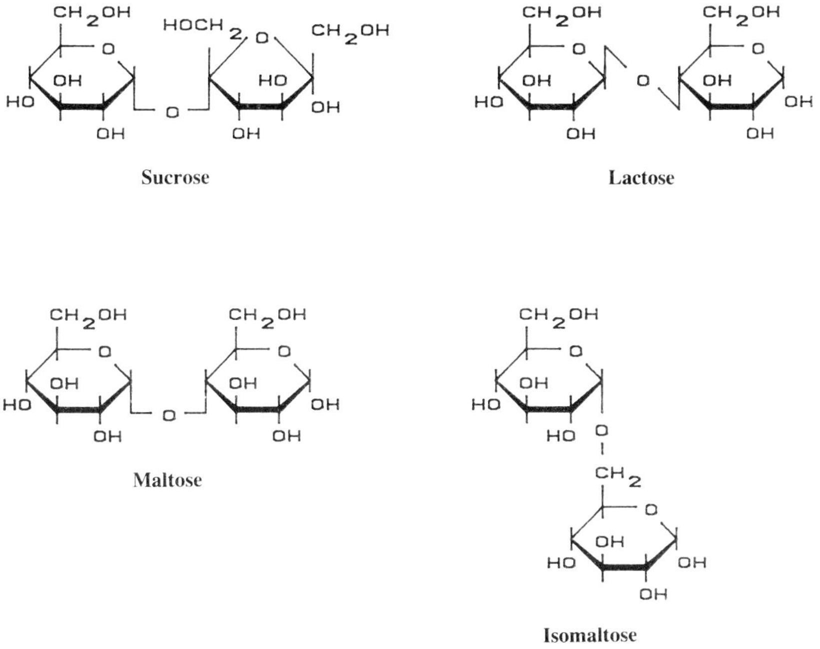

Figure 4.3 The common disaccharides: sucrose, lactose, maltose and isomaltose
Sucrose is ordinary cane or beet sugar. It is a dimer of glucose and fructose. Lactose is the sugar of milk. It is a dimer of glucose and galactose. Maltose and isomaltose arise from the digestion of starch. They are both dimers of two molecules of glucose, and differ in the position of the linkage between the two glucose units.

Sugar alcohols, formed by the reduction of the aldehyde group of a monosaccharide to a hydroxyl (–OH) group, are also important, especially **sorbitol**, formed by the reduction of glucose. It is only slowly absorbed from the intestinal tract and metabolized, so that it has very much less effect on the concentration of glucose in the bloodstream than other carbohydrates. It is widely used in preparation of foods suitable for use by diabetics. However, sorbitol is metabolized as a metabolic fuel, with an energy yield approximately equal to that of glucose, so that it is not suitable for the replacement of carbohydrates in weight-reducing diets.

Xylitol is the sugar alcohol formed by reduction of the five-carbon sugar, xylose. It is of interest because, far from promoting dental caries, as do other sugars (see p. 23), xylitol has an anti-cariogenic action. The reasons for this are not well understood, but sucking sweets made from xylitol results in a significant reduction in the incidence of caries.

Disaccharides

The four common disaccharides are shown in Figure 4.3. They are:
(a) **sucrose**, cane or beet sugar, which is a dimer of glucose and fructose;
(b) **maltose**, the sugar originally isolated from malt, which is a dimer of glucose;
(c) **isomaltose**, which is also a dimer of glucose, but linked differently from the linkage in maltose; both maltose and isomaltose arise from the digestion of starch;
(d) **lactose**, the sugar of milk, which is a dimer of glucose and galactose.

Reducing and non-reducing sugars

The aldehyde group of glucose is a chemical reducing agent. That is, it can readily react to reduce another compound, itself being oxidized to an acid group (–COOH) in the process. This forms the basis of a simple test for glucose. Under appropriate conditions, glucose reacts with copper ions, reducing them to elemental copper, and itself being oxidized. The original solution of copper ions has a blue colour; the elemental copper forms a yellow-brown precipitate. This is the basis of Clinitest[R], which is used to detect the presence of glucose in urine.

This reaction is not specific for glucose. Other sugars with a free aldehyde group at carbon-1 are also reducing agents, and can undergo the same reaction. This lack of specificity can cause problems when a positive result of such a test is interpreted as meaning the presence of glucose. Some monosaccharides (including vitamin C, see p. 273) and several disaccharides (including maltose and lactose, but not sucrose) will all react with copper ions and give a positive result. While copper reagents are sometimes used, there are more specific tests, using the enzyme glucose oxidase, which measure only glucose.

It is important to realize that when we talk about reducing sugars, we are talking about a chemical reaction of the sugars – the ability to reduce a suitable acceptor such as copper ions. It has nothing to do with weight reduction and slimming, although some people erroneously believe that reducing sugars somehow help you to reduce excessive weight. This is not correct, the energy yield from reducing sugars and non-reducing sugars is exactly the same, and excess of either will contribute to obesity.

Polysaccharides: starches and glycogen

Starch is a polymer of glucose, containing a large, but variable, number of glucose units. It is thus impossible to quote a relative molecular mass for starch; it is highly variable, and if we want to talk about amounts of starch then we have to talk in grams, not mol. We can, however, hydrolyse starch to its constituent glucose molecules, and express the results in terms of mol of glucose.

The simplest form of starch is just a straight chain of glucose molecules, joined "end to end", with glycoside links between carbon-1 of one glucose unit and carbon-4 of the next. This is **amylose** (see Fig. 4.4). Some types of starch have a branched structure, where every so often one glucose molecule has glycoside links to three others instead of just two. The branch is formed by linkage between carbon-1 of one glucose unit and carbon-6 of the next. This is **amylopectin** (see Fig. 4.5).

Starches are the storage carbohydrates of plants, and the relative amounts of amylose and amylopectin differ in starches from different sources, as indeed does the size of the overall starch molecule. On average, about 20–25% of starch in foods is the straight-chain polymer, amylose, and the remaining 75–80% is amylopectin.

Glycogen is the storage carbohydrate of mammalian muscle and liver. It is synthesized from glucose in the fed state, and is broken down to allow its constituent glucose units to be used as a metabolic fuel in the fasting state. Like amylopectin, glycogen is a branched polymer, and has the same structure as shown in Figure 4.5 for amylopectin.

Other polysaccharides in foods are collectively known as **non-starch polysaccharides**, the major components of dietary fibre (see p. 23). None of the non-starch polysaccharides is digested by human enzymes, although all can be fermented to some extent by intestinal bacteria, and the products of bacterial fermentation may be absorbed and metabolized as metabolic fuels.

The non-starch polysaccharides include:

(a) **cellulose** – a polymer of glucose in which the configuration of the glycoside bond between the glucose units is in the opposite configuration from that in starch, and cannot be hydrolysed by human enzymes;

(b) **hemicelluloses** – branched polymers of pentose (five-carbon) and hexose (six-carbon) sugars;

(c) **inulin** – a polymer of fructose, which is the storage carbohydrate of Jerusalem artichoke and some other root vegetables;

(d) **pectin** – a complex polymer of a variety of monosaccharides, including some methylated sugars;

(e) **plant gums** such as gum Arabic, gum Tragacanth, acacia, carob and

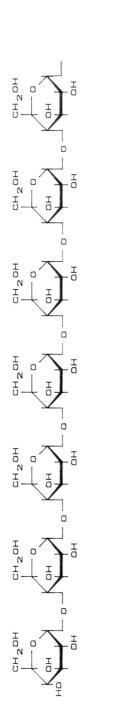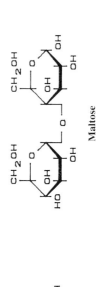

Glucose

Maltose

Figure 4.4 Amylose – the straight-chain form of starch

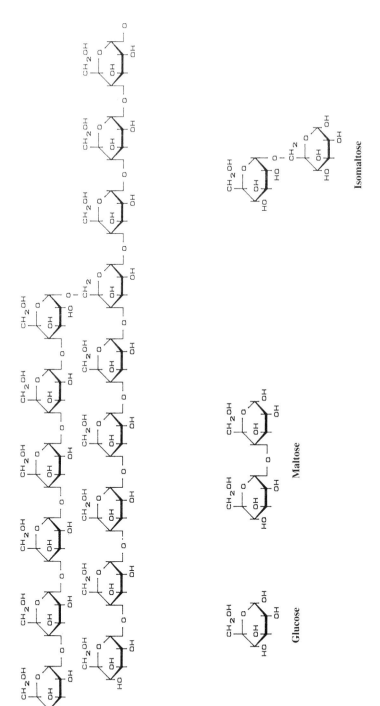

Figure 4.5 Amylopectin – the branched form of starch

Glycogen, the storage carbohydrate of mammalian muscle and liver has the same branched structure as amylopectin (see also Fig. 6.14 on p. 152).

guar gums – complex polymers of mixed monosaccharides;

(f) **mucilages** such as alginates, agar and carrageen – complex polymers of mixed monosaccharides found in seaweeds and other algae.

Cellulose, hemicelluloses and inulin are insoluble non-starch polysaccharides, while pectin and the plant gums and mucilages are soluble non-starch polysaccharides. The other major constituent of dietary fibre, **lignin**, is not a carbohydrate, but a polymer of aromatic alcohols.

Lipids: fats and oils

Three groups of metabolically important compounds can be considered under the heading of lipids:

(a) **triacylglycerols** – the common oils and fats of the diet;

(b) **phospholipids** – chemically similar to triacylglycerols, but with a phosphate group in the molecule;

(c) **steroids**, including cholesterol (see p. 84), the steroid hormones (see p. 219) and vitamin D (see p. 242). Chemically these are completely different from triacylglycerols and phospholipids.

Triacylglycerols

Triacylglycerols have the general structure shown in Figure 4.6. They

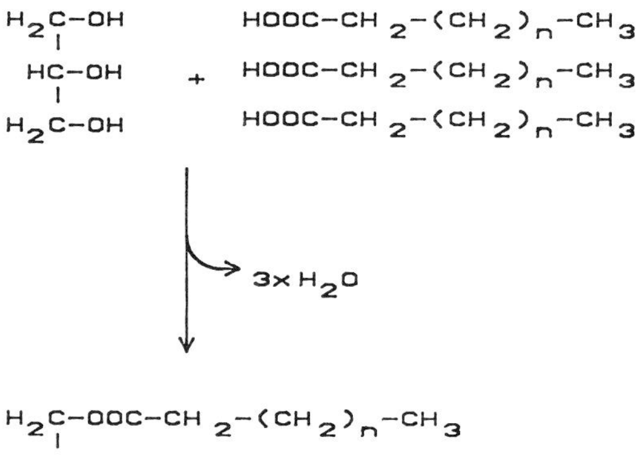

Figure 4.6 Triacylglycerols
Triacylglycerols are formed by a condensation reaction between a molecule of glycerol and three molecules of fatty acids. The three fatty acids in each molecule of any triglyceride need not be the same (see also Fig. 6.13 on p. 150).

consist of a molecule of the three-carbon-sugar derivative **glycerol** esterified to three **fatty acid** molecules (acyl groups). They are sometimes called **triglycerides**.

Triacylglycerols provide a major tissue reserve of metabolic fuel, within specialized tissue known as **adipose tissue**. Cells of adipose tissue contain only a relatively small amount of cytoplasm; the vast majority of the cell is triacylglycerol. As discussed on p. 150, fatty acids and triacylglycerols are synthesized, and added to adipose tissue reserves, after a meal. They are hydrolysed and the resultant free fatty acids and glycerol are released for use as metabolic fuels in the fasting state.

Fatty acids Fatty acids differ in both the length of the carbon chain and whether or not they have one or more double bonds (–CH=CH–) in the chain. Those with no double bonds are known as **saturated fatty acids** – the carbon chain is completely saturated with hydrogen. Those with double bonds are known as unsaturated fatty acids – the carbon chain is not completely saturated with hydrogen (see p. 38). Fatty acids with just one double bond are known as **mono-unsaturated**, while those with two or more double bonds are known as **polyunsaturated** (see Fig. 4.7).

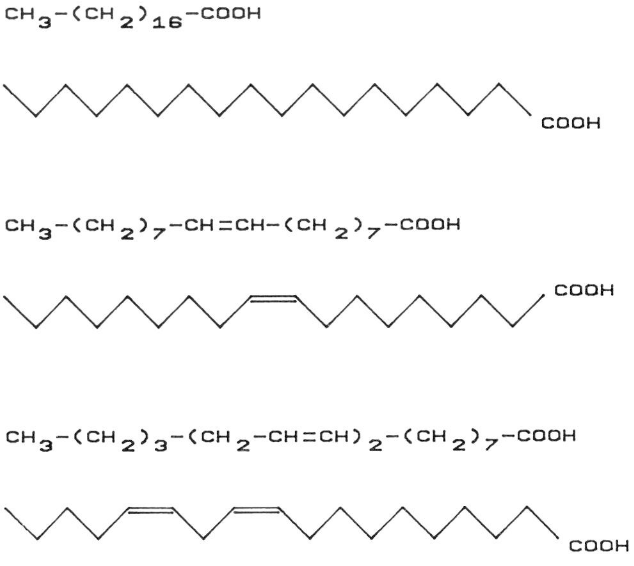

$$CH_3-(CH_2)_{16}-COOH$$

$$CH_3-(CH_2)_7-CH=CH-(CH_2)_7-COOH$$

$$CH_3-(CH_2)_3-(CH_2-CH=CH)_2-(CH_2)_7-COOH$$

Figure 4.7 Types of fatty acid: saturated, mono-unsaturated and polyunsaturated
The fatty acids shown here all 18 carbon atoms, and are: stearic acid (C18:0), oleic acid (C18:1 ω-9) and linoleic acid (C18:2 ω-6) (see Table 4.1 for the naming of fatty acids).

Note that while correctly it is the fatty acids that are saturated or unsaturated, we frequently talk about saturated and unsaturated fats. This is not really correct, and indeed it is unlikely that all three positions on the glycerol of a triacylglycerol would contain unsaturated fatty acids. Most are a mixture of different types of fatty acid. Nevertheless, it is a useful shorthand to talk about some fats being more less or saturated or unsaturated than others. What we really mean is that different fats contain different proportions of saturated and unsaturated fatty acids, as shown in Table 2.7 on p. 21.

Table 4.1 The naming of fatty acids.

	C atoms	Double bonds		1st double bond
Saturated fatty acids				
Butyric	4	0		C4:0
Caproic	6	0		C6:0
Caprylic	8	0		C8:0
Capric	10	0		C10:0
Lauric	12	0		C12:0
Myristic	14	0		C14:0
Palmitic	16	0		C16:0
Stearic	18	0		C18:0
Arachidic	20	0		C20:0
Mono-unsaturated fatty acids				
Palmitoleic	16	1	6	C16:1 n-6
Oleic	18	1	9	C18:1 n-9
Poly-unsaturated fatty acids				
Linoleic	18	2	6	C18:2 n-6
α-Linolenic	18	3	3	C18:3 n-3
γ-Linolenic	18	3	6	C18:3 n-6
Arachidonic	20	4	6	C20:4 n-6
Eicosapentaenoic	20	5	3	C20:5 n-3
Docosatetraenoic	22	4	6	C22:4 n-6
Docosapentaenoic	22	5	3	C22:5 n-3
Docosapentaenoic	22	5	6	C22:5 n-6
Docosahexaenoic	22	6	3	C22:6 n-3

There are three different ways of naming the fatty acids:

(a) many of them have trivial names, often derived from the name of the source from which they were originally isolated; thus, oleic acid was first isolated from olive oil, stearic acid from beef tallow, palmitic acid from palm oil, etc.;

(b) all of them have systematic chemical names, based on the number of carbon atoms in the chain and the number of double bonds (if any);

(c) we often use a shorthand to show simply the number of carbon atoms in the molecule, followed by a colon and the number of double bonds

(Table 4.1). The position of the first double bond from the methyl group of the fatty acid is shown by n- or ω- (the ω-carbon is the furthest from the α-carbon, which is the one to which the –COOH group is attached; ω is the last letter of the Greek alphabet).

This is the reverse of the "correct" systematic chemical way of naming compounds. Systematic nomenclature starts at the carbon atom containing the functional group for which the compound is named (see p. 64). By systematic chemical nomenclature, the positions of carbon–carbon double bonds in fatty acids would be numbered from the carboxylic acid end. Biochemically, what is important in unsaturated fatty acids is the position of the carbon–carbon double bond which is nearest to the methyl group. Therefore for nutritional and biochemical purposes we number carbon atoms from this end.

Polyunsaturated fatty acids The polyunsaturated fatty acids have two or more –CH=CH– double bonds in the molecule, and in the nutritionally important polyunsaturated fatty acids this is always in an alternating arrangement with –CH_2– units, as:

$$-CH_2-CH=CH-CH_2-CH=CH-CH_2-.$$

The –CH_2– grouping is a methylene group, and this arrangement is known as "methylene-interrupted".

In the nutritionally important unsaturated fatty acids, and in membrane structure, the carbon–carbon double bonds are in the *cis*-configuration, as shown in Figure 4.7. The *trans*-isomers of unsaturated fatty acids do occur in foods to some extent, but they do not have the desirable biological actions of the *cis*-isomers, and indeed *trans*-isomers of unsaturated fatty acids have deleterious effects, since they distort the structure of cell membranes (see p. 83). It is recommended that average consumption of *trans*-unsaturated fatty acids should not increase above the present 2% of energy intake.

The polyunsaturated fatty acids have two main functions in the body: in cell membranes (see p. 83), and as precursors for the synthesis of a group of compounds which includes prostaglandins, prostacyclins and thromboxanes. These function as local hormones, being secreted by cells into the extracellular fluid, and acting on nearby cells. Prostaglandins and the other compounds derived from polyunsaturated fatty acids are important in the regulation of the normal adhesiveness of blood cells, inflammation reactions, etc.

The polyunsaturated fatty acids can be interconverted to a limited extent in the body, but we are reliant on a dietary intake of **linoleic acid** (C18:2 ω-6) and **linolenic acid** (C18:3 ω-3), since these two, which can each be considered to be the parent of a family of related fatty acids, cannot be synthesized in the body. An intake of polyunsaturated fatty acids greater than the amount to meet physiological requirements confers benefits in terms of lowering the plasma concentration of cholesterol and reducing the risk of atherosclerosis and ischaemic heart disease. The **requirement** is less than 1% of energy intake, but it is **recommended** that 6% of energy intake should come from polyunsaturated fatty acids.

Phospholipids

Phospholipids are, as their name suggests, lipids which also contain the element phosphorus, as a phosphate group. They consist of glycerol esterified to two fatty acid molecules, one of which (esterified to carbon-2 of glycerol) is normally a polyunsaturated fatty acid. The third hydroxyl group of glycerol is not esterified to a fatty acid as in triacylglycerols, but to phosphate. The phosphate, in turn, is esterified to one of a variety of compounds, including the amino acid serine (see p. 87), ethanolamine (which is formed from serine), choline (which is formed from ethanolamine), inositol or one of a variety of other compounds (Fig. 4.8).

A phospholipid lacking the group esterified to the phosphate is known

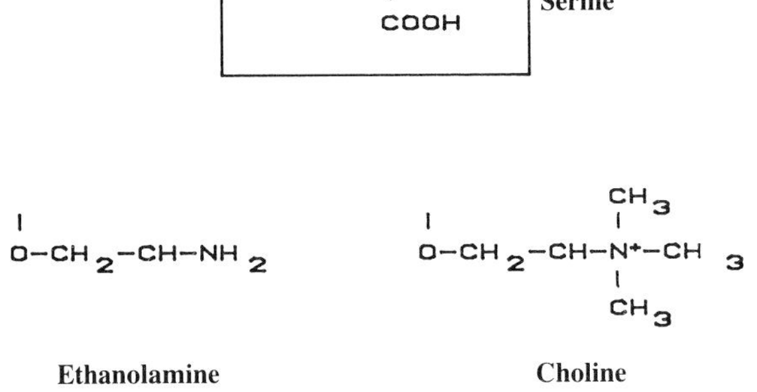

Figure 4.8 The structure of phospholipids
Phospholipids consist of glycerol, esterified to two fatty acids (as in triacylglycerols, see Fig. 4.6). The third hydroxyl group of glycerol is esterified to phosphate. In turn, the phosphate is esterified to one of several different compounds. In this example, the compound in the box is the amino acid serine, and the resultant phospholipid is phosphatidyl serine. Two further phospholipids can be derived from phosphatidyl serine, by modification of serine to give ethanolamine or choline.

as a phosphatidic acid, and the complete phospholipids are called phosphatidyl serine, phosphatidyl ethanolamine, phosphatidyl choline (also called lecithin), phosphatidyl inositol, etc.

A specific type of phosphatidyl choline, in which both the fatty acids are palmitate, is the major constituent of **lung surfactant**. Failure to synthesize lung surfactant is the cause of respiratory distress in premature infants.

In addition to its rôle in the structure of cell membranes (discussed below), phosphatidyl inositol has a specialized rôle in membranes, acting to release inositol triphosphate and diacylglycerol as intracellular second messengers in response to the actions of hormones, etc., binding to the outer surface of cell membranes (see p. 224).

The arrangement of lipids to form cell membranes We have already seen that fatty acids can interact with both lipid and water, because they have both hydrophobic and hydrophilic regions in the molecule (see Fig. 3.8 on p. 54). Phospholipids can interact with both lipid and water in the same way; the phospholipid molecule has two hydrophobic chains from its two fatty acids, and a very hydrophilic region formed by the phosphate and the attached group.

Phospholipids readily form a double layer (known as a **lipid bilayer**), with the hydrophobic chains of two layers of molecules interacting with each other in the centre of the bilayer. Both faces of the bilayer are made up of the hydrophilic groups, which interact with water. This is the basis of the structure of membranes around and within cells (see Fig. 4.9).

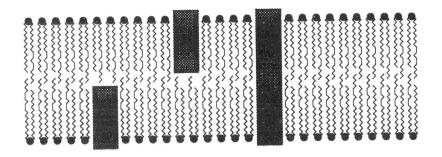

Figure 4.9 The arrangement of phospholipids to form cell membranes
Membranes consist of a bilayer of phospholipids, with the hydrophobic fatty acids inside and the hydrophilic groups outside, interacting with water. Proteins are also found as a part of the structure of membranes. Such proteins have a hydrophobic region which is embedded in the lipid, and a hydrophilic region which interacts with water.

In addition to phospholipids, the lipid inner part of the membrane bilayer contains cholesterol (see below) and vitamin E (see p. 247). The presence of *cis*-polyunsaturated fatty acids in the membrane phospholipids is essential for the close packing of the lipids to form the membrane and maintain its fluidity. *Trans*-isomers cannot take up the same arrangement in the membrane, and they distort the structure.

Membranes also contain **proteins**. These may be located at the outer or inner face of the membrane, and some of the most important membrane proteins span the whole width of the membrane, and interact with water at both surfaces. All membrane-associated proteins have hydrophobic regions, which interact with the lipids, and hydrophilic regions, which stick out from the lipid layer and interact with water. (See p. 88 for a discussion of protein structure and p. 222 for the rôle of membrane proteins in the responses to hormones.)

Membranes, both those within the cell and those surrounding the cell, are not rigid static structures, but have a considerable degree of **fluidity**. The proteins can move around in the lipid bilayer, and regions of membrane can form vesicles for the transport of compounds into and out of the cell. A region of cell membrane can invaginate, to form a depression in the cell surface. This deepens, and the space which communicates with the outside closes off, until a separate membrane-enclosed vesicle has been formed inside the cell. This is the process of **endocytosis**.

The reverse process occurs in the **secretion** of proteins, hormones and neurotransmitters from the cell. The compounds to be exported are synthesized or accumulated in membrane-enclosed vesicles. These vesicles then migrate to the surface of the cell, where the membrane of the vesicle fuses with the cell membrane, leading to the formation of a pore in the membrane through which the contents of the vesicle can be exported into the extracellular fluid.

Cholesterol and the steroids

As can be seen from Figure 4.10, steroids are chemically completely different from triacylglycerols or phospholipids. However, steroids are also hydrophobic molecules, and share some chemical and physical properties with other lipids.

The parent compound of all the steroids in the body is **cholesterol**; different steroids are then formed by replacing one or more of the hydrogens with hydroxyl groups or oxo-groups, and in some cases by shortening the side-chain.

Apart from cholesterol, which has a major rôle in membrane structure and the synthesis of bile salts (see p. 133) the steroids are **hormones** – compounds synthesized in one tissue, then released into the circulation to act on a variety of other tissues. Some of the important steroid hormones include cortisol, and the sex steroids, oestrogens and progesterone (which are important in the control of reproductive biology in females) and testosterone (which is the major male sex hormone). Vitamin D is a derivative of cholesterol, and can also be considered to be a steroid hormone (see p. 242). The mechanism steroid hormone action is discussed on p. 226.

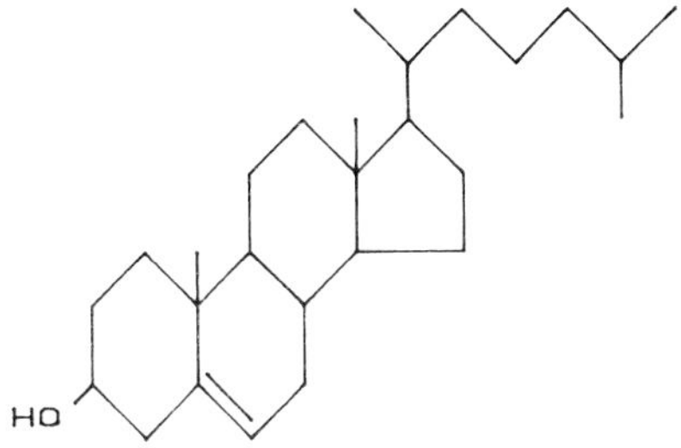

Cholesterol

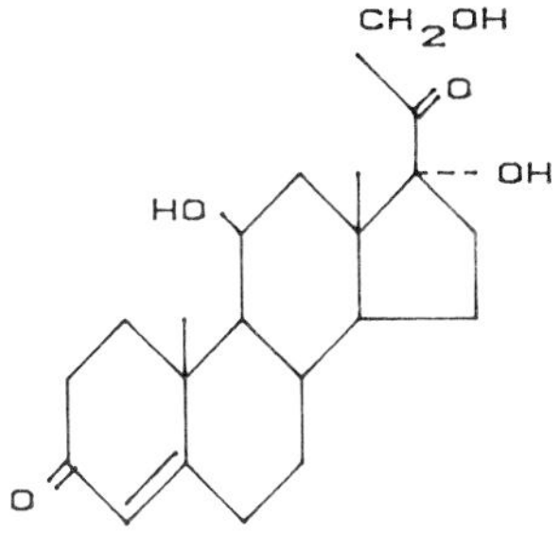

Cortisol

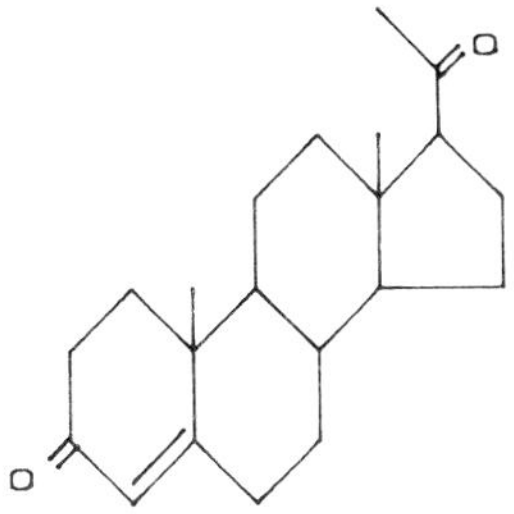

Progesterone

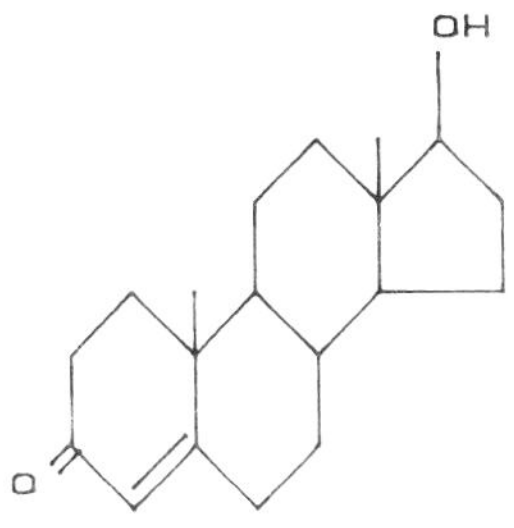

Testosterone

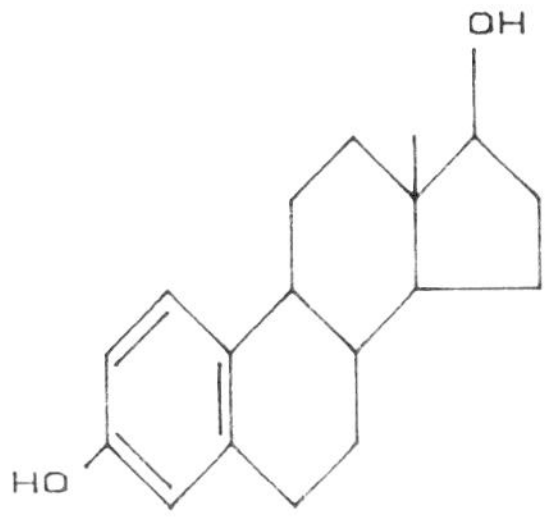

Oestradiol

Figure 4.10 Cholesterol and some steroid hormones
The various steroid hormones are all synthesized from cholesterol. Relatively subtle changes (such as the addition of a hydroxyl- or oxo-group) have major effects on the ability of different steroids to interact with tissue-specific receptors, and thus on the physiological actions of the hormones (see p. 226).

The cholesterol which is required for cell-membrane synthesis, and the very much smaller amount which is required for the synthesis of steroid hormones, can either be synthesized in the body or provided by the diet. There is no requirement for cholesterol in the diet.

A raised concentration of cholesterol in plasma is a risk factor for atherosclerosis and ischaemic heart disease; concentrations of cholesterol above 5.2 mmol/l are associated with increased risk, and between 4 and 4.5 mmol/l with least risk.

There is little evidence that for most healthy people the dietary intake of cholesterol has any significant effect on the plasma concentration of cholesterol. Several factors, including the total intake of dietary fat, and the relative amounts of saturated and unsaturated fatty acids, can affect the amount of cholesterol which is formed in the liver. Saturated fatty acids generally increase the rate of cholesterol synthesis and unsaturated fatty acids reduce it. This is the basis for the recommendation that fat should provide 30% of energy intake, with only 10% from saturated fatty acids (see p. 19).

In general, if the dietary intake of preformed cholesterol is relatively high, then synthesis in the liver will be reduced. It is only in people with genetic defects of the control of cholesterol synthesis (familial hyperlipid-aemia) that the dietary intake of cholesterol has any significant effect on plasma cholesterol. However, the main sources of preformed cholesterol in the diet are the same animal fats that are the main sources of saturated fatty acids (which tend to increase cholesterol synthesis). A lower intake of these foods will reduce the intake of preformed cholesterol and, more importantly, will reduce the synthesis of cholesterol in the body.

Amino acids, peptides and proteins

Proteins are large polymers. Unlike starch and glycogen, which are poly-mers of only a single type of monomer unit (glucose), proteins consist of 20 different amino acids. There is an almost infinite variety of proteins, composed of different numbers of the different amino acids (between 50 and 1,000 amino acids in a single protein molecule), in different orders. There are some 50,000 different proteins and polypeptides in the human body.

Each protein has a specific sequence of amino acids. This means that if we are considering an individual protein, we can determine its relative molecular mass, and can talk about mol of that protein. For the complex mixtures of proteins which make up tissues and foods, we obviously cannot define a molecular mass, and hence we still have to talk about

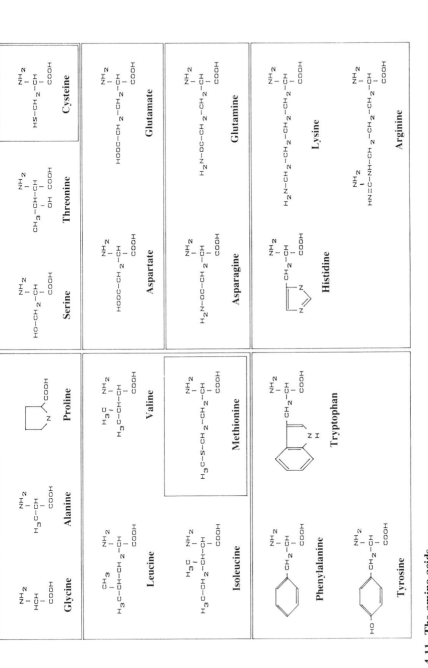

Figure 4.11 The amino acids

Twenty amino acids are involved in proteins. They can be classified according to the chemistry of their side-chains. The amino acids in the boxes on the left have hydrophobic side-chains (although tyrosine has a hydroxyl group, and can therefore interact with water to some extent), while those in the boxes on the right are hydrophilic.

grams of protein. Small proteins have a relative molecular mass of about 50×10^3 – 100×10^3, while some of the large complex proteins have a relative molecular mass of up to 10^6. In addition to proteins, smaller polymers of amino acids, containing up to about 50 amino acids, are important in the regulation of metabolism. Collectively these are known as **polypeptides**.

The amino acids

There are 20 amino acids which are involved in the formation of proteins, and several more which are metabolic intermediates, but are not involved in proteins. A few additional amino acids are found in proteins as a result of chemical modification after the protein has been synthesized. Chemically the amino acids all have the same basic structure, an amino group ($-NH_2$) and a carboxylic acid group ($-COOH$) attached to the same carbon atom (the α-carbon). As shown in Figure 4.11, what differs between the amino acids is the nature of the other group that is attached to the α-carbon. In the simplest amino acid, glycine, there are two hydrogen atoms, while in all other amino acids there is one hydrogen atom and one side-chain, varying in chemical complexity from the simple methyl group ($-CH_3$) of alanine to the aromatic ring structures of phenylalanine, tyrosine and tryptophan.

We can classify the amino acids according to the chemical nature of the side-chain; whether it is hydrophobic (on the left of Fig. 4.11) or hydrophilic (on the right of Fig. 4.11) and the nature of the group:
(a) small hydrophobic amino acids: glycine, alanine and proline;
(b) branched-chain amino acids: leucine, isoleucine and valine;
(c) aromatic amino acids: phenylalanine, tyrosine and tryptophan;
(d) sulphur-containing amino acids: cysteine and methionine;
(e) neutral hydrophilic amino acids: serine and threonine;
(f) acidic amino acids: glutamic and aspartic acids;
(g) amides of the acidic amino acids: glutamine and asparagine;
(h) basic amino acids: lysine, arginine and histidine.

Protein structure

Proteins are composed of linear chains of amino acids, joined by condensation of the carboxyl group of one with the amino group of another, to form a **peptide bond** (see Fig. 4.12). Chains of amino acids linked in this way are known as polypeptides.

Primary structure   The sequence of amino acids in a protein is its primary structure. It is different for each protein, although proteins which are closely related to each other often have similar primary structures. The primary structure of a protein is determined by the gene containing the information for that protein (see pp. 93 & 204).

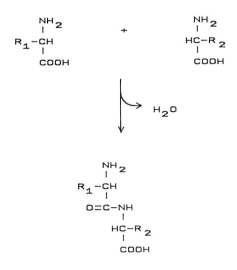

Figure 4.12 The peptide bond between two amino acids
The peptide bond is formed by a condensation reaction between the carboxyl (–COOH) group of one amino acid and the amino (–NH₂) group of another. Note how we can show an amino acid by using "–R" to represent the side-chain when it is not important which amino acid we are considering. If we wish to show that two different amino acids are involved, we can represent their side-chains as "–R₁" and "–R₂".

Secondary structure   Polypeptide chains fold up in a variety of ways. Two main types of chemical interaction are responsible for this folding: hydrogen bonds between the oxygen of one peptide bond and the nitrogen of another (see p. 51) and interactions between the side-chains of the amino acids. Depending on the nature of the side-chains, different regions of the chain may fold into one of the following patterns:

(a) **α-helix**, in which the peptide backbone of the protein adopts a spiral (helix) form (see Figure 4.13a);

(b) **ß-pleated sheet**, in which regions of the polypeptide chain lie alongside one another, forming a "corrugated" or pleated surface (see Fig. 4.13b). There are two different types of pleated sheet, with the adjacent chains of the polypeptide running in the same direction (parallel pleated sheet) or in opposite directions (anti-parallel pleated sheet).

These two types of secondary structure are mainly due to hydrogen bonding between the C=O group of one peptide bond (the oxygen is electronegative and has a δ^- partial charge) and the H–N of another peptide bond (nitrogen is also electronegative, so the hydrogen has a δ^+ partial charge). In the α-helix the hydrogen bonds are formed between peptide bonds which are near each other in the primary sequence. In the ß-pleated sheet the hydrogen bonds are between peptide bonds in different parts of the primary sequence.

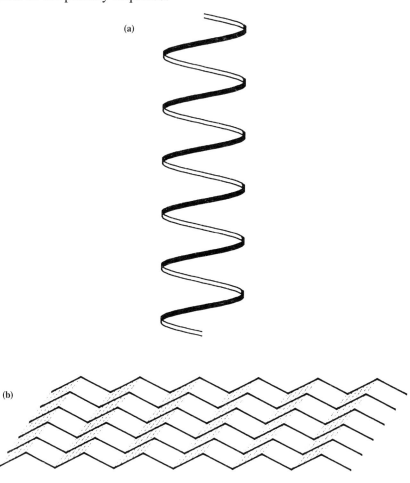

Figure 4.13 The secondary structure of proteins
(a) In the α-helix, shown on the left, a single chain of amino acids is wound into a helix; (b) in the ß-pleated sheet, shown on the right, several strands of amino acids come to lie alongside each other, forming a pleated or corrugated surface.

In addition, we see two further types of secondary structure:
(a) **hairpins and loops**, in which small regions of the polypeptide chain form very tight bends;

(b) **random coil**, in which there is no recognizable organized structure. Although this appears to be random, in that it is not an organized structure, for any one protein the shape of a random coil region will always be the same.

A protein may have several regions of α-helix, ß-pleated sheet (parallel and/or anti-parallel), hairpins and random coil, all in the same molecule.

Tertiary structure Having formed regions of secondary structure, the whole protein molecule then folds up into a compact shape. This is the third (tertiary) level of structure.

This is largely the result of interactions of the side-chains of the amino acids, both with each other and with the environment. Proteins which are in an aqueous medium in the cell generally adopt a tertiary structure in which hydrophobic amino acid side-chains are inside the molecule and can interact with each other, while hydrophilic side-chains are exposed to interact with water. By contrast, proteins which are embedded in membranes (see Fig. 4.9) have a hydrophobic region on the outside, to interact with the membrane lipids.

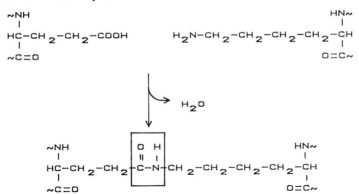

Figure 4.14 Cross-linking between peptide chains in proteins: the formation of peptide bridges
The carboxyl group of the side-chain of glutamate in one region of a protein can undergo a condensation with the side-chain amino group of lysine in another region, forming a peptide bond between the two side-chains, so linking the two regions of the protein together.

Two further interactions between amino acid side-chains may be involved in the formation of tertiary structure:
(a) The amino group on the side-chain of lysine can form a peptide bond with the carboxyl group of aspartate or glutamate (see Fig. 4.14);
(b) the sulphydryl (–SH) groups of two cysteine molecules may be oxidized, to form a disulphide bridge between two parts of the protein chain (see Fig. 4.15).

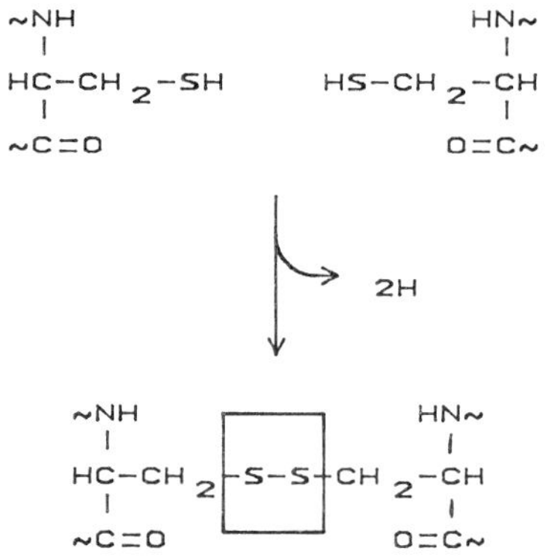

Figure 4.15 Cross-linking between peptide chains in proteins: the formation of disulphide bridges
The sulphydryl (–SH) groups of two cysteine molecules in different regions of a protein can undergo an oxidation reaction (the loss of 2H to an acceptor of some kind) to form a disulphide (–S–S–) bridge between the two side-chains, so linking the two regions of the protein together.

Since the way in which a protein chain folds is determined by interactions between amino acid side-chains, it obviously depends on both the sequence of amino acids (the primary structure) and the way in which different regions are brought near each other by the secondary structure. The shape adopted is characteristic of the particular protein and is essential for its structural and catalytic (enzymic) functions.

Quaternary structure Some proteins consist of more than one polypeptide chain. Quaternary structure is the way in which these polypeptide chains interact with each other after they have separately coiled up into their secondary and tertiary structures. Interactions between the subunits of complex proteins, involving changes in quaternary structure, are important in haemoglobin and some enzymes (see p. 111).

Denaturation of proteins Apart from covalent links formed by reaction between the side-chains of lysine and aspartate or glutamate, and disulphide bridges, the structure of proteins is maintained by relatively weak non-covalent forces: ionic interactions, hydrogen bonding and van der Waals forces.

Like all molecules, proteins vibrate, and as the temperature increases, so the vibration increases. Eventually, this vibration disrupts the weak non-covalent forces which hold the protein in its organized structure. When this happens, proteins frequently become insoluble. We call this process **denaturation** – a loss of the native structure of the protein. We can see denaturation most readily when we watch the clear, liquid white of an egg become solid and opaque as it is cooked; the proteins in the egg white are becoming denatured, and insoluble. (See also the discussion of denaturation of enzymes by heat on p. 108.)

Denaturation of proteins is important in nutrition. The compact structure of proteins means that they are relatively resistant to the action of digestive enzymes, which act to hydrolyse the peptide bonds between individual amino acids (see p. 134). Proteins which have been denatured have lost their compact structure, and many more peptide bonds are accessible to the digestive enzymes. Cooked proteins are generally more readily digested. The acid of the gastric juice is also important, since relatively strong acid will also disrupt hydrogen bonds and so denature proteins.

The nucleic acids

Purines and pyrimidines: the nucleic acid bases

Two groups of heterocyclic compounds are especially important in biochemistry: the purines adenine and guanine, and the pyrimidines uracil, cytosine and thymine (see Fig. 4.16).

All five of these compounds form **nucleosides** by reaction with sugars, either ribose or deoxyribose. These nucleosides are then known as adeno-

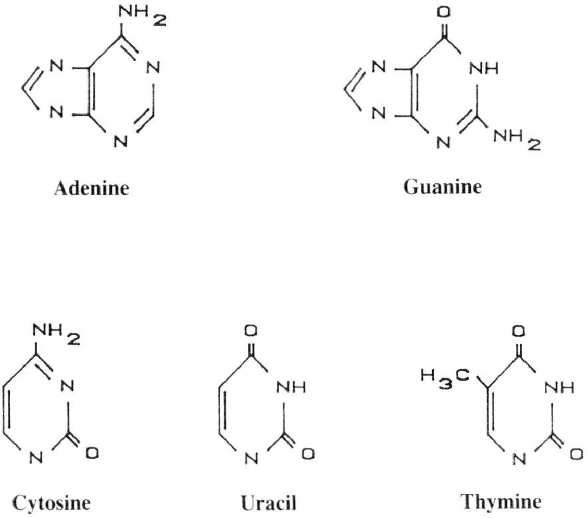

Figure 4.16 The purines and pyrimidines (the nucleic acid bases)
The purines are adenine and guanine; the pyrimidines are cytosine, uracil and thymine.

sine, guanosine, uridine, cytidine and thymidine. When the sugar is deoxyribose, the nucleosides (correctly known as deoxynucleosides) are known as deoxyadenosine, etc.

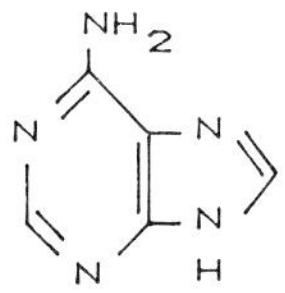

Adenine

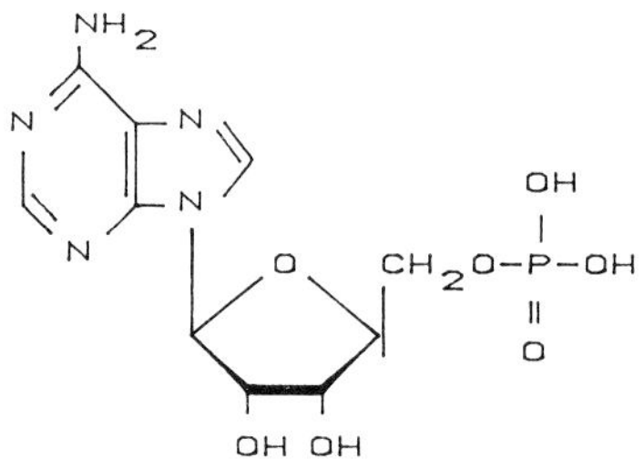

AMP

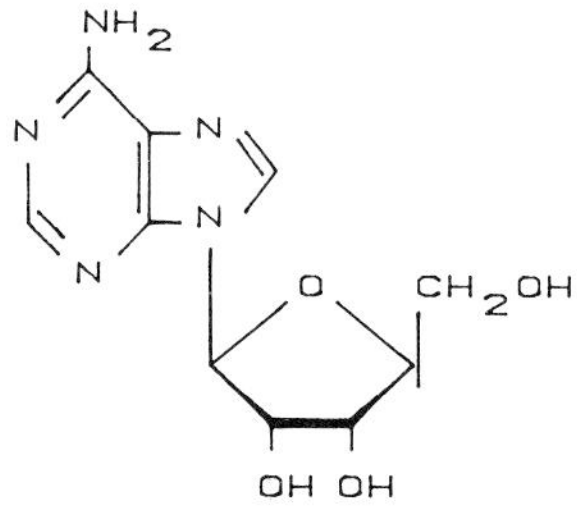

Adenosine

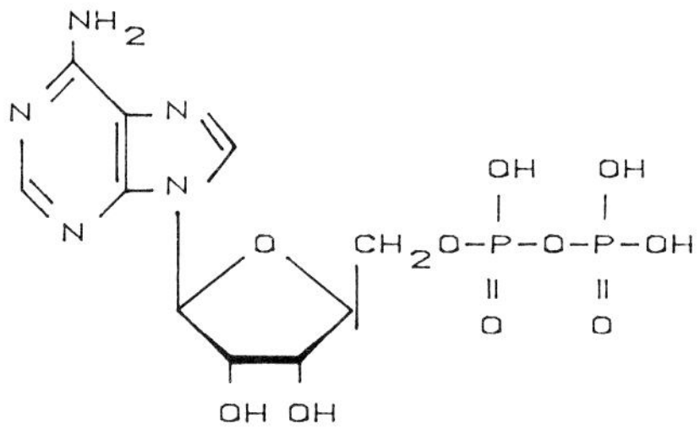

ADP

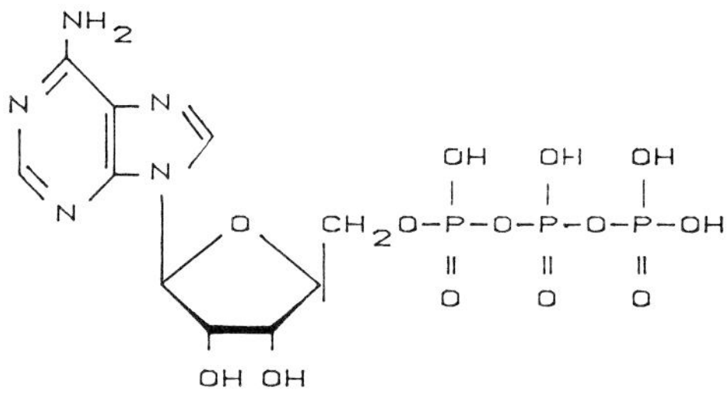

ATP

Figure 4.17 Adenine, adenosine and the adenine nucleotides
Adenine can be bound to ribose or deoxyribose, to form the nucleoside adenosine. When the sugar is phosphorylated, the result is a nucleotide: with one phosphate, the product is adenosine monophosphate, AMP; with two phosphates, the product is adenosine diphosphate, ADP; with three phosphates, the product is adenosine triphosphate, ATP. The other purines and pyrimidines can similarly form nucleosides and deoxynucleosides:

Base	*Nucleoside*	*Nucleotides*
adenine	adenosine	AMP, ADP, ATP
guanine	guanosine	GMP, GDP, GTP
cytosine	cytidine	CMP, CDP, CTP
uracil	uridine	UMP, UDP, UTP
thymine	thymidine	TMP, TDP, TTP

The sugar part of the nucleoside can be esterified to phosphate (phosphorylated), to form a **nucleotide** (or deoxynucleotide if the sugar is deoxyribose). Nucleotides may have one, two or three phosphate groups. The adenine nucleotides are shown in Figure 4.17. We generally abbreviate the names, so that adenosine triphosphate is ATP, adenosine diphosphate is ADP and adenosine monophosphate is AMP. We use similar abbreviations for the other nucleotide phosphates: GTP, GDP and GMP for guanine nucleotides; and similarly, U for uridine; C for cytidine and T for thymidine.

The adenine nucleotides (and to some extent also the guanine nucleotides) have a central rôle in metabolism, as coenzymes in a wide variety of reactions. They provide the link between the oxidation of metabolic fuels and the expenditure of metabolic energy. The oxidation of metabolic fuels is linked to the phosphorylation of ADP to form ATP, while biosynthetic reactions, the pumping of ions across cell membranes and muscle contraction are linked to the hydrolysis of ATP to yield ADP and phosphate (see p. 125).

Adenine and guanine nucleotides are also important in intracellular signalling in response to the actions of hormones and neurotransmitters on cell-surface receptor proteins. This is discussed on p. 223.

The nucleic acids: RNA and DNA

The nucleic acids are linear polymers of purine and pyrimidine nucleotides, linked by phosphate diester bonds. When the sugar is ribose, the resultant nucleic acid is **ribonucleic acid, RNA**. When the sugar is deoxyribose, the resultant nucleic acid is **deoxyribonucleic acid, DNA**.

The sequence of purines and pyrimidines in DNA carries the information for the synthesis of the 50,000 proteins and polypeptides which make up the body and control its metabolic functions.

RNA: ribonucleic acid   The structure of a short region of RNA is shown in Figure 4.18; it consists of a "backbone" of alternating ribose and phosphate units, with the phosphate groups forming links from carbon-3 of one ribose to carbon-5 of the next. At one end of the chain is a ribose with a free hydroxyl group on carbon-3, while at the other end is a ribose with a free hydroxyl group on carbon-5. We refer to these ends of the RNA chain as the 3' end (with a free hydroxyl group on carbon-3) and the 5' end (with a free hydroxyl group on carbon-5).

The purines and pyrimidines (collectively called **bases**) project from the ribose-phosphate chain. RNA contains the purines adenine and guanine, and the pyrimidines uracil and cytosine. It does not contain thymidine.

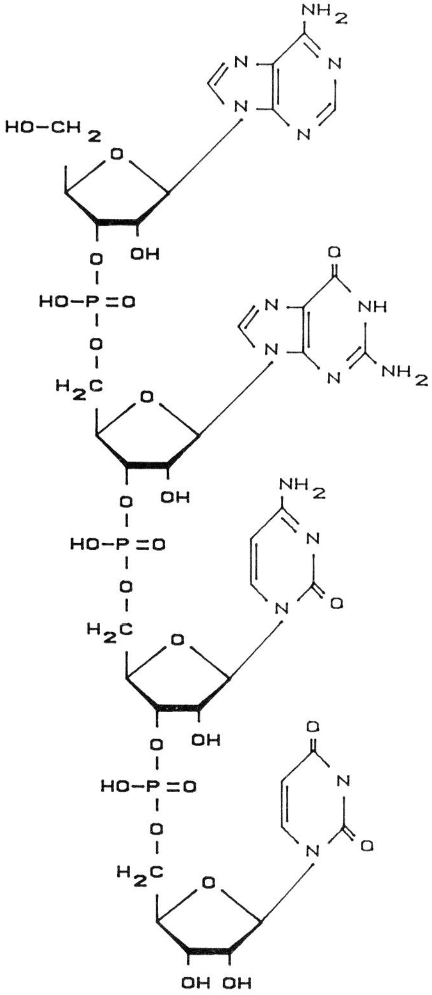

Figure 4.18 The structure of RNA (ribonucleic acid)
RNA is a linear polymer of nucleotides, linked by a phosphodiester bridge from carbon-3 of one ribose to carbon-5 of the next. The purine and pyrimidine bases of the nucleotides "stick out" from this sugar–phosphate backbone of the molecule. The 3′ end of the molecule, with a free –OH group on C-3 of ribose is shown at the top, and the 5′ end at the bottom of the diagram.

There are three main types of RNA in the cell:

(a) **Messenger RNA (mRNA)** is made in the nucleus, as a copy of one strand of DNA (the process of **transcription**, see p. 205). After some editing of the message, it is transferred into the cytosol, where it binds to ribosomes. The information carried by the mRNA is then **translated** into the amino acid sequence of proteins – the process of

96

protein synthesis (see p. 212).
(b) **Ribosomal RNA (rRNA)** is part of the structure of the ribosomes on which protein is synthesized (see p. 208).
(c) **Transfer RNA (tRNA)** provides the link between mRNA and the amino acids required for protein synthesis on the ribosome (see p. 209).

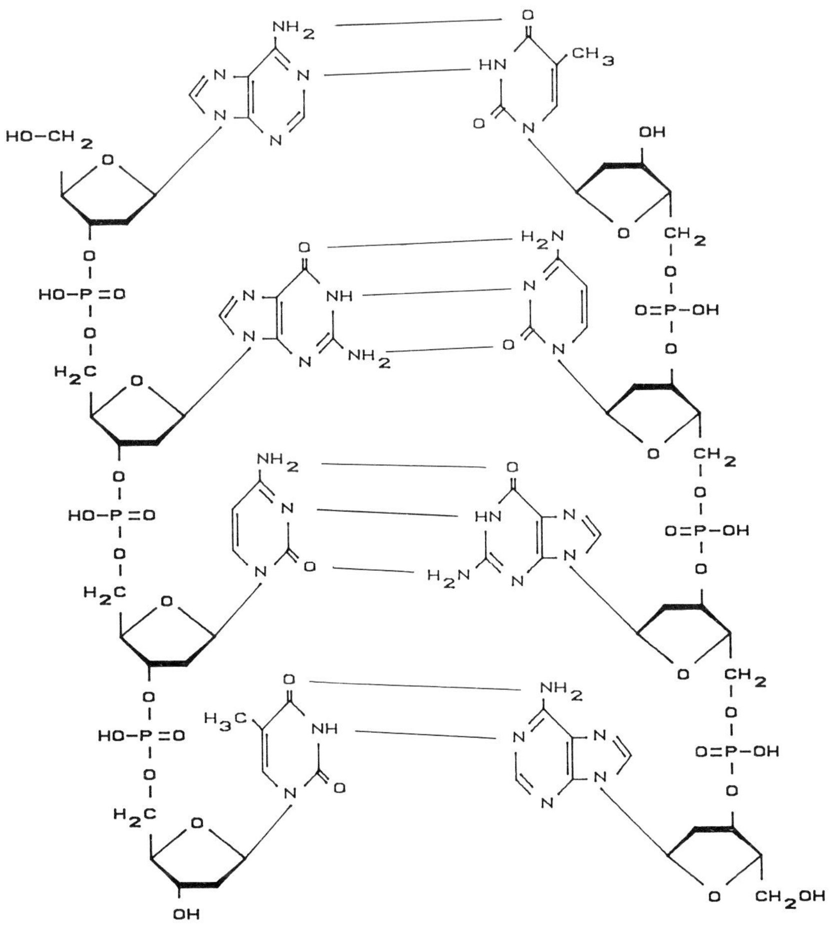

Figure 4.19 The structure of DNA (deoxyribonucleic acid)
DNA is a linear polymer of deoxynucleotides linked by a phospho-diester bridge from carbon-3 of one deoxyribose to carbon-5 of the next. The purine and pyrimidine bases of the nucleotides "stick out" from this sugar–phosphate backbone of the molecule. DNA normally exists as two parallel strands of deoxynucleotides, held together by hydrogen bonds between the purine and pyrimidine bases. In each case a purine forms hydrogen bonds to a pyrimidine (or vice versa): adenine forms two hydrogen bonds to thymine (A...T); guanine forms three hydrogen bonds to cytosine (G...C).

DNA: deoxyribonucleic acid The structure of a short region of DNA is shown in Figure 4.19. Like RNA, it consists of a "backbone" of alternating sugar and phosphate units, with the phosphate groups forming links from carbon-3 of one sugar to carbon-5 of the next. The sugar in DNA is deoxyribose. Like RNA, the strand of DNA has a free 3'-hydroxyl at one end and a free 5'-hydroxyl group at the other. Again the bases project from the sugar–phosphate backbone of the molecule.

In DNA the purines are adenine and guanine, as in RNA. The pyrimidines are cytosine (as in RNA) and thymine (rather than uracil as in RNA). Chemical analysis of DNA shows that two pairs of bases always occur in the same proportions:

the amount of adenine = the amount of thymine;
the amount of guanine = the amount of cytosine.

The relative amounts of [A + T] and [G + C] differ from one species of organism to another, but are constant for any one species, and are the same in all cells of the body.

This equality in the amounts of [A + T], and of [G + C], is due to the structure of DNA. Unlike RNA, it does not exist as a single strand of nucleotides, but as two strands which interact with each other. As shown in Figure 4.19, the bases in DNA form hydrogen bonds between the two strands. Each molecule of A forms two hydrogen bonds to T, and each G forms three hydrogen bonds to C. These hydrogen bonds serve to keep the two strands together. Although individually hydrogen bonds are relatively weak (see p. 41), the sum of the very large number in a molecule of DNA results in a very strong force to maintain the structure of the molecule.

The two strands of a DNA molecule run in opposite directions. In other words, where one strand has a 3'-hydroxyl group at the end, on the complementary chain there is a free 5'-hydroxyl group. The information of DNA is always read from the 3' end towards the 5' end.

We can draw a simplified representation of the structure of DNA, using complementary shapes to represent the complementary bases which form hydrogen bonds to each other, as shown on the left in Figure 4.20. As shown on the right in Figure 4.20, the two strands of DNA are coiled around a common axis to form a helical structure. Because the helix is formed from a double strand of DNA, it is known as the **double helix**.

The DNA in a human cell contains some 1.2×10^{10} base-pairs. The total length in each cell would about $2\,m$ if it were stretched out. Obviously, since it is to be contained within a nucleus which is only $5\,\mu m$ in diameter, the DNA must be folded tightly. The double helix can be bent into smooth curves, or supercoiled upon itself, with little or no disruption of the underlying conformation of the helix itself. This is exactly the same as coiling, twisting and knotting a rope which is made up of twisted strands. The arrangement of the strands relative to each other is unaffected, but a considerable length of rope (or DNA) can be fitted into quite a small space.

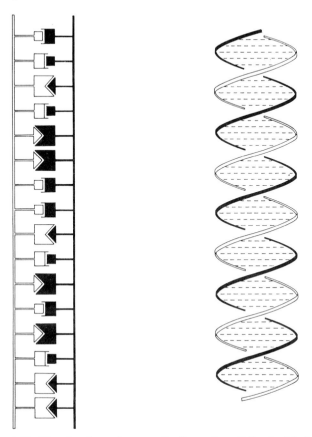

Figure 4.20 The structure of DNA – the formation of the double helix
We can simplify the representation of the structure of DNA shown in Figure 4.19, just drawing a line to represent the sugar–phosphate backbone, and shapes to represent the purines and pyrimidines, as shown on the left in this diagram. The two strands of DNA, held together by the hydrogen bonds between the purines and pyrimidines, form a spiral structure, or helix, shown on the right in this diagram.

The DNA in the nucleus is not only coiled upon itself, but is wrapped around a variety of proteins. At the beginning of cell division, when DNA is about to undergo replication (see below) we can see the DNA–protein complexes under the microscope as densely staining "bodies" inside the nucleus – the **chromosomes**. Altogether there are 46 chromosomes in human cells; two copies of each of 22 chromosomes, and one pair which are known as the **sex chromosomes** – two X-chromosomes in females or an X plus a Y in males. Ova and sperm cells contain only one copy of each chromosome, and only one sex chromosome: always X in the ovum, and either X or Y in the sperm.

Not all of the DNA carries information for genes. Indeed, only 10% of the DNA in a human cell actually carries information for the 50,000 genes which make up the human genome. The remainder is made up of:

(a) **Control regions**, which promote or enhance the expression of individual genes, and include regions which respond to hormones and other factors which modulate gene expression (see p. 226), as well as sites for the initiation and termination of DNA replication (see below).

(b) **Spacer regions**, both between and within genes, which carry no translatable message, but serve to link those regions which do carry a translatable message. When such regions occur within a gene sequence, they are called **introns** (see p. 208).

(c) **Pseudo-genes**, which seem to be genes that have undergone mutation in our evolutionary past, and are now untranslatable. We presume that they are simply a reminder of our evolutionary history.

The replication of DNA Cells replicate by division. The single cell of the fertilized ovum grows and undergoes repeated divisions to yield the approximately 2×10^{12} cells in the body of the new-born infant. Cell division then continues throughout life, both for growth and because there is turnover and replacement of cells after growth has ceased.

When cells divide, each of the two new cells has a complete copy of the DNA of the parent cell. This means that prior to cell division the whole of the DNA of the cell has to be copied.

The replication of DNA requires an extremely high degree of precision and fidelity. Any changes in the information carried by DNA will be transmitted to future generations of cells. Considering the number of cell divisions which must occur throughout life, it is obvious that mistakes in replicating DNA could result in garbling of the information.

The key to the very high fidelity in replicating DNA is the base-pairing which is responsible for the double helical structure of the molecule. As shown in Figure 4.21, replication involves the unwinding of a section of DNA, separation of the hydrogen-bonded base pairs, then binding of complementary bases onto each strand of the parent DNA. The result of this process is that each the two copies of the DNA that are formed (one of which will end up in the nucleus of each new cell) has one newly synthesized strand and one from the parent molecule.

As the strands of DNA are unwound for replication, so the nucleotide triphosphates with bases complementary to those present on the strand to be copied form hydrogen bonds. If the hydrogen bonding to form base pairs is correct (A pairs with T and G pairs with C) then the phosphates undergo a condensation reaction, forming the sugar–phosphate backbone of the new strand of DNA. If the base-pairing is not correct, this will dis-

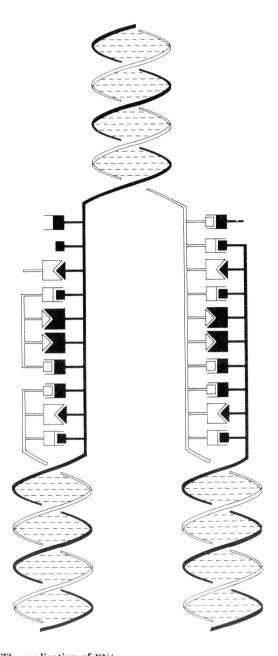

Figure 4.21 The replication of DNA
A small region of the double strand of DNA is unwound at a time, by breaking the hydrogen bonds between the purines and pyrimidines which hold the two strands together. Each base then forms hydrogen bonds to the complementary deoxynucleoside triphosphate: adenine binds thymidine triphosphate; guanine binds cytidine triphosphate; cytosine binds guanosine triphosphate; thymine binds adenosine triphosphate. As each base is matched by a deoxynucleoside triphosphate, so a phosphate bond is formed to the adjacent deoxyribose, with the elimination of pyrophosphate.

tort the shape of the molecule, and the sugar–phosphate bonds cannot be formed. The mistaken base must be removed and replaced by the correct one before the formation of the phosphate bond can occur.

The synthesis of DNA always proceeds in the same direction, from the 3' end of the strand being copied, and hence the 5' end of the strand being synthesized. For one strand this presents no problem, since it can be copied in one go, starting from its 3' end, as shown on the right in Figure 4.21. The complementary strand (shown on the left in Fig. 4.21) runs in the opposite direction. This strand is copied in short pieces, which are then joined together.

Despite the "checking" before the formation of the sugar–phosphate bonds, and "proof-reading" of the newly synthesized DNA, the rate of replication is of the order of 30,000 nucleotides incorporated/minute. This may seem an impressive rate of reaction, until we remember that the total human DNA to be replicated consists of some 1.2×10^{10} base-pairs. If DNA replication simply started at one end of the molecule, it would take some 6,700 hours to make a complete copy. Even allowing for the fact that the 46 chromosomes could be copied simultaneously, it would take about 6 days to make a complete set of copies. What happens is that replication starts at several hundred sites in each molecule of DNA, so that at any time during replication there are several hundred areas of unwinding and replication like that shown in Figure 4.21. In this way replication of the whole of the DNA of a cell can occur in only about 7 hours.

Mistakes do occur in DNA replication. Even a rate of only one mistake in a thousand million base pairings would mean 12 mistakes every time DNA was replicated. As well as occasional mistakes in replication, changes in the base sequence of DNA can occur as a result of the effects of various chemical agents and free radicals produced by radiation, which cause chemical changes to the bases. This means that a base other than the one which was intended will form an appropriate base pair, and so be incorporated into the new strand of DNA. The alteration to the base sequence of DNA will then be perpetuated in future replications.

Such changes in DNA, accumulating gradually over a life-time, constitute one of the mechanisms involved in the causation of **cancer**, and chemicals which cause DNA damage in this way are **carcinogens** – cancer-causing chemicals. If the changes in DNA occur in cells which give rise to ova or sperm, then the altered DNA is inherited by the next generation; now we have a **mutation**. Most mutations are undesirable, and are the basis of inherited diseases (see p. 286), but we must also bear in mind that the process of evolution is based on the (relatively few) mutations which have resulted in beneficial changes.

Frequently, the chemical changes which might lead to incorrect base-pairing in replication also lead to a distortion of the structure of DNA, and activate a series of DNA **repair enzymes**, which remove the base causing the distortion, and replace it with one which forms a correct base-pair with the complementary strand. The importance of these DNA repair mechanisms is seen in the disease **xeroderma pigmentosum**, which results from genetic defects of the DNA repair mechanism. Patients are unusually sensitive to ultraviolet light, leading to atrophy of the dermis and the development of skin cancer, frequently with fatal metastasis before the age of 30.

The genetic code It is difficult at first sight to understand how a code made up of only four letters (A, G, C and T) can carry the large amount of information which we know must be contained in the nucleus of the cell, for the 50,000 different proteins which are to be synthesized.

The answer is that the bases are read in groups of three, not singly. Since each group of three can contain any one of the four bases in each position, there are 64 possible combinations. This means that four bases give a code consisting of 64 words. Each group of three nucleotides is called a **codon** – a single unit of the genetic code.

While 64 codons might not seem much to carry complex information, there is a need for only 22 codons. The information which has to be coded for in DNA is the sequence of the 20 amino acids in proteins, together with codes for the beginning and end of messages. If you consider how 26 letters of the alphabet can carry the information for the whole of literature and our written knowledge, you can see how a simple code, based on 64 possible combinations of three out of four nucleotides, can similarly form the basis of a very large information store. The genetic code is shown in Tables 9.6 and 9.7, with a discussion of the rôles of DNA and RNA in protein synthesis.

DNA fingerprinting It is obvious from the discussion above that there can be many differences in the detailed sequence of bases in DNA between individuals. Apart from identical twins, who develop from the same fertilized ovum, no two individuals have identical DNA sequences, regardless of how similar the information contained in that DNA is.

We do not have to read the complete sequence of bases in DNA to see these differences. Indeed, this would be an almost impossible task. We can take the DNA from a small sample of tissue, and break it into several thousand fragments, using specific enzymes which cleave DNA at defined sequences. We can then separate the fragments chemically on a gel, and see a pattern. If we have fragmented the DNA enough, we can see that every individual has a unique pattern. This is like the use of fingerprints to distinguish between individuals, and the process is known as DNA fingerprinting.

DNA fingerprinting has two important applications:

(a) In police work, where the DNA in body fluids (for example at the site of a crime) can be compared with that of suspects, in the same way as ordinary fingerprints can be used to establish identity.

(b) In the establishment of paternity. A child receives one set of chromosomes (and hence one copy of DNA) from each parent. This means that we can compare the DNA fingerprints of the child, its mother and the presumed father, to see whether or not the pattern the child has inherited matches that of the presumed father.

CHAPTER FIVE

Enzymes and metabolic pathways

Enzymes are proteins that catalyse metabolic reactions. Since all of metabolism depends on enzyme-catalysed reactions, an understanding of enzyme action and the ways in which the activity of enzymes can be altered is obviously essential for an understanding of nutrition and metabolism.

A **catalyst** increases the rate at which a chemical reaction comes to equilibrium. While it may be involved in the processes of breaking and making chemical bonds during the reaction, the catalyst itself is unchanged at the end of the reaction.

The folding of the peptide chain of a protein results in reactive groups from a variety of amino acid side-chains, which may be widely separated in the primary sequence of the protein, coming close to each other (see p. 89). This creates a site on the surface of the protein which has a defined shape and array of chemically reactive groups, formed by the side-chains of the amino acids. This is the **active site** of the enzyme. It is the site that both binds the compounds which are to undergo reaction (the **substrates**) and catalyses the reaction.

The binding of substrates to enzymes involves interactions between the substrate and reactive groups of the amino acid side-chains which make up the active site of the enzyme. This means that enzymes show a considerable degree of **specificity** for the substrates they bind. Normally, several different interactions occur before the substrate can bind in the correct orientation to undergo reaction. Enzymes distinguish between the D- and L-isomers, and between the *cis*- and *trans*-isomers, of the substrate, because they have a different shape or spatial arrangement, although in non-enzymic chemical reactions the isomers may behave identically. The shape and conformation of the substrate are critically important for binding to an enzyme.

Enzymes are not just passive surfaces which bind the substrates. The active site of the enzyme plays an important part in the reaction process. Various amino acid side-chains of the enzyme molecule at the active site provide chemically reactive groups which can facilitate the making or breaking of specific chemical bonds in the substrate by donating or withdrawing electrons. In this way the enzyme can lower the activation energy of a chemical reaction (see p. 49). Rather than needing an input of energy to excite the electrons in a bond, the enzyme achieves this excitation by interactions between the substrate and reactive groups at the active site.

This means that an enzyme can achieve a very much greater increase in the rate at which a reaction attains equilibrium than a simple chemical catalyst, and frequently under very much milder conditions. If we want to hydrolyse a protein into its constituent amino acids in the laboratory, we normally use concentrated acid as a catalyst, and heat the sample at 105°C overnight to provide the activation energy of the hydrolysis. As discussed on p. 134, this is the process of digestion of proteins, which occurs in the human gut under only slightly acid or alkaline conditions, at 37°C, and is complete within a few hours of eating a meal.

We can write the sequence of events in an enzyme catalysed reaction as follows: $E + S \rightleftharpoons E\text{-}S \rightleftharpoons E\text{-}P \rightleftharpoons E + P$
where E is the enzyme, S the substrate and P the product. The reaction occurs in three stages, all of which are reversible:

(a) binding of the substrate to the enzyme, to form the enzyme–substrate complex $E + S \rightleftharpoons E\text{-}S$;
(b) reaction of the enzyme–substrate complex to form the enzyme–product complex $E\text{-}S \rightleftharpoons E\text{-}P$;
(c) breakdown of the enzyme–product complex, with release of the product $E\text{-}P \rightleftharpoons E + P$.

The fact that enzymes not only bind the substrates, but also participate in the reaction (although they emerge unchanged at the end of the reaction) means that as well as conferring specificity for the substrates, an enzyme also confers specificity for the reaction which is followed. Consider a reaction between two substrates, A and B, which can proceed to give two different sets of products, X and Y or P and Q. With a chemical catalyst, we would expect a complex mixture at equilibrium, containing A, B, P, Q, X and Y. Both reactions occur at the same time, and each comes to its own equilibrium. With an enzyme, we find that only one reaction occurs: A and B react to form only P and Q with one enzyme, and only X and Y with a different enzyme.

Factors which affect the activity of enzymes

When an enzyme has been purified, it is possible to express the amount of that enzyme in tissues, etc., as the number of mol present. However, what is more important is not how much of the enzyme protein is present in the cell, but how much catalytic activity there is; how much substrate can be converted to product in a given time. Therefore amounts of enzyme are usually expressed in terms of units of activity:

1 unit of activity $= 1\ \mu$mol of substrate converted/min determined under specified optimum conditions for that enzyme.

pH

Both the binding of the substrate to the enzyme and the catalysis of the reaction depend on interactions between the substrates and reactive groups in the amino acid side-chains which make up the active site. This means that both the substrates and these various reactive groups have to be in the appropriate ionized form for binding and reaction to occur. The state of ionization depends on the pH of the medium. This means that an enzyme will have maximum activity at a specific pH. This is the **optimum pH** for that enzyme; obviously, it will be different for different enzymes. As the pH rises or falls away from the optimum, so the activity of the enzyme will decrease. Most enzymes have little or no activity 2–3 pH units away from their pH optimum. This is shown for three different enzymes, with different pH optima, in Figure 5.1.

There is very precise control over pH in the body. As discussed on p. 46, a relatively small change in the pH of blood plasma away from the

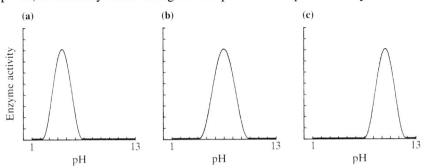

Figure 5.1 The effect of pH on enzyme activity
The pH of the medium affects the activity of enzymes. For any enzyme, there is a relatively narrow range of pH in which it has maximum activity. In these examples enzyme (a) has a pH optimum of 4.5, which is relatively acidic; enzyme (b) has a pH optimum of 7, which is neutral, while enzyme (c) has a pH optimum of 9.5, which is alkaline.

normal value of 7.4 results in serious problems of acidosis (when the plasma pH is below 7.2) or alkalosis (when the plasma pH is above 7.6). Nevertheless, enzymes with pH optima very different from 7.4, and which may have no significant activity at pH 7.4, are important in the body. This is because the pH within different regions and compartments of the cell can be very different from the average pH of the cell as a whole, or the pH of plasma.

Temperature

Chemical reactions proceed faster at higher temperatures. The rate of reaction generally doubles for each 10°C rise in temperature. This is because molecules move faster at higher temperatures, and hence have a greater chance of colliding to undergo reaction. At a higher temperature it is also easier for electrons to gain activation energy, and hence become excited into unstable orbitals to undergo reaction.

Enzymes also have a faster rate of reaction at higher temperatures. However, because they are proteins, enzymes are also denatured at high temperatures (see p. 93). This means that while small increases in temperature increase the rate of reaction, as the enzyme begins to be denatured (as the temperature rises above about 50°C), so there is a sudden decrease in the rate of reaction (see Fig. 5.2). Denaturation is irreversible, so once an enzyme has been denatured by heat it is permanently inactivated.

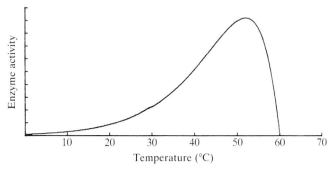

Figure 5.2 The effect of temperature on the rate of an enzyme reaction

In the body, this effect of temperature is not normally important. Body temperature is normally 37°C. However, some fever effects (when temperature may rise to 40°C) may be due to changes in the enzyme reaction rates. Because different enzymes respond to changes in temperature in different ways, there can be a considerable loss of the normal integration between different enzymic reactions and metabolic pathways.

We take advantage of slowing rates of enzymic reactions as the temperature falls in open-heart surgery, for example, when the patient's body temperature is deliberately lowered, to reduce the metabolic rate.

The concentration of substrate

In a simple chemical reaction, the rate at which a product is formed increases in a linear fashion as the concentration of the substrate increases (see Fig. 5.3a). There is more substrate available to undergo the reaction, and as the concentration increases, so there is a greater chance for molecules to come together to react.

With enzymic reactions, the change in the rate of formation of product with increasing concentration of substrate is not linear, but curved, as shown in Figure 5.3b. At relatively low concentrations of substrate (region (i) in Fig. 5.3b), the catalytic site of the enzyme may be empty at times, until more substrate binds and undergoes reaction. Under these conditions, what limits the rate of formation of product is the time taken for another molecule of substrate to bind to the enzyme. Adding more substrate shortens this time, and so increases the rate of formation of product . A relatively small change in the concentration of substrate has a large effect on the rate at which product is formed in this region of the curve.

At high concentrations of substrate (region (ii) in Fig. 5.3b), as soon as the product leaves the catalytic site, another molecule of substrate binds. Under these conditions, when the enzyme is saturated with substrate, it is acting as fast as it can. The limiting factor in the formation of product is now that rate at which the enzyme can catalyse the reaction, and not the availability of substrate. The enzyme is acting at its **maximum rate**. Even a relatively large change in the concentration of substrate has little effect on the rate of formation of product in this region of the curve. The maximum rate or velocity of an enzyme reaction is usually abbreviated to V_{max}. It is an innate property of the enzyme.

From a graph of the rate of formation of product versus the concentration of substrate (Fig. 5.3b & c), it is easy to see what is the maximum rate of reaction that an enzyme can achieve (V_{max}) when it is saturated with substrate. However, it is not possible to determine from this graph the concentration of substrate required to achieve saturation, because the enzyme gradually approaches its maximum rate of reaction as the concentration of substrate increases.

It is easy to find the concentration of substrate at which the enzyme is has half its maximum rate of reaction. The concentration of substrate to achieve half V_{max} is called the Michaelis constant of the enzyme (abbreviated to K_m), to commemorate Michaelis, who, together with Menten, first

109

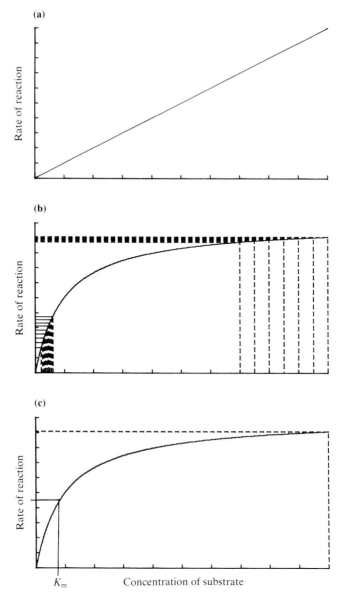

Figure 5.3 The effect of substrate concentration on the rate of reaction
(a) In a simple chemical reaction the rate at which a product is formed increases linearly
with the amount of substrate available to undergo the reaction. (b) With an enzyme-
catalysed reaction there is a non-linear dependence of the rate of reaction on the
concentration of substrate available to undergo reaction: (i) at low concentrations of
substrate, the limiting factor is the time taken for the enzyme to "find" a molecule of
substrate to act on, and therefore the amount of substrate available; (ii) at high
concentrations of substrate, as soon as a molecule of substrate has been converted to
product, and the product has left the enzyme, another molecule of substrate is available
to bind to the enzyme and undergo reaction. Under these conditions, the enzyme is
saturated with substrate. The limiting factor here is the activity of the enzyme itself. Even
relatively large changes in the concentration of substrate in this region have little effect
on the rate of formation of product. (c) The determination of V_{max}, the maximum rate of
reaction of an enzyme, and K_m, the concentration of substrate at which it has half its
maximum rate of reaction

formulated a mathematical model of the dependence of the rate of enzymic reactions on the concentration of substrate.

The K_m of an enzyme is an innate property of the enzyme and is not affected by the amount of the enzyme that is present. It is an (inverse) index of the ease with which an enzyme can bind substrate. An enzyme which has a high K_m has a relatively poor ability to bind its substrate compared with an enzyme which has a lower K_m. The higher the value of K_m, the greater is the concentration of substrate required to achieve half-saturation of the enzyme.

In general, enzymes which have a low K_m compared with the normal concentration of substrate in the cell are likely to be acting at or near their maximum rate, and hence to have a more or less constant rate of reaction despite (modest) changes in the concentration of substrate. By contrast, an enzyme which has a high K_m compared with the normal concentration of substrate in the cell will show a large change in the rate of reaction with relatively small changes in the concentration of substrate.

If two enzymes in a cell can both act on the same substrate, catalysing different reactions, the enzyme with the lower K_m will be able to bind more substrate, and therefore its reaction will be favoured at relatively low concentrations of substrate.

Co-operative (allosteric) enzymes Not all enzymes have the simple dependence of rate of reaction on substrate concentration shown in Figure 5.3. Some enzymes consist of several separate protein chains, each with an active site. In many such enzymes, the binding of substrate to one active site causes changes in the quaternary structure (i.e. the conformation of the whole assembly, see p. 92). This alters the ease with which substrate can bind to the other active sites. This is called **co-operativity**: the different sub-units of the complete enzyme co-operate with each other. Because there is a change in the conformation (or shape) of the enzyme molecule, the phenomenon is also called **allostericity** (from the Greek for "different shape"), and such enzymes are called **allosteric enzymes**.

Figure 5.4a shows the change in rate of reaction with increasing concentration of substrate for an enzyme which displays substrate co-operativity. At low concentrations of substrate the enzyme has little activity. As one of the binding sites is occupied, this causes a conformational change in the enzyme, and so increases the ease with which the other sites can bind substrate. Therefore there is a steep increase in the rate of reaction with increasing concentration of substrate. Of course, as all the sites become saturated, so the rate of reaction cannot increase any further with increasing concentration of substrate; the enzyme achieves its maximum rate of reaction.

Enzymes which display substrate co-operativity are frequently important

111

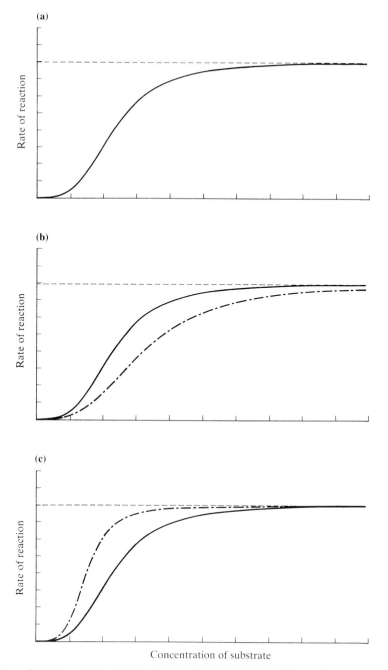

Figure 5.4 The relationship between substrate concentration and rate of reaction for an enzyme which shows co-operative binding of substrate
(a) At low concentrations of substrate the enzyme has very little activity. However, binding of substrate to one site on the enzyme facilitates binding at the other sites and, as the first site becomes saturated, so binding to the other sites increases, and the rate of formation of product increases very sharply with increasing concentration of substrate. As the concentration of substrate increases further, all the sites become saturated, and the limiting factor is the activity of the enzyme. (b) The dotted line shows the effect of adding a compound which impairs the co-operativity between the sites on the enzyme. (c) The dotted line shows the effect of adding a compound which enhances the co-operativity between the sites of the enzyme.

in controlling the overall rate of metabolic pathways. They are very sensitive to the concentration of substrate, and, perhaps more importantly, their sensitivity can easily be modified. A variety of compounds can bind the specific regulator sites on the enzyme and affect its conformation. End-products and precursors of metabolic pathways frequently act in this way to modify the activity of key enzymes.

As shown in Figure 5.4b, some compounds can reduce the co-operativity between the active sites, so reducing the activity of the enzyme at the same concentration of substrate. The graph of rate of reaction versus substrate concentration is shifted to the right. The enzyme is inhibited; it has lower activity at a given concentration of substrate in the presence of the inhibitor.

Other compounds can increase the activity of the enzyme, by mimicking the co-operativity normally associated with a high concentration of substrate. When such compounds bind to the enzyme, they cause the same conformational change as is achieved by increasing the concentration of substrate. As shown in Figure 5.4c, in the presence of such a compound all of the active sites have increased affinity for the substrate, and the enzyme has higher activity at low concentrations of substrate.

Inhibition of enzymes

Compounds which are structurally similar to the substrate can often compete with the substrate for the active site of the enzyme, although they do not undergo reaction to form products. Such compounds are called **competitive inhibitors** of the enzyme. They reduce its rate of reaction, simply because at any moment in time some molecules of the enzyme have bound the inhibitor, and therefore are not free to bind the substrate. We can write the sequence of events in the presence of a competitive inhibitor as:

$$E{-}S \rightleftharpoons E{-}P \rightleftharpoons E + P$$
$$E + I + S$$
$$E{-}I$$

where E is the enzyme, S the substrate, P the product and I the inhibitor. The enzyme can form either the enzyme–substrate complex, E-S, which goes on to form products, or the enzyme–inhibitor complex, E-I, which does nothing useful.

If the concentration of substrate is increased, it will compete more effectively with the inhibitor for the active site of the enzyme. This means that at high concentrations of substrate the enzyme will achieve the same maximum rate of reaction (V_{max}) in the presence or absence of inhibitor. It is simply that in the presence of inhibitor the enzyme requires a higher

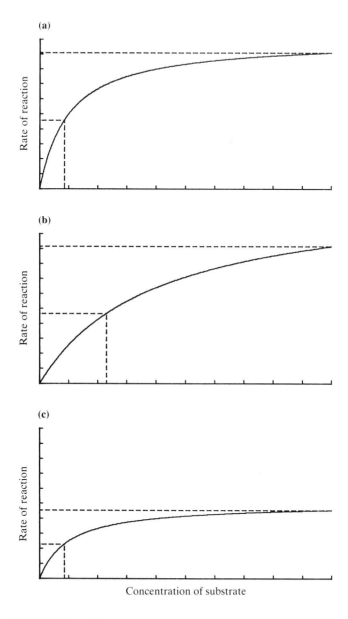

Figure 5.5 Inhibition of enzymes
(a) The relationship between the concentration of substrate and rate of formation of product in the absence of inhibitor. (b) The effect of adding a competitive inhibitor. As the concentration of substrate increases, so it can compete with the inhibitor. The V_{max} is the same as when there was no inhibitor present, but the K_{m} is higher. (c) The effect of adding a non-competitive inhibitor. The V_{max} of the enzyme is reduced by addition of the inhibitor, but the K_{m} is unaffected.

concentration of substrate to achieve saturation; in other words, the K_m of the enzyme is higher in the presence of a competitive inhibitor (see Fig. 5.5b).

Other compounds can bind to the enzyme together with the substrate, and slow down the rate at which the enzyme catalyses the formation of product. These are called **non-competitive inhibitors**. We can write the sequence of events in the presence of a non-competitive inhibitor as:

$$E + I + S \rightleftharpoons E\text{-}S + I \rightleftharpoons E\text{-}S\text{-}I \rightleftharpoons E\text{-}P\text{-}I \rightleftharpoons E + I + P$$

The reaction of the enzyme–substrate–inhibitor complex (E–S–I) to form the enzyme–product–inhibitor complex (E–P–I) is slower than the reaction of E–S to form E–P, and therefore the rate of reaction is slower in the presence of the inhibitor.

In the presence of a non-competitive inhibitor, the maximum rate of reaction of the enzyme (V_{max}) is reduced. Because there is no competition between the inhibitor and the substrate for binding to the enzyme, increasing the concentration of substrate has no effect on the activity of the enzyme in the presence of a non-competitive inhibitor. The K_m of the enzyme is unaffected by a non-competitive inhibitor (see Fig. 5.5c).

Some metabolic intermediates can act as inhibitors of enzymes, and so can act to regulate metabolic processes. Many of the drugs used to treat various diseases are inhibitors of enzymes. Some act by inhibiting the activity of the patient's enzymes, and so altering metabolic regulation; others act by preferentially inhibiting the enzymes of bacteria or other micro-organisms which are causing disease.

Coenzymes and prosthetic groups

Although enzymes are proteins, many contain small non-protein molecules as an integral part of their structure. These may be organic compounds, which are known as **coenzymes**, or they may be metal ions. In either case, they are essential to the function of the enzyme, and the enzyme has no activity in the absence of the metal ion or coenzyme.

Coenzymes may be relatively loosely bound to the enzyme, so that they can be lost or exchanged between different enzymes, or they may be very tightly bound. When a coenzyme is covalently bound to the protein, as a result of a chemical reaction between the coenzyme and the enzyme protein, it is sometimes called a **prosthetic group**. Like the enzyme itself, the coenzyme or prosthetic group participates in the reaction, but at the end emerges unchanged. Sometimes the coenzyme is chemically modified in one reaction, then restored to its original state by reaction with a second enzyme.

Many of the coenzymes are derived from vitamins; despite their importance, they cannot be made in the body, but must be provided in the diet. Table 5.1 shows the major coenzymes, the vitamins they are derived from and their principal metabolic functions. Vitamins and minerals are discussed in Chapter 11.

Table 5.1 The major coenzymes.

	Name	Source	Functions
CoA	coenzyme A	pantothenic acid	acyl transfer reactions
FAD	flavin adenine dinucleotide	vitamin B_2	oxidation reactions
FMN	flavin mononucleotide	vitamin B_2	oxidation reactions
NAD	nicotinamide adenine dinucleotide	niacin	oxidation and reduction reactions
NADP	nicotinamide adenine dinucleotide phosphate	niacin	oxidation and reduction reactions
PLP	pyridoxal phosphate	vitamin B_6	amino acid metabolism

There are other coenzymes, which are discussed as they are relevant to specific metabolic pathways. In addition to those shown in this table, most of the other vitamins also function as coenzymes; see Chapter 11.

The rôle of coenzymes and metals in oxidation and reduction reactions

Metabolic reactions involving the oxidation and reduction of substrates involve an acceptor for the hydrogen (or electrons) removed from the substrate in oxidation, or a donor for the hydrogen (or electrons) added in reduction reactions (see p. 55). In some cases the hydrogen acceptor or donor is an integral part of the molecule of the enzyme which catalyses the reaction; in other cases the hydrogen acceptor or donor is an alternative substrate.

The electron acceptor or donor may be a metal ion which can have two different stable electron configurations. Commonly iron (which can form Fe^{2+} or Fe^{3+} ions) and copper (which can form Cu^+ or Cu^{2+} ions) are involved, although other metal ions, including molybdenum, may be involved in some systems. In some enzymes the metal ion is simply bound to the enzyme; in others it is incorporated in an organic molecule, which in turn is attached to the enzyme. For example, haem is an organic compound containing iron which is the coenzyme for a variety of enzymes collectively known as the cytochromes (see p. 128). Haem is also the prosthetic group of haemoglobin, the protein in red blood cells which binds and transports oxygen between the lungs and other tissues.

The nicotinamide nucleotide coenzymes, NAD and NADP   As shown in

116

Figure 5.6, there are two closely related compounds which, together, we refer to as the nicotinamide nucleotide coenzymes. These are nicotinamide adenine dinucleotide (NAD) and nicotinamide adenine dinucleotide phosphate (NADP). They differ only in that NADP has an additional phosphate

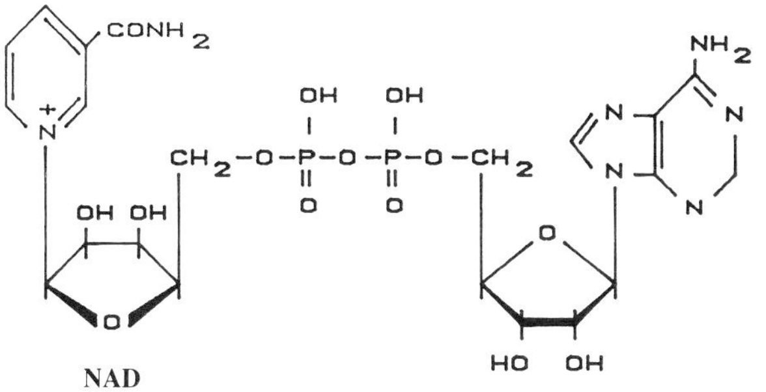

NAD

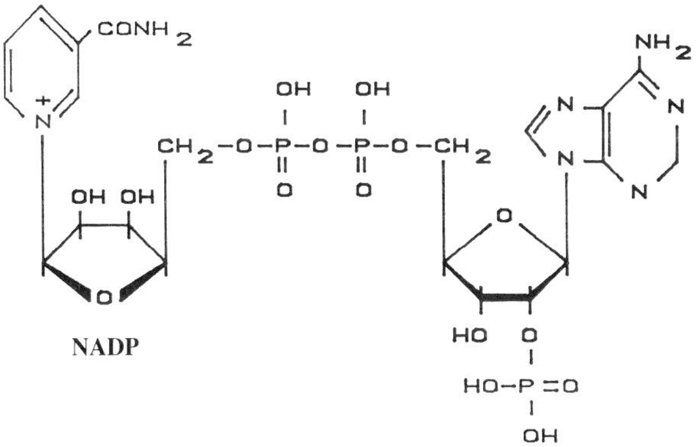

NADP

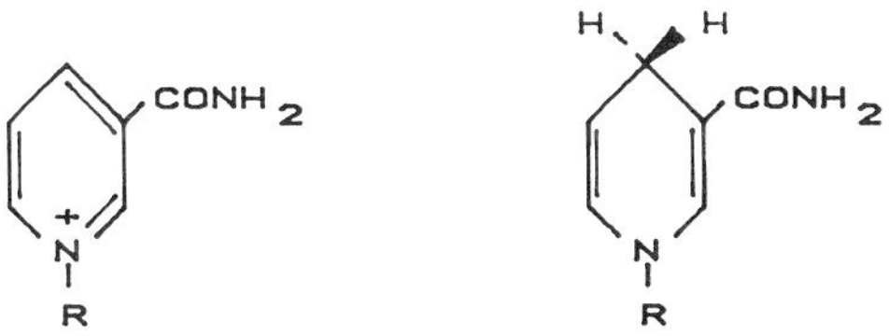

Oxidized Reduced

Figure 5.6 The nicotinamide nucleotide coenzymes, NAD and NADP
Two coenzymes are derived from the vitamin niacin; they differ in that NADP (nicotinamide adenine dinucleotide phosphate) has an additional phosphate group. The functionally important part of both coenzymes is the nicotinamide ring; the oxidized form is shown on the left, and the reduced form on the right.

group attached to the ribose. The whole of the coenzyme molecule is essential for binding to enzymes, and most enzymes can bind and use only one of these two coenzymes, either NAD or NADP, despite the overall similarity in their structures.

The functionally important part of the nicotinamide nucleotide coenzymes is the nicotinamide ring, which is derived from the vitamin niacin (see p. 259). As shown in Figure 5.6, this can undergo reduction. In the oxidized coenzymes there is a positive charge associated with the nitrogen atom in the nicotinamide ring. We sometimes write the oxidized forms of the coenzymes as NAD^+ and $NADP^+$ to show this. Reduction involves the transfer of two electrons and two hydrogen ions (H^+) from the substrate to the coenzyme. One electron neutralizes the positive charge on the nitrogen atom. The other, with its associated H^+ ion, is incorporated into the ring as a second hydrogen at carbon-4. In the oxidized coenzyme there was one hydrogen at carbon-4, but we do not normally show this when we draw chemical structures. In the reduced coenzymes we show both hydrogens, as in Figure 5.6. We generally draw a dotted bond to one hydrogen, and a bold bond to the other, to show that the ring as a whole is flat, and lies in the plane of the page, with one hydrogen at carbon-4 above the plane of the ring, and the other below.

The second H^+ ion removed from the substrate remains associated with the coenzyme. This means that we can write the reaction as:

$$X\text{-}H_2 + NAD^+ \rightleftharpoons X + NADH + H^+$$

where $X\text{-}H_2$ is the substrate and X is the product (the oxidized form of the substrate).

Note that the reaction is reversible, and NADH can act as a reducing agent:

$$X + NADH + H^+ \rightleftharpoons X\text{-}H_2 + NAD^+$$

where X is now the substrate and $X\text{-}H_2$ is the product (the reduced form of the substrate).

We do not always show the positive charge on the nicotinamide ring of the oxidized coenzymes, or the H^+ associated with the reduced coenzyme. In general in this book we will show the oxidized coenzymes as NAD and NADP, and the reduced coenzymes as NADH and NADPH.

The flavins: riboflavin and flavoproteins   Vitamin B_2 (riboflavin, see p. 257) is also important in a very great number of oxidation and reduction reactions. It is generally covalently bound to enzymes, and the resultant enzymes with attached riboflavin are collectively known as **flavoproteins**. As shown in Figure 5.7, riboflavin (or the riboflavin part of flavoproteins) can undergo two reductions. It can accept one hydrogen, to form the flavin radical (generally written as flavin-H·), followed by a second hydrogen forming fully reduced flavin-H_2.

Some reactions involve the transfer of a single hydrogen to a flavin, forming flavin-H·, which is then recycled in a separate reaction. Sometimes two molecules of flavin each accept one hydrogen atom from the substrate to be oxidized. Other reactions involve the sequential transfer of two hydrogens onto the flavin, forming first the flavin-H· radical, then fully reduced flavin-H$_2$.

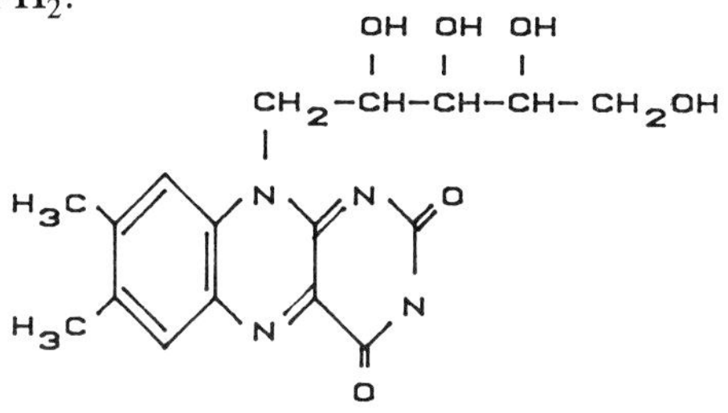

Riboflavin (oxidized)

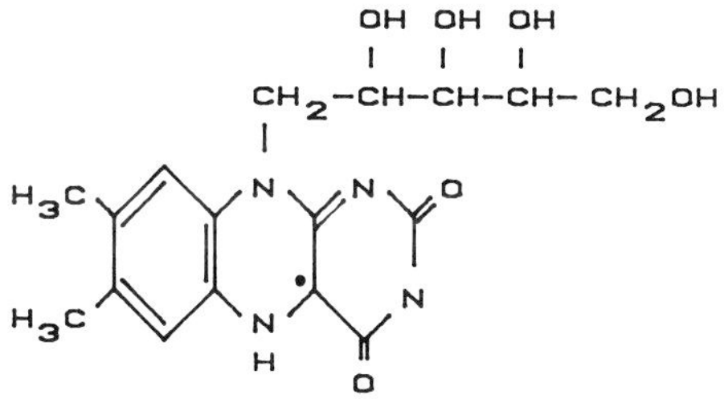

Riboflavin radical (flavin-H•)

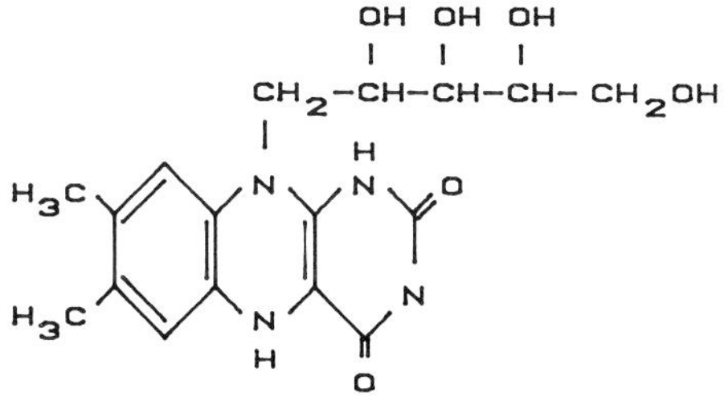

Fully reduced riboflavin (flavin-H$_2$)

Figure 5.7 The rôle of riboflavin as a coenzyme in oxidation and reduction reactions
Riboflavin is vitamin B$_2$. It may be incorporated into enzymes as riboflavin itself, as the phosphate or as flavin adenine dinucleotide. Oxidized riboflavin, shown at the top of the diagram, may undergo reduction by a single electron (together with a hydrogen ion), to yield the flavin-H · radical, shown in the middle diagram, or reduction by two electrons (together with two hydrogen ions) to form the fully reduced flavin-H$_2$, shown in the lower diagram.

119

The rôle of ATP in enzyme reactions

We have already seen that enzymes lower the activation energy of the reactions they catalyse. However, as discussed on p. 48, some chemical reactions, especially those which are synthetic reactions, forming larger compounds from small substrates, are endergonic. In the test tube they require a considerable input of energy, usually as heat.

As discussed on p. 50, the position of the equilibrium between substrates and products in any reaction is determined by two factors:
(a) the extent to which the reaction is endergonic (in one direction, and exergonic in the other);
(b) the relative concentrations of the substrates and products.

ATP (adenosine triphosphate, see Fig. 4.17 on p. 94) provides a link between the exergonic reactions of the oxidation of metabolic fuels and the various endergonic reactions of the body. The hydrolysis of ATP:
$$ATP + H_2O \rightarrow ADP + phosphate$$
is exergonic, while the reverse reaction, the phosphorylation of ADP (the condensation reaction between ADP and phosphate to form ATP):
$$ADP + phosphate \rightarrow ATP + H_2O$$
is endergonic. If we consider a reaction
$$A \rightarrow X$$
which is endergonic, we would not normally expect much formation of X from A at body temperature. If we can link this reaction to the hydrolysis of ATP, in such a way that both reactions *must* occur at the same time:
$$ATP + H_2O \rightarrow ADP + phosphate$$
$$A \rightarrow X$$
then if the concentration of ATP is very much higher than that of ADP, this will shift the equilibrium of both reactions to the right. Under these conditions we would expect to see a significant formation of X from A, linked to the hydrolysis of ATP to ADP and phosphate.

Such linkage between two apparently unrelated reactions is quite easy in enzyme systems. The reaction might, for example, involve the intermediate formation of a complex between substrate A and phosphate, or might involve transfer of a phosphate group from ATP onto the enzyme as a transient step.

The concentration of ATP in cells is always very much higher than that of ADP (the ratio of ATP:ADP is about 500:1), so that in the example shown above the equilibrium of the linked reactions will indeed lie to the right. Many of the reactions discussed in later chapters are linked to the hydrolysis of ATP to ADP and phosphate in this way, so that reactions which might, at first sight, appear to be unfavoured can proceed under physiological conditions.

Not only is the concentration of ADP in cells very much lower than that of ATP, but it is kept low by the rapid rephosphorylation of ADP to ATP, linked to the oxidation of metabolic fuels (see p. 126). Therefore as long as there is a supply of metabolic fuels to be oxidized, the ratio ATP:ADP remains high and ATP is available to shift the equilibrium of otherwise unfavoured reactions.

The classification and naming of enzymes

There is a formal system of enzyme nomenclature, in which each enzyme has a number, and the various enzymes are classified according to the type of reaction catalysed and the substrates, products and coenzymes of the reaction. This is used in research publications, when there is a need to identify an enzyme unambiguously, but for general use we use a less formal system of naming enzymes. Almost all enzyme names end in "-ase", and many are derived simply from the name of the substrate acted on, with the suffix "-ase". In some cases, the type of reaction catalysed is also included.

Although the variety of metabolic pathways, and hence the number of different enzymes in human metabolism, seems enormous at first sight, we can classify the enzymes into only six groups, depending on the types of chemical reaction they catalyse:
(a) oxidation and reduction reactions;
(b) transfer of a reactive group from one substrate onto another;
(c) hydrolysis of bonds;
(d) addition across carbon–carbon double bonds;
(e) rearrangement of groups within a single molecule of substrate;
(f) formation of bonds between two substrates, frequently linked to the hydrolysis of ATP to ADP and phosphate.
This classification of enzymes is expanded in Table 5.2, to give some examples of the types of reactions catalysed.

Metabolic pathways

Most important metabolic reactions do not occur in a single step, but as a series of linked reactions, each resulting in a small change in the substrate. The product of each individual reaction is the substrate for the next enzyme. Such a group of linked reactions constitutes a metabolic pathway.

We can divide metabolic pathways into two broad groups:
(a) **Catabolic pathways**, in which relatively complex compounds are

broken down, often involving oxidation to water, carbon dioxide and other end-products which are excreted. Catabolic pathways generally involve the breaking of chemical bonds, often by hydrolysis, and they are usually linked to the phosphorylation of ADP to ATP. These are the pathways for the oxidation of metabolic fuels.

(b) **Biosynthetic (or anabolic) pathways**, which result in the formation of the specialized compounds required in the body, both relatively simple small molecules and large complex molecules such as DNA, RNA and proteins.

Biosynthetic reactions are frequently reductions, often involve the elimination of water (condensation reactions) and are generally linked to the hydrolysis of ATP to ADP and phosphate.

Biosynthetic reactions are also involved in the metabolism of drugs and other foreign compounds, and hormones and neurotransmitters, to yield unreactive compounds which can be excreted in the urine.

Linear and branched pathways

The simplest type of metabolic pathway is a single sequence of reactions in which the starting material is converted to the end-product with no possibility of alternative reactions or branches in the pathway.

Table 5.2 The classification of enzymes by the reactions catalysed.

Class	Reaction catalysed
Oxidoreductases	oxidation and reduction reactions
dehydrogenases	addition or removal of H
oxidases	two-electron transfer to O_2 forming H_2O_2
	two-electron transfer to $\frac{1}{2}O_2$ forming H_2O
oxygenases	incorporate O_2 into product
hydroxylases	incorporate $\frac{1}{2}O_2$ into product as $-OH$ and form H_2O
peroxidases	use H_2O_2 as oxygen donor, forming H_2O
Transferases	transfer a chemical group from one substrate to the other
kinases	transfer phosphate from ATP onto substrate
Hydrolases	hydrolysis of C–O, C–N, O–P and C–S bonds
	(e.g. esterases, proteases, phosphatases, deamidases)
Lyases	addition of groups across a carbon–carbon double bond
	(e.g. dehydratases, hydratases, decarboxylases)
Isomerases	intramolecular rearrangements
Ligases (synthetases)	formation of bonds between two substrates frequently
	linked to utilisation of ATP, with intermediate
	formation of phosphorylated enzyme or substrate

Simple linear pathways are rare, since many of the intermediate compounds in metabolism can be used in a variety of different pathways, depending on the body's need for various end-products. Many metabolic pathways involve branch points, where an intermediate may proceed down one branch or another. The enzymes catalysing reactions at such branch points are frequently subject to regulation, so as to "direct" substrates down one branch or the other.

Looped reaction sequences

Sometimes a complete metabolic pathway involves repeating a series of similar reactions several times over. Thus, the synthesis of fatty acids (see Fig. 6.12 on p. 149) involves the repeated addition of two-carbon units until the final chain length (commonly 14, 16 or 18 carbon units) has been achieved. The addition of each two-carbon unit involves four separate reaction steps, which are repeated each time. Similarly, the oxidation of fatty acids proceeds by the sequential removal of two-carbon units (see Fig. 6.9 on p. 145). Again, the removal of each two-carbon unit involves a repeated sequence of reactions.

Cyclic pathways

The third type of metabolic pathway is cyclic – the end-product is the same compound as the starting material. Thus, in the synthesis of urea (see Fig. 9.7 on p. 203), the molecule of urea is built up in a series of stages as part of a larger carrier molecule. At the end of the reaction sequence, the urea is released by hydrolysis, resulting in the formation of the starting material to undergo a further cycle of reaction. Similarly, in the citric acid cycle (see Fig. 6.8 on p. 142) the four-carbon compound oxaloacetate can be considered to be the beginning of the pathway. It reacts with the two-carbon compound, acetate, to form a six-carbon compound, citrate. Two carbon atoms are lost as carbon dioxide in the reaction sequence, so that at the end oxaloacetate is reformed.

The intermediates in a cyclic pathway can be considered to be catalysts, in that they participate in the reaction sequence, but at the end they emerge unchanged.

A note on metabolic pathways

A metabolic pathway is no more than a map showing you the steps by which one compound is converted to another. Along the way are points of interest: key steps which allow for the regulation and integration of different pathways; enzymes which are targets for drugs or poisons; enzymes which are affected by disease, etc.

There is no more point in "learning" a metabolic pathway than there is "learning" a road map.

What is important is to be able to read the pathways in the same way as you read a map. In this way you can see how metabolic intermediates are related to each other, how changes in one system affect other systems, and which are the points of interest.

In subsequent chapters of this book, the diagrams show metabolic pathways in considerable detail. The text describes the key features and should serve to guide you through the pathways represented in the diagrams.

CHAPTER SIX

Energy nutrition

The prime nutritional requirement of the body is a source of metabolically usable energy. This is provided by the oxidation of metabolic fuels: carbohydrates, fats, proteins and alcohol, linked to the formation of ATP from ADP and phosphate ions.

The expenditure of metabolic energy – the biosynthesis of body constituents, to replace those continuously being broken down and replaced; the maintenance of ion gradients across nerve and muscle membranes; transport of compounds into and out of cells; and the contraction of muscle for the performance of physical work – all result in the hydrolysis of ATP to ADP and phosphate.

We saw on p. 120 how the maintenance of a high ratio of ATP:ADP permits apparently unfavoured biosynthetic reactions to proceed, by linking the reaction to the hydrolysis of ATP to ADP and phosphate. Since the ratio of ATP:ADP is 500:1, the equilibrium of this reaction lies well over towards the hydrolysis of ATP. This means that the equilibrium of the linked reaction will be shifted by the hydrolysis of ATP to ADP and phosphate.

The **pumping of ions** across cell membranes, so that there is a higher concentration of potassium ions (K^+) inside cells than in the extracellular fluid, and a higher concentration of sodium ions (Na^+) outside cells than inside, is linked to the hydrolysis of ATP to ADP and phosphate in the same way. This gradient of sodium ions across the cell membrane can be used for the transport of substrates into, and products out of, cells. Compounds are transported inwards together with sodium, while other compounds are transported outwards in exchange for sodium which is transported inwards (see Fig. 6.1).

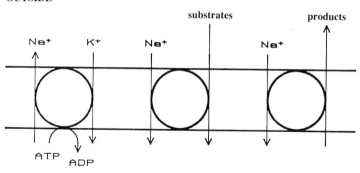

Figure 6.1 The rôle of ATP in transport across cell membranes
The sodium pump transports sodium (Na^+) ions out of the cell, exchanging them for potassium (K^+) ions, which are pumped inwards, linked to the hydrolysis of ATP to ADP and phosphate. Sodium ions re-enter the cell either together with substrates such as amino acids and glucose, or in exchange for metabolic products secreted by the cell.

The **contraction of muscle** is also linked to the hydrolysis of ATP to ADP and phosphate. The proteins of muscle are arranged in filaments, which slide over each other when the muscle is contracted. This movement of the filaments occurs by the formation of phosphate bridges between two proteins; the phosphate is provided by transfer from ATP. As shown in Figure 6.2, the phosphate bridge is between one reactive group in each protein, and forming the bridge brings the two reactive groups closer to each other. This means that as each bridge is formed, it causes the two proteins to move slightly. Once this has happened, the phosphate bridge is hydrolysed, releasing free phosphate, and another bridge can be formed, causing the chains to move slightly further.

Oxidative phosphorylation: the phosphorylation of ADP to ATP linked to the oxidation of metabolic fuels

A few reactions are linked directly to the phosphorylation of ADP to ATP, transferring a phosphate group from the substrate of the reaction onto ADP. However, of the 37 mol of ADP phosphorylated to ATP for each mol of glucose which is oxidized to carbon dioxide and water, only 2 mol are phosphorylated in this manner (see Fig. 6.4). The rest are phosphorylated in the mitochondria, by the process of **oxidative phosphorylation**.

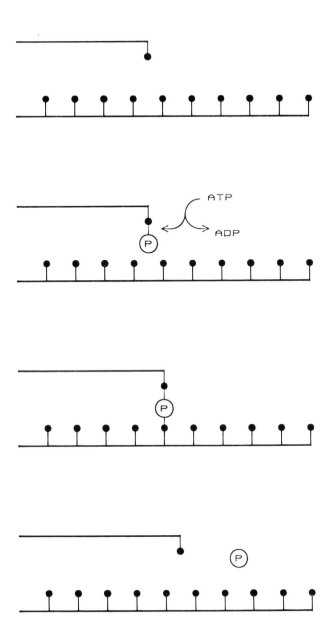

Figure 6.2 The rôle of ATP in muscle contraction
The contractile proteins of muscle slide over one another in a series of small movements during muscle contraction. One of the proteins is phosphorylated by ATP (releasing ADP). This phosphorylated protein then forms a phosphodiester linkage to the other protein. This process causes the proteins to move relative to each other. Finally, the phospho-diester linkage is hydrolysed, releasing phosphate, and leaving the two protein molecules ready to undergo another cycle of phosphorylation and movement.

127

Many of the reactions in the metabolism of carbohydrates, fats and amino acids result in the reduction of NAD to NADH, or the reduction of flavoproteins. These reduced coenzymes are then reoxidized in the mitochondria. Within the inner membrane of the mitochondrion there is a series of coenzymes which are able to undergo reduction and oxidation. The first coenzyme in the chain is reduced by reaction with NADH, and is then reoxidized by reducing the next coenzyme. In turn, each coenzyme in the chain is reduced by the preceding coenzyme, and then reoxidized by reducing the next one. The final step is the oxidation of a reduced coenzyme by oxygen, resulting in the formation of water.

This stepwise oxidation of NADH and reduction of oxygen to water is linked to the phosphorylation of ADP to ATP. For each mol of NADH oxidized, 3 mol of ATP are formed. Flavoproteins reduce an intermediate coenzyme in the chain, and 2 mol of ADP are phosphorylated to ATP for each mol of reduced flavoproteins which is oxidized.

The reaction between ADP and phosphate to form ATP is a condensation reaction, just as the reverse reaction, from ATP to ADP and phosphate is a hydrolysis:

$$ADP + phosphate \rightarrow ATP + H_2O.$$

We can consider that the water takes part in the reaction as H^+ and OH^- ions, rather than simply as unionized H_2O:

$$ADP + phosphate \rightarrow ATP + H^+ + OH^-.$$

The enzyme that catalyses this reaction is a part of the membrane of the mitochondrion. The H^+ ions which are formed leave the enzyme on the inside of the membrane, while the OH^- ions leave on the outside of the membrane. This means that the enzyme tends to create a pH gradient across the mitochondrial membrane, with an accumulation of H^+ ions inside and OH^- ions outside. This is unlikely to proceed to any significant extent under resting conditions, and anyway the equilibrium of the reaction between ADP and phosphate is such that the phosphorylation of ADP to ATP is unfavoured. Therefore this equilibrium needs to be shifted towards the formation of ATP from ADP and phosphate.

We have already seen that the position of the equilibrium in a chemical reaction can be shifted by removing one or more of the products as they are formed (see p. 50). If a source of H^+ ions were to exist on the outside of the membrane, they would react with the OH^- ions produced in the reaction between ADP and phosphate, forming H_2O. Similarly, a source of OH^- ions on the inside of the membrane would react with the H^+ ions formed by reaction between ADP and phosphate, again forming H_2O. This would shift the equilibrium in the direction of ATP formation as long as there was a source of ADP and phosphate, since two of the products, H^+ and OH^-, are removed as they are formed. This is what occurs.

Some of the coenzymes in the mitochondrial membrane which link the oxidation of NADH or reduced flavoproteins with the reduction of oxygen to water carry hydrogen atoms (i.e. H^+ ions and electrons), while others carry only electrons. Two hydrogen ions and two electrons are removed from NADH in the process of oxidizing it back to NAD. These are carried across the mitochondrial membrane as hydrogen atoms. At the outer surface they react with an electron carrier, which transports the electrons back to the inner surface of the mitochondrial membrane, leaving two H^+ ions on the outside.

At the inner surface of the mitochondrial membrane, this electron carrier interacts with a hydrogen carrier, which transports hydrogen atoms back to the outer surface. These hydrogen atoms arise from reaction with water at the inner face of the membrane, providing H^+ ions to be transported with the electrons and leaving OH^- ions inside.

This sequence of reactions is repeated twice more, so that altogether three H^+ ions are transported to the outer surface of the mitochondrial membrane, and three OH^- ions are left at the inner surface for each mol of NADH oxidized. Reduced flavin coenzymes react with an intermediate carrier, resulting in the transport of two H^+ for each flavin-H_2 oxidized. At the final stage, the last hydrogen carrier reacts with oxygen to form water (see Fig. 6.3).

Thus, the oxidation of NADH or reduced flavins results in the creation of a separation of the ions of water across the mitochondrial membrane, with a gradient of H^+ and OH^- in the opposite direction from that produced by the reaction between ADP and phosphate in which ATP is formed. The net result is the formation of water by reaction between H^+ and OH^- ions on both sides of the mitochondrial membrane. This results in a continuous shifting of the equilibrium of the reaction between ADP + phosphate $\rightarrow$ ATP, towards the formation of ATP.

The two processes of the oxidation of NADH or reduced flavins and the phosphorylation of ADP to ATP are normally tightly **coupled**. ADP phosphorylation cannot occur in mitochondria unless the gradient of H^+ ions across the membrane is created as a result of the oxidation of NADH or reduced flavins.

Equally, if there is little or no ADP available, the oxidation of NADH and reduced flavins is inhibited, because the H^+ gradient builds up and inhibits the transport reactions. This means that NADH and reduced flavoproteins are only oxidized when there is ADP available.

In turn, metabolic fuels can only be oxidized when NAD and oxidized flavoproteins are available. Therefore, if there is little or no ADP available in the mitochondria (i.e. it has all been phosphorylated to ATP), there will be an accumulation of reduced coenzymes, and hence a slowing down of the rate of oxidation of metabolic fuels. In other words, *metabolic fuels are oxidized only when there is a need for the phosphorylation of ADP to*

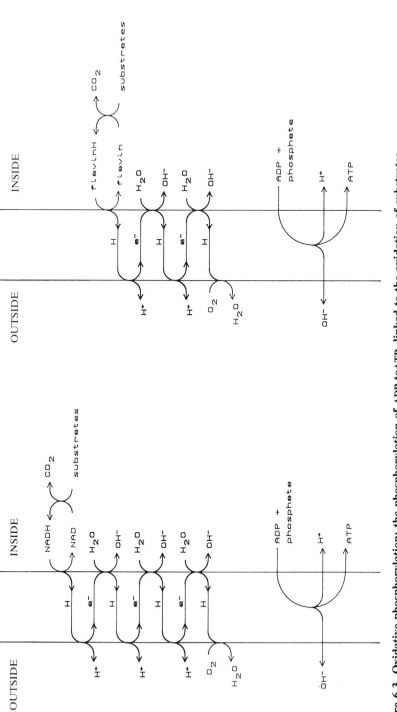

Figure 6.3 Oxidative phosphorylation: the phosphorylation of ADP toATP, linked to the oxidation of substrates

Inside the mitochondrion, substrates are oxidized to carbon dioxide, with the reduction of either NAD to NADH (in the left-hand diagram) or flavin to flavin-H_2 (in the right-hand diagram). The oxidation of NADH or flavin-H_2 is linked to the reduction of oxygen to water by a series of carriers which span the mitochondrial membrane, and transport H^+ ions to the outside, leaving OH^- ions inside. The reaction between ADP and phosphate to form ATP is a condensation; the water is eliminated in such a way that for each mol of ATP formed, an OH^- ion is transferred to the outer surface of the membrane, and an H^+ ion to the inner surface.

ATP. This means that metabolic fuels are only oxidized when ATP has been hydrolysed to ADP and phosphate by linkage to synthetic reactions, transport of compounds across cell membranes or muscle contraction.

It is possible to break this tight coupling between electron transport and ADP phosphorylation, by adding compounds which render the mitochondrial membrane freely permeable to H^+ ions. In the presence of such compounds, the H^+ ions transported out do not accumulate, but cross back to the inside, where they react with the OH^- ions, forming water. Under these conditions ADP is not phosphorylated to ATP, and the oxidation of NADH and reduced flavins can continue unimpeded.

The result of this **uncoupling** of electron transport from the phosphorylation of ADP is that a great deal of substrate is oxidized, with little production of ATP, although heat is produced. This is one of the physiological mechanisms for heat production to maintain body temperature without performing physical work, so-called **non-shivering thermogenesis**. The process is especially important in babies, but also occurs to a limited extent in adults. Brown fat tissue in various parts of the body can, under appropriate conditions, uncouple the processes of electron transport and phosphorylation of ADP to a limited extent, and so oxidize substrates for heat production without the normal control by the availability of ADP.

Digestion and absorption of metabolic fuels

The major components of the diet are starches, sugars, fats and proteins. These have to be hydrolysed to their constituent smaller molecules for absorption and metabolism. Starches and sugars are absorbed as monosaccharides; fats may either be absorbed intact or as free fatty acids and glycerol; proteins are absorbed as their constituent amino acids or small peptides.

Carbohydrate digestion

There are three groups of carbohydrate in the diet which function as metabolic fuels: starches, disaccharides and monosaccharides (see p. 69). Non-starch polysaccharides are important for the normal healthy functioning of the gastrointestinal tract (see p. 75), but are not metabolized to any significant extent. A small proportion of the non-starch polysaccharide in the diet is fermented by gut bacteria, and some of the products of this fermentation may be absorbed and contribute to energy intake.

Starch digestion As discussed on p. 75, starches are polymers of glucose, either as straight or branched chains (see Fig. 4.4 on p. 76 and Fig. 4.5 on p. 77). The process of digestion is simply a matter of hydrolysing the bonds between adjacent molecules to liberate free glucose, which can then be absorbed. Some maltose is also formed by the hydrolysis of starch. Where the starch molecule has a branch point, the disaccharide isomaltose is released. The digestion of disaccharides is considered below.

The enzymes which catalyse the hydrolysis of starch are amylases. Amylase is secreted both in the saliva, and also by the pancreas into the small intestine. This means that the digestion of starch begins when food is chewed, and continues, at least for a time, in the stomach. However, the gastric juice is very acid (about pH 1.5–2), and amylase is inactive at this pH. This means that although the digestion of starch continues in the middle of the food bolus in the stomach, as the contents are mixed with gastric juice, so the digestion of starch comes to a halt. When the food leaves the stomach and enters the small intestine, it is neutralized by the alkaline pancreatic juice (pH 8.8) and bile (pH 8). Amylase secreted by the pancreas continues the digestion of starch begun by salivary amylase.

Free glucose released from starch digestion (as well as any free glucose, fructose and other monosaccharides in food) is absorbed throughout the small intestine, being carried across the intestinal mucosa into the bloodstream by specific transport proteins in the membranes of the mucosal cells.

Not all of the dietary starch is digested by amylase. Uncooked starch is especially resistant to amylase action, because it is present as small insoluble granules. The process of cooking swells the starch granules, resulting in a gel on which amylase can act. A proportion of the starch in foods is still enclosed in plant cells walls, which are mainly composed of cellulose. Cellulose is not digested by human enzymes, and again this starch is protected against digestion. Some of the **resistant starch** is metabolized by bacteria in the large intestine, and a proportion of the products of bacterial metabolism, including fatty acids, may be absorbed and metabolized.

Digestion of disaccharides As shown in Figure 4.3 on p. 73, the nutritionally important disaccharides are sucrose (ordinary cane or beet sugar), maltose and isomaltose (arising from the digestion of starch), and lactose (the sugar of milk). These enter the brush border of the intestinal mucosal cells, where they are hydrolysed to their constituent monosaccharides: **maltose and isomaltose** are hydrolysed by the enzyme maltase to yield two molecules of glucose; **sucrose** is hydrolysed by the enzyme sucrase to yield glucose and fructose; **lactose** is hydrolysed by the enzyme lactase to yield glucose and galactose.

132

Disaccharide intolerances Deficiency of the enzyme lactase is common. Indeed, it is only in people of European origin that lactase persists after childhood. In most other people, and in some Europeans, lactase is gradually lost through adolescence, so-called **alactasia**. The result of this is that lactose cannot be absorbed. It remains in the intestinal lumen, where it is a substrate for bacterial fermentation. The result of the bacterial fermentation is an explosive watery diarrhoea and severe abdominal pain. Even the relatively small amounts of lactose in milk may upset people with a complete deficiency of lactase. Such people can normally tolerate yoghurt and other fermented milk products, since much of the lactose has been converted to lactic acid. Fortunately for people who suffer from alactasia, milk is the only significant source of lactose in the diet, so it is relatively easy to avoid consuming lactose.

A distinct condition, which is treated in the same way by exclusion of lactose from the diet, is **galactosaemia**. This is an inability to metabolize the galactose moiety of lactose, and leads to mental retardation and the development of liver failure and cataracts. It is a rare inborn error of metabolism, occurring about 1/40,000 live births.

Rarely, people may lack sucrase and/or maltase. This may either be a genetic lack of the enzyme, or an acquired loss as a result of intestinal infection. They are intolerant of sucrose and/or maltose, and suffer in the same way as alactasic subjects given lactose. It is relatively easy to avoid maltose, since there are few sources of it in the diet; the small amount formed in the digestion of starch does not seem to cause any significant problems. People who lack sucrase have a more serious problem, since as well as the obvious sugar in cakes and biscuits, jams, etc., many manufactured foods contain added sucrose.

Fat digestion and absorption

The major fats in the diet are triacylglycerols and, to a lesser extent, phospholipids (see Fig. 4.6 on p. 78 and Fig. 4.8 on p. 82). The problem with the digestion and absorption of fats is that they are not miscible with the watery contents of the intestinal lumen. Therefore the first stage is **emulsification**, breaking the fat up into small droplets which can then be dispersed in water. This is the function of the bile salts. Like fatty acids and phospholipids, bile salts have both hydrophobic and hydrophilic regions, and can thus emulsify lipids by forming small water-dispersible micelles (see p. 54).

Some of the dietary fat is hydrolysed in the intestinal lumen by the enzyme **lipase**, which is secreted by the pancreas. The products are glycerol and free fatty acids. Glycerol is water-soluble, and is readily absorbed throughout the small intestine. The fatty acids dissolve in lipid droplets, and aid the process of emulsification.

The emulsified lipid droplets, containing intact triacylglycerol, phospholipids and free fatty acids, are absorbed across the intestinal wall into the lymphatics, forming **chylomicrons** which enter the bloodstream and are removed from the circulation by the liver and adipose tissue. The fat-soluble vitamins, A, D, E and K, as well as carotene (see Ch. 11), are absorbed dissolved in the lipid of chylomicrons; thus, as well as being a metabolic fuel, dietary fat is essential for the absorption of these vitamins.

Protein digestion

Protein digestion can be said to start in the cooking pot, where the proteins are denatured by heat; this renders them more susceptible to hydrolysis by enzymes. The acid in the stomach has a similar effect, continuing the denaturation of proteins, and also releasing some of the protein-bound vitamins, especially vitamin B_{12} (see p. 264).

Protein digestion occurs by hydrolysis of the peptide bonds between amino acids (see Fig. 4.12 on p. 89). There are two main classes of protein digestive enzymes: the **endopeptidases**, which cleave proteins by hydrolysing peptide bonds between specific amino acids in the middle of the molecule, and the **exopeptidases**, which remove amino acids one at a time from the end of the molecule, again by the hydrolysis of the peptide bond (see Table 6.1).

The first enzymes to act on dietary proteins are the endopeptidases: **pepsin** in the gastric juice and **trypsin**, **chymotrypsin** and **elastase** secreted by the pancreas into the small intestine. The result of the combined action of these enzymes is that the large protein molecules are broken down into medium-sized polypeptides, with many ends for the exopeptidases to act on.

There are two classes of exopeptidase: **carboxypeptidases** are secreted in the pancreatic juice, and release amino acids sequentially from the free carboxyl terminal of peptides; **aminopeptidases** are secreted by the intestinal mucosal cells and release amino acids sequentially from the amino terminal of peptides.

The end-product of the action of these various peptidases is a mixture of free amino acids, dipeptides and tripeptides. Free amino acids are absorbed across the intestinal mucosa by specific carriers. Dipeptides and tripeptides enter the brush border of the intestinal mucosal cells, where they are hydrolysed to free amino acids, which are then transported into the bloodstream together with free amino acids absorbed directly from the intestinal lumen.

Table 6.1 The major protein digestive enzymes.

	Secreted by	Specificity
Endopeptidases		
pepsin	gastic mucosa	adjacent to aromatic amino acid, leucine or methionine
trypsin	pancreas	lysine or arginine esters
chymotrypsin	pancreas	aromatic esters
elastase	pancreas	neutral aliphatic esters
enteropeptidase	intestinal mucosa	trypsinogen → trypsin
Exopeptidases		
carboxypeptidases	pancreas	carboxy-terminal amino acids
aminopeptidases	intestinal mucosa	amino-terminal amino acids
tripeptidases	intracellular in intestinal mucosa	tripeptides
dipeptidases	intracellular in intestinal mucosa	dipeptides

The various protein digestive enzymes are secreted as inactive enzyme precursors or **zymogens**; this is essential if they are not to digest themselves and each other, as well as tissue proteins, before they are secreted. In each case the active site of the enzyme is masked by a small length of protein which has to be removed for the enzyme to have activity. This is achieved by hydrolysis of a specific peptide bond in the precursor molecule, releasing the blocking peptide and revealing the active site of the enzyme.

Pepsin is secreted in the stomach as pepsinogen, which is activated by the action of gastric acid, and also by the action of already activated pepsin. In the small intestine, trypsinogen, the precursor of trypsin, is activated by the action of a specific enzyme, enteropeptidase, secreted by the duodenal epithelial cells; trypsin can then activate the precursors of other protein digestive enzymes, and also trypsinogen.

Energy-yielding metabolism

The metabolism of glucose: glycolysis

The overall reaction for the metabolism of glucose is oxidation to carbon dioxide and water:

$$C_6H_{12}O_6 + 6\ O_2 \rightarrow 6\ CO_2 + 6\ H_2O.$$

In the process, NAD is reduced to NADH, and it is the re-oxidation of this NADH which results in the phosphorylation of ADP to ATP, as discussed on p. 126. In addition, there are steps where a phosphate group is transferred directly from an intermediate onto ADP, yielding further ATP.

As shown in Figure 6.4, although the aim of glucose oxidation is to phosphorylate ADP to ATP, the pathway involves two steps in which ATP is used, one to form glucose-6-phosphate and the other to form fructose bisphosphate. In other words, there is a modest cost of ATP to start the metabolism of glucose. The final yield of ATP is great enough for this investment to be worthwhile; overall, there is a net yield of 37 mol of ATP for each mol of glucose oxidized to carbon dioxide and water.

Fructose bisphosphate is split into two three-carbon compounds, which are interconvertible. The metabolism of these three-carbon sugars is linked to both the reduction of NAD to NADH, and direct phosphorylation of ADP to ATP. The result is the formation of 2 mol of pyruvate from each mol of glucose.

The oxidation of glucose to pyruvate thus requires the utilization of 2 mol of ATP (giving ADP) per mol of glucose metabolized, but yields 4 × ATP by direct phosphorylation of ADP, and 2 × NADH (formed from NAD), which is equivalent to a further 6 × ATP when oxidized in the electron transport chain (see p. 126). There is thus a net yield of 8 × ADP + phosphate → ATP from the oxidation of 1 mol of glucose to 2 mol of pyruvate.

This pathway provides a route for the metabolism not only of glucose, but also of:

(a) **glycogen**, which is broken down to yield glucose-1-phosphate (see p. 150) (glucose-1-phosphate and glucose-6-phosphate are readily interconvertible);

(b) **fructose**, which can be phosphorylated directly to fructose-6-phosphate;

(c) **glycerol**, from the hydrolysis of triacylglycerols: glycerol can be phosphorylated and oxidized to dihydroxy-acetone phosphate.

The overall sequence of reactions from glucose to pyruvate is known as **glycolysis** – the process of splitting glucose. As discussed on p. 153, the reverse of this pathway is important as a means of glucose synthesis, i.e. the process of **gluconeogenesis**. Most of the reactions of glycolysis are readily reversible, but at three points (reactions a, c and j in Fig. 6.4) there are separate enzymes involved in glycolysis and gluconeogenesis.

For both hexokinase (reaction a) and phosphofructokinase (reaction c) the equilibrium of the reaction is towards glycolysis, because of the utilization of ATP in the reaction and the high ratio of ATP:ADP in the cell (see p. 120). These two reactions are reversed in gluconeogenesis by sim-

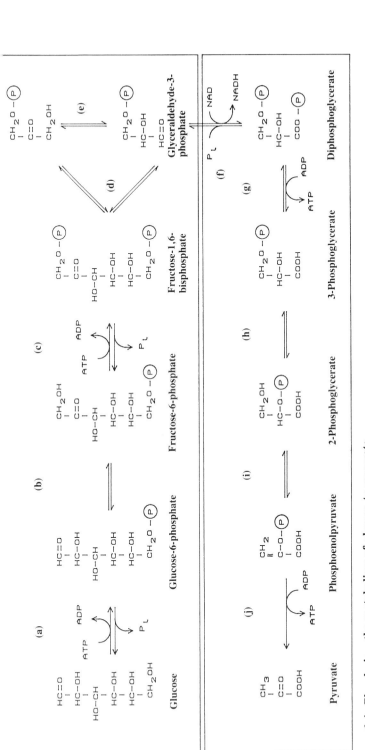

Figure 6.4 Glycolysis – the metabolism of glucose to pyruvate

Overall, 1 mol of glucose is split to give 2 mol of the three-carbon compound pyruvate, with a net yield of 2 mol of ADP phosphorylated to ATP directly, and 2 mol of NAD reduced to NADH (equivalent to $2 \times 3 = 6$ mol of ADP phosphorylated to ATP). At three steps there are separate enzymes involved in the synthesis of glucose from pyruvate (reactions a, c and j). The reactions in the upper box (reactions a–e) occur once and those in the lower box (reactions f–j) twice, for each molecule of glucose metabolized. (a) *Hexokinase*: the first step is the phosphorylation of glucose by the enzyme *glucose-6-phosphatase*. (b) *Phosphoglucomutase*: isomerization of glucose-6-phosphate to glucose-6-phosphate. In the reverse direction, glucose-6-phosphate is hydrolysed to release free glucose and phosphate by the enzyme *glucose-6-phosphatase*. (c) *Phosphofructokinase*: fructose-6-phosphate is phosphorylated to fructose-1,6-bisphosphate. In the reverse direction, fructose-1,6-bisphosphate is hydrolysed to fructose-6-phosphate and phosphate by the enzyme *fructose bisphosphatase*. (d) *Aldolase*: fructose-bisphosphate is cleaved to give two three-carbon compounds: dihydroxyacetone phosphate and glyceraldehyde-3-phosphate. (e) *Triose phosphate isomerase*: dihydroxyacetone phosphate is isomerized to glyceraldehyde-3-phosphate. (f) *Glyceraldehyde-3-phosphate dehydrogenase*: glyceraldehyde-3-phosphate is oxidized and phosphorylated by reaction with phosphate, forming 2,3-diphosphoglyceric acid. (g) *Phosphoglycerate kinase*: 2,3-diphosphoglyceric acid reacts with ADP, transferring a phosphate to form ATP, leaving 3-phosphoglyceric acid. (h) *Phosphoglyceromutase*: 3-phosphoglyceric acid is isomerized to 2-phosphoglyceric acid. (i) *Enolase*: 2-phosphoglyceric acid is isomerized to phosphoenol-pyruvate. (j) *Pyruvate kinase*: phosphoenolpyruvate transfers its phosphate onto ADP, forming ATP, and undergoes isomerization to pyruvate (see also Fig. 6.5).

simple hydrolysis of fructose bisphosphate to fructose-6-phosphate and phosphate (fructose bisphosphatase), and of glucose-6-phosphate to glucose and phosphate (glucose-6-phosphatase).

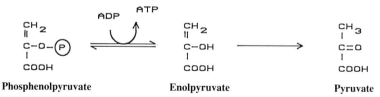

Phosphenolpyruvate   Enolpyruvate   Pyruvate

Figure 6.5 The reaction of pyruvate kinase
The immediate product of the enzyme reaction is enolpyruvate. The reaction between ADP and phosphoenolpyruvate to yield ATP and enolpyruvate is freely reversible. However, enolpyruvate is chemically unstable, and rapidly undergoes non-enzymic isomerization to pyruvate.

The equilibrium of pyruvate kinase (reaction j) is also strongly towards glycolysis. In this case it is because the immediate product of the reaction is enolpyruvate, which is chemically unstable. As shown in Figure 6.5, enolpyruvate undergoes a rapid non-enzymic reaction to yield pyruvate. This means that the product of the enzymic reaction is not available to any significant extent to undergo the reverse reaction in the direction of gluco-neogenesis. The reversal of the pyruvate kinase reaction in gluconeogenesis is discussed on p. 154.

The metabolism of pyruvate

Pyruvate can be metabolized in three different ways, depending on the metabolic state of the body:
(a) reduction to lactate;
(b) complete oxidation to carbon dioxide and water;
(c) as a substrate for glucose synthesis (gluconeogenesis, see p. 153).

The reduction of pyruvate to lactate: anaerobic glycolysis As shown in Figure 6.4, the oxidation of glucose to pyruvate results in the reduction of 2 mol of NAD to NADH. This is normally reoxidized to NAD in the mitochondrial electron transport chain, linked to the phosphorylation of $3 \times$ ADP to ATP for each NADH oxidized (see p. 126). However, under conditions of **maximum exertion**, for example in sprinting, the rate at which oxygen can be taken up into the muscle is not great enough to allow for the re-oxidation of all the NADH which is being formed. In order to maintain the oxidation of glucose, and the net yield of $2 \times$ ATP per mol of glucose oxidized, NADH is oxidized back to NAD by the reduction of pyruvate to lactate (see Fig. 6.6).

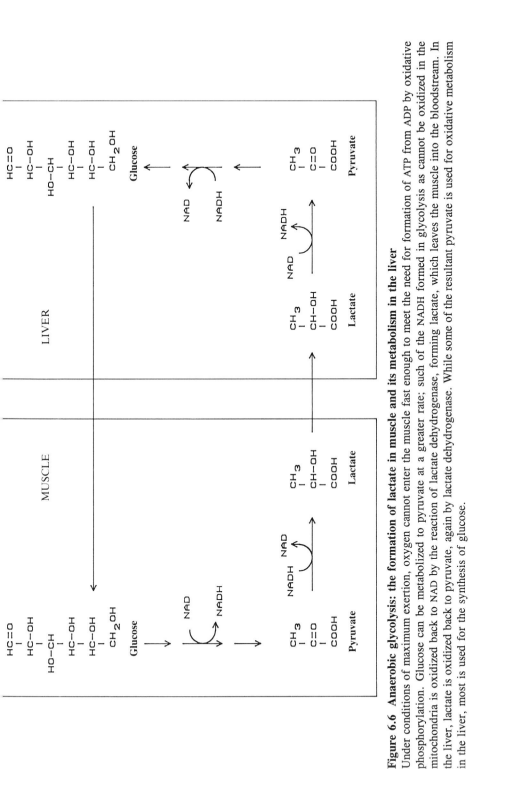

Figure 6.6 Anaerobic glycolysis: the formation of lactate in muscle and its metabolism in the liver

Under conditions of maximum exertion, oxygen cannot enter the muscle fast enough to meet the need for formation of ATP from ADP by oxidative phosphorylation. Glucose can be metabolized to pyruvate at a greater rate; such of the NADH formed in glycolysis as cannot be oxidized in the mitochondria is oxidized back to NAD by the reaction of lactate dehydrogenase, forming lactate, which leaves the muscle into the bloodstream. In the liver, lactate is oxidized back to pyruvate, again by lactate dehydrogenase. While some of the resultant pyruvate is used for oxidative metabolism in the liver, most is used for the synthesis of glucose.

The resultant lactate is exported from the muscle and taken up by the liver, where it is used to resynthesize glucose (see p. 153). Lactate can also be taken up by other tissues, where oxygen availability is not a limiting factor under these conditions, such as the heart. Here it is oxidized to pyruvate, and the resultant NADH is oxidized in the mitochondrial electron transport chain, yielding $3 \times$ ATP. The pyruvate is then a substrate for complete oxidation to carbon dioxide and water, as discussed below.

The conversion of glucose to lactate is called **anaerobic glycolysis**, since it does not require oxygen. However, it is not true to say that human metabolism is ever anaerobic. The formation of lactate is the fate of *some* of the pyruvate formed from glucose under conditions of maximum muscle exertion when oxygen is limiting, but as much as possible will continue to undergo complete oxidation.

Truly anaerobic glycolysis does occur in micro-organisms which are capable of living in the absence of oxygen. Here there are two possible fates for the pyruvate formed from glucose, both of which involve the oxidation of NADH to NAD:

(a) reduction to lactate, as occurs in human muscle – this is the pathway in lactic acid bacteria, which are responsible for the fermentation of lactose in milk to form yoghurt and cheese;

(b) decarboxylation and reduction to ethanol – the pathway of fermentation in yeast, which is exploited to produce alcoholic beverages.

The oxidation of pyruvate The first step in the complete oxidation of pyruvate is a complex reaction in which carbon dioxide is lost, and the resulting two-carbon compound is oxidized to acetate. The oxidation involves the reduction of NAD to NADH. Since 2 mol of pyruvate are formed from each mol of glucose, this step represents the formation of 2 mol of NADH, equivalent to $6 \times$ ATP for each mol of glucose metabolized. The acetate is released from the enzyme esterified to coenzyme A, as acetyl CoA (Fig. 6.7).

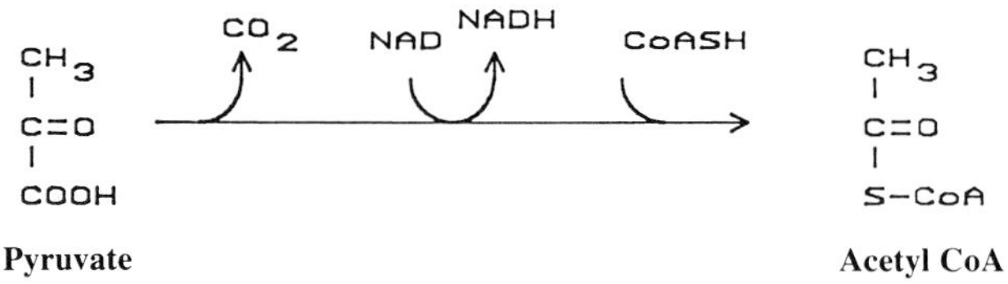

Figure 6.7 The reaction of pyruvate dehydrogenase
Pyruvate undergoes a three-step reaction in which it is decarboxylated to enzyme-bound acetaldehyde. This is then oxidized to enzyme-bound acetate, with the reduction of NAD to NADH. The acetate is released from the enzyme after reaction with CoA, as acetyl CoA. Since 2 mol of pyruvate are formed from each mol of glucose, this step represents the formation of 2 mol of NADH (equivalent to $2 \times 3 = 6$ mol of ATP) for each mol of glucose metabolized.

140

The decarboxylation and oxidation of pyruvate to form acetyl CoA requires the coenzyme thiamin diphosphate, which is formed from vitamin B_1 (thiamin, see p. 255). In **thiamin deficiency** this reaction is impaired, and deficient subjects are unable to metabolize glucose normally. Especially after a test dose of glucose or moderate exercise they develop high blood concentrations of pyruvate and lactate. In some cases this may be severe enough to result in life-threatening acidosis.

Oxidation of acetyl CoA: the citric acid cycle

The acetate part of acetyl CoA undergoes a stepwise oxidation to carbon dioxide and water in a cyclic pathway, the citric acid cycle, shown in Figure 6.8. For each mol of acetyl CoA oxidized in this pathway, there is a yield of:

$3 \times$ NAD reduced to NADH, equivalent to $9 \times$ ATP;
$1 \times$ flavoprotein reduced, equivalent to $2 \times$ ADP;
$1 \times$ GDP phosphorylated to GTP, equivalent to $1 \times$ ATP.

This is a total of $12 \times$ ATP for each mol of acetyl CoA oxidized; since two mol of acetyl CoA are formed from each mol of glucose, this cycle yields $24 \times$ ATP for each mol of glucose oxidized.

Although it appears complex at first sight, the citric acid cycle is a relatively simple pathway. A four-carbon compound, oxaloacetate, reacts with acetyl CoA to form a six-carbon compound, citric acid. The cycle is then a series of steps in which these two carbon atoms are oxidized and released as carbon dioxide, eventually reforming oxaloacetate. The CoA of acetyl CoA is released, and is available for further formation of acetyl CoA from pyruvate.

The citric acid cycle is also involved in the oxidation of acetyl CoA arising from other sources, mainly from the oxidation of fatty acids (see p. 144), but also from the oxidation of ketones in fasting and starvation (see p. 147); and the metabolism of some amino acids gives rise to acetyl CoA.

This cycle is an important central metabolic pathway, providing the link between carbohydrate, fat and amino acid metabolism. Many of the intermediates can be used for the synthesis of other compounds, for example oxoglutarate and oxaloacetate can give rise to the amino acids glutamate and aspartate, respectively; citrate is used as the source of acetyl CoA for fatty acid synthesis in the cytosol in the fed state (see p. 148); and oxaloacetate is an important precursor for glucose synthesis in the fasting state (see p. 153).

Obviously, if oxaloacetate is removed from the cycle for glucose synthesis, it must be replaced, since if there is not enough oxaloacetate

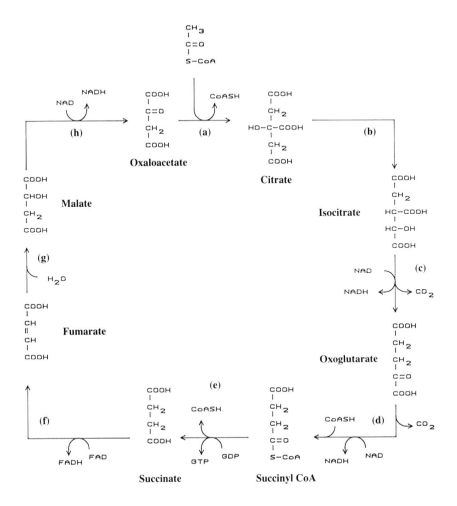

Figure 6.8 The citric acid cycle

This provides a cyclic pathway for the oxidation of acetate to carbon dioxide, linked to the reduction of $3 \times$ NAD to NADH and 1 FAD to FADH for each mol of acetate oxidized. In addition, 1 mol of GDP is phosphorylated to GTP. Since each mol of glucose gives rise to 2 mol of acetyl CoA, this means that this pathway yields $2 \times 3 \times 3 = 18$ ATP from the oxidation of NADH, plus $2 \times 2 = 4$ ATP from the oxidation of FADH, plus the equivalent of $2 \times$ ATP from the GTP formed in reaction (e) $= 24 \times$ ATP per mol of glucose. (a) *Citrate synthase*: the first reaction is between the four-carbon compound oxaloacetate and acetyl CoA to form the six-carbon compound citrate, with the release of CoA. (b) *Isomerase*: citrate undergoes isomerization to isocitrate. (c) *Isocitrate dehydrogenase*: isocitrate undergoes an oxidative decarboxylation, with the reduction of NAD to NADH and the release of carbon dioxide. The product is oxoglutarate. (d) *Oxoglutarate dehydrogenase*: oxoglutarate undergoes an oxidative decarboxylation, with the reduction of NADH to NAD, release of carbon dioxide and the incorporation of CoA to form succinyl CoA. This reaction is essentially the same as the reaction of pyruvate dehydrogenase, which results in the formation of acetyl CoA from pyruvate (see Fig. 6.7). (e) *Succinyl CoA synthase*: succinyl CoA undergoes hydrolysis to succinate, releasing CoA, in a reaction which is coupled to the phosphorylation of GDP to GTP.

available to form citrate, the rate of acetyl CoA metabolism will slow down. Although the cycle acts to interconvert the various intermediates, it cannot act as a net source of compounds unless there is some source of one of the intermediates (any one of them will do) to replace what is being lost. A variety of amino acids give rise to citric acidcycle intermediates such as oxoglutarate, fumarate and oxaloacetate.

The metabolism of fats

Triacylglycerols may arise either from the diet (in the fed state) or from adipose tissue reserves (in the fasting state). In either case they are metabolized in the same way:

(a) hydrolysis of the triacylglycerol to yield three molecules of fatty acids and a molecule of glycerol (see Fig. 4.6 on p. 78);

(b) glycerol is converted to dihydroxyacetone phosphate (see Fig. 6.4) and so is available for either onward oxidation, via pyruvate to acetyl CoA, in the fed state, or conversion to glucose in the fasting state (see p. 153);

(c) the fatty acids are oxidized by the ß-oxidation pathway, in which two carbon atoms at a time are removed from the fatty acid chain as acetyl CoA. This acetyl CoA then enters the citric acid cycle, together with that arising from the metabolism of pyruvate.

The ß-oxidation of fatty acids Fatty acids are oxidized inside the mitochondria. The first step is the formation of a CoA derivative, fatty acyl CoA. This then undergoes a series of four reactions, as shown in Figure 6.9, which result in the cleavage of the fatty acid molecule to give acetyl CoA and a new fatty acyl CoA which is two carbons shorter than the one we started with. This new, shorter, fatty acyl CoA is then a substrate for the same sequence of reactions, which is repeated until the final result is cleavage to yield two molecules of acetyl CoA.

The reactions of ß-oxidation are simple:

(a) The first step is the removal of two hydrogens from the fatty acid, to form a carbon–carbon double bond – an oxidation reaction. The hy-

---

(Note that this enzyme is named for the reverse reaction, the synthesis of succinyl CoA from succinate and CoA.) (f) *Succinate dehydrogenase*: succinate is oxidized, to form the unsaturated compound fumarate, in a reaction linked to the reduction of FAD to FADH.
(g) *Fumarase*: the carbon–carbon double bond of fumarate is hydrated, to form malate.
(h) *Malate dehydrogenase*: the hydroxyl group of malate is oxidized to an oxo-group, with the reduction of NAD to NADH. The product of this reaction is oxaloacetate, which is therefore available to react with a further molecule of acetyl CoA to restart the cycle.

hydrogens are transferred onto a flavoprotein, and so for each double bond formed in this way there is a yield of $2 \times$ ATP.

(b) The newly formed double bond in the fatty acyl CoA then reacts with water, yielding a hydroxyl group – a hydration reaction.

(c) The hydroxylated fatty acyl CoA undergoes a second oxidation in which the hydroxyl group transfers hydrogen onto a flavoprotein (hence again a yield of $2 \times$ ATP per cycle of reaction). The result of this second oxidation is the formation of an oxo-fatty acyl CoA.

d) This is then cleaved by reaction with CoA, to form acetyl CoA and the shorter fatty acyl CoA, which undergoes the same sequence of reactions.

Almost all of the metabolically important fatty acids have an even number of carbon atoms, so that the final cycle of ß-oxidation is the conversion of a four-carbon fatty acyl CoA (butyryl CoA) to two molecules of acetyl CoA.

Ketone bodies   In the fasting state, the liver is capable of forming considerably more acetyl CoA from fatty acids than is required for its own metabolism. It takes up fatty acids from the circulation and oxidizes them to acetyl CoA, then exports four-carbon "ketones" formed from acetyl CoA for other tissues (especially muscle) to use as a metabolic fuel.

The reactions involved are shown in Figure 6.10. Acetoacetyl CoA is formed by reaction between two molecules of acetyl CoA. This is essentially the reverse of the final reaction of fatty acid ß-oxidation (see Fig. 6.9). Acetoacetyl CoA then reacts with a further molecule of acetyl CoA to form hydroxymethyl-glutaryl CoA. Hydroxymethyl-glutaryl CoA then undergoes cleavage to release acetyl CoA and acetoacetate.

As well as being an intermediate in the synthesis of ketone bodies, hydroxymethyl-glutaryl CoA is the precursor for the synthesis of cholesterol and the other steroids (see p. 85). Inhibitors of the enzyme which commits hydroxymethyl-glutaryl CoA to cholesterol synthesis (hydroxymethyl-glutaryl CoA reductase) are commonly used in the treatment of patients with dangerously high plasma concentrations of cholesterol as a result of genetic defects in the regulation of cholesterol synthesis.

Acetoacetate is chemically unstable, and much is reduced to hydroxybutyrate before being released from the liver. Hydroxybutyrate and acetoacetate are metabolic fuels for tissues outside the liver in the fasting state (see Fig. 6.11).

A small amount of acetoacetate undergoes a non-enzymic reaction to yield acetone, which is metabolically useless. There is no pathway for its utilization; it is excreted in the urine and in exhaled air.

Acetoacetate, hydroxybutyrate and acetone are collectively known as the **ketone bodies**, and the occurrence of increased concentrations of these

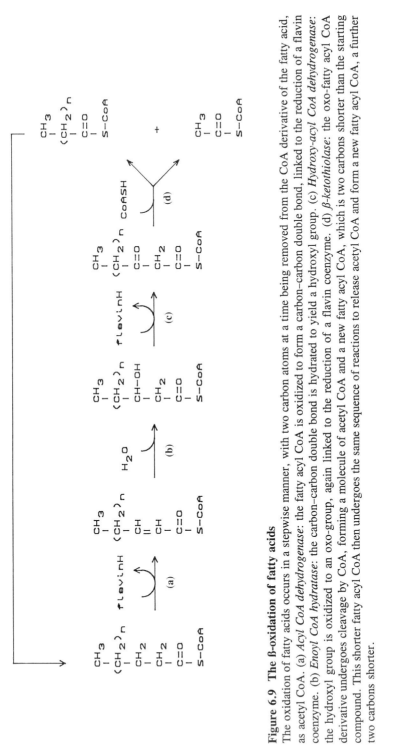

Figure 6.9 The β-oxidation of fatty acids

The oxidation of fatty acids occurs in a stepwise manner, with two carbon atoms at a time being removed from the CoA derivative of the fatty acid, as acetyl CoA. (a) *Acyl CoA dehydrogenase*: the fatty acyl CoA is oxidized to form a carbon–carbon double bond, linked to the reduction of a flavin coenzyme. (b) *Enoyl CoA hydratase*: the carbon–carbon double bond is hydrated to yield a hydroxyl group. (c) *Hydroxy-acyl CoA dehydrogenase*: the hydroxyl group is oxidized to an oxo-group, again linked to the reduction of a flavin coenzyme. (d) *β-ketothiolase*: the oxo-fatty acyl CoA derivative undergoes cleavage by CoA, forming a molecule of acetyl CoA and a new fatty acyl CoA, which is two carbons shorter than the starting compound. This shorter fatty acyl CoA then undergoes the same sequence of reactions to release acetyl CoA and form a new fatty acyl CoA, a further two carbons shorter.

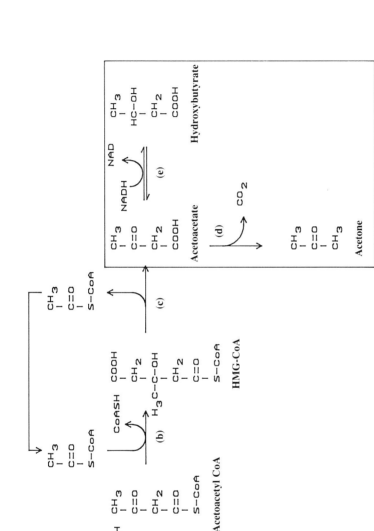

Figure 6.10 The formation of ketone bodies from acetyl CoA

The two metabolically important ketone bodies are acetoacetate and hydroxybutyrate, shown in the box on the right of the diagram. (a) *β-ketothiolase*: two molecules of acetyl CoA react together to form acetoacetyl CoA, with the release of free CoA. (b) *HMG CoA synthase*: acetoacetyl CoA reacts with a further molecule of acetyl CoA to form hydroxymethylglutaryl CoA (HMG-CoA), with the release of a molecule of CoA. (c) *HMG-CoA lyase*: HMG-CoA undergoes a cleavage reaction which releases a molecule of acetyl CoA, and results in the formation of acetoacetate. (d) Acetoacetate is chemically unstable, and undergoes a non-enzymic reaction to form acetone. There is no pathway for the metabolism of acetone, which is thus a useless (and wasteful) side-product. (e) *Hydroxybutyrate dehydrogenase*: most acetoacetate is reduced to hydroxybutyrate, in a reaction in which NADH is the hydrogen donor, and it is mainly hydroxybutyrate which is released from the liver as a metabolic fuel for other tissues.

three compounds in the bloodstream is known as **ketosis**. In fact, although acetone and acetoacetate are chemically ketones, having the $-C=O$ grouping, hydroxybutyrate is not a ketone. It is classified with the other two because of its metabolic relationship.

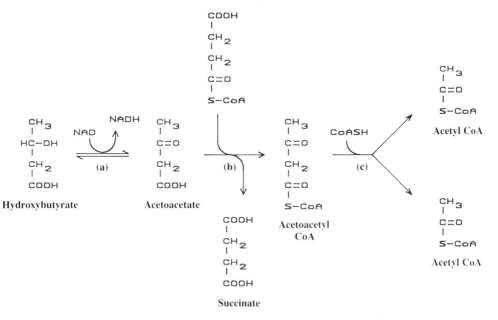

Figure 6.11 The utilization of ketone bodies in tissues outside the liver
(a) *Hydroxybutyrate dehydrogenase*: hydroxybutyrate is oxidized to acetoacetate in a reaction linked to the reduction of NAD to NADH. (b) *Acetoacetate-succinyl CoA transferase*: CoA is transferred onto acetoacetate, forming acetoacetyl CoA. The CoA donor is succinyl CoA, an intermediate in the citric acid cycle, and the product is succinate. (c) *β-Ketothiolase*: acetoacetyl CoA is cleaved by reaction with CoA, to form two molecules of acetyl CoA.

Tissue reserves of metabolic fuels

In the fed state, as well as providing for immediate energy needs, substrates are converted into storage forms for use later, in the fasting state. There are two main stores of metabolic fuels:
(a) triacylglycerols in adipose tissue;
(b) glycogen as a carbohydrate reserve in liver and muscle.
In addition, there is an increase in the synthesis of tissue proteins in response to a meal, so that there is some increase in the total body content of protein. This can also be used as a metabolic fuel in the fasting state.

In the fasting state, which is the normal state between meals, these reserves are mobilized and used. Glycogen is a source of glucose, while

147

adipose tissue provides both fatty acids and glycerol from triacylglycerol. Some of the relatively labile protein laid down in response to meals is also mobilized in fasting.

Synthesis of fatty acids and triacylglycerols Fatty acids are synthesized by the successive addition of two-carbon units from acetyl CoA. The process of fatty acid synthesis occurs in the cytosol, while the source of acetyl CoA is inside the mitochondria. Acetyl CoA cannot cross the mitochondrial membrane. Citrate is formed inside the mitochondria by reaction between acetyl CoA and oxaloacetate (see Fig. 6.8). Citrate can be transported out of the mitochondria, to undergo cleavage in the cytosol to yield acetyl CoA and oxaloacetate. The acetyl CoA is used for fatty acid synthesis, while the oxaloacetate (indirectly) returns to the mitochondria to maintain citric acid cycle activity.

The chemical reactions involved in the synthesis of fatty acids are essentially the same as those in the oxidation of fatty acids to acetyl CoA (see Fig. 6.9), but in the reverse order. As shown in Figure 6.12, two-carbon units are added sequentially; the resultant oxo-fatty acid derivative then undergoes:
(a) reduction to the hydroxy-derivative;
(b) dehydration to yield a carbon–carbon double bond;
(c) reduction of the double bond to give the saturated fatty acid chain.
There are two main differences between fatty acid synthesis and oxidation:
(a) ß-Oxidation occurs inside the mitochondria, while fatty acid synthesis occurs in the cytosol.
(b) ß-Oxidation occurs with acyl CoA derivatives, while fatty acid synthesis involves the formation of more tightly enzyme-associated intermediates, which are bound to the enzyme by an acyl carrier protein (generally abbreviated to ACP). Fatty acid synthesis occurs in a large multi-enzyme complex, in which the growing fatty acid moves from one enzyme active site to the next, at the end of the rotating "arm" provided by the ACP. Like CoA, the functionally important part of the ACP is derived from the vitamin pantothenic acid (see p. 272).

Although each turn of the reaction sequence shown in Figure 6.12 involves the addition of a two-carbon unit to the growing fatty acid chain, what is actually added each time is the three-carbon compound, malonyl-ACP. This is formed from acetyl-ACP by reaction with carbon dioxide (a carboxylation reaction), and undergoes decarboxylation (the loss of carbon dioxide) as it condenses with the growing fatty acid chain. The vitamin **biotin** (see p. 271) acts as the intermediate carrier of carbon dioxide in the carboxylation of acetyl CoA to malonyl CoA.

Figure 6.12 The synthesis of fatty acids

The synthesis of fatty acids involves the stepwise addition of two-carbon units, from acetyl CoA, to build up the complete fatty acid molecule. (a) *Acetyl CoA carboxylase*: acetyl CoA is carboxylated to malonyl CoA, in a reaction linked to the hydrolysis of ATP to ADP and phosphate. (b) *Acyl transferase*: malonyl CoA reacts with the acyl carrier protein (ACP) of the multi-enzyme complex to form malonyl-ACP. The functional group of the acyl carrier protein is the same as that of CoA. (c) *β-Keto-acyl ACP synthase*: malonyl-ACP reacts with the growing fatty acyl ACP attached to the enzyme, releasing its ACP, and losing the carbon dioxide which was added in reaction (a). The result is an oxo-fatty acyl ACP derivative. (d) *β-Keto-acyl ACP reductase*: the oxo-group of the oxo-fatty acyl ACP is reduced to a hydroxyl group, in a reaction in which NADPH is the hydrogen donor. (e) *β-Hydroxy-acyl ACP dehydratase*: the hydroxy-fatty acyl ACP undergoes a dehydration reaction to yield a carbon–carbon double bond. (f) *Enoyl ACP reductase*: the carbon–carbon double bond is reduced to a saturated single bond, again in a reaction in which the hydrogen donor is NADPH. The result is a saturated fatty acyl ACP derivative which is two carbons longer than the starting compound. It now undergoes the same sequence of reactions again, until the final product is the 18-carbon fatty acid, stearic acid.

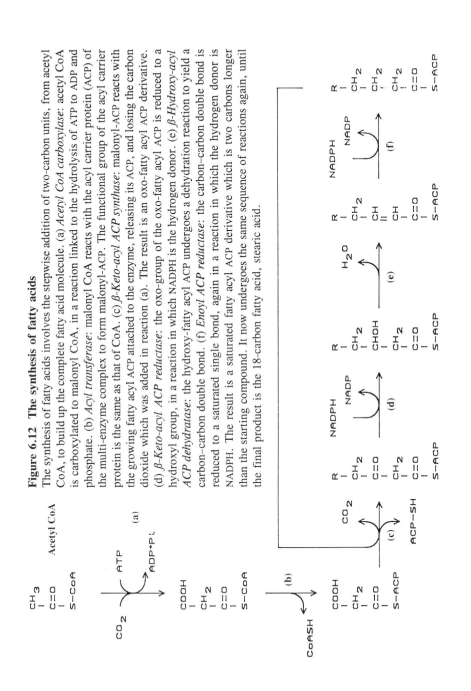

Unsaturated fatty acids   Although fatty acid synthesis involves the formation of an unsaturated intermediate, the next step, reduction to the saturated fatty acid derivative, is an obligatory part of the reaction sequence, and cannot be omitted. Man and other animals can synthesize some unsaturated fatty acids from saturated fatty acids, by the removal of hydrogen to yield a carbon–carbon double bond.

The polyunsaturated fatty acids cannot be synthesized in human tissues. There is considerable interconversion of polyunsaturated fatty acids in tissues, but two of them, **linoleic** and **linolenic acids**, must be provided in the diet. These are the so-called **essential fatty acids.**

Synthesis of triacylglycerols   The storage lipids in adipose tissue are triacylglycerols: glycerol esterified with three molecules of fatty acid (see Fig. 4.6 on p. 78). The three fatty acids in a triacylglycerol molecule are not always the same as each other.

Triacylglycerols are synthesized in the liver and adipose tissue, using both fatty acids synthesized in these tissues and also fatty acids arising from dietary lipids. As shown in Figure 6.13, glycerol phosphate is esterified with fatty acids; this may either be formed by phosphorylation of glycerol, or may arise from the reduction of dihydroxyacetone phosphate formed from fructose bisphosphate (see Fig. 6.4).

Two molecules of fatty acid are esterified to the free hydroxyl groups of glycerol phosphate, by transfer from fatty acyl CoA, forming monoacylglycerol phosphate and then diacylglycerol phosphate (or phosphatidic acid). The resultant diacylglycerol phosphate can act as the precursor for the synthesis of **phospholipids** (see Fig. 4.8 on p. 82), or it can react with a further molecule of fatty acyl CoA to form a triacylglycerol, releasing phosphate.

Glycogen   Glycogen is a branched polymer of glucose (see Fig. 4.5 on p. 77). In the fed state glycogen is synthesized from glucose in both liver and muscle. The reaction is a step-wise addition of glucose units onto the glycogen that is already present.

As shown in Figure 6.14, glycogen synthesis involves the intermediate formation of UDP-glucose by reaction between glucose-1-phosphate and UTP. As each glucose unit is added to the growing glycogen chain, so UDP is released, and must be rephosphorylated to UTP by reaction with ATP. There is thus a significant cost of ATP in the synthesis of glycogen: 2 mol of ATP are converted to ADP and phosphate for each glucose unit added.

Glycogen synthetase forms only the straight chains of glycogen. The branch points are introduced by the transfer of 6–10 glucose units in a chain from carbon-4 to carbon-6 of the glucose unit at the branch point.

In the fasting state, glycogen is broken down by the removal of glucose

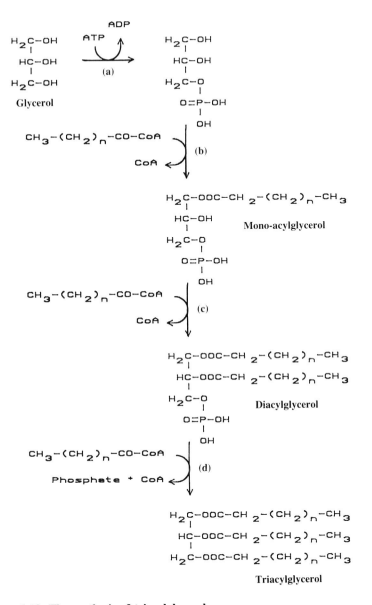

Figure 6.13 The synthesis of triacylglycerol

(a) *Glycerol kinase*: glycerol is phosphorylated to glycerol phosphate. Glycerol phosphate can also be formed by reduction of dihydroxyacetone phosphate formed by the cleavage of fructose-1,6-bisphosphate (reaction (d) in Fig. 6.4). (b) Glycerol phosphate then reacts with a fatty acyl CoA to form the fatty acid ester at carbon-1 of glycerol phosphate, and release CoA. The product is a mono-acylglycerol phosphate. (c) Mono-acylglycerol phosphate reacts with a second molecule of fatty acyl CoA, to form a fatty acid ester at carbon-2 of glycerol and release CoA. The product is a diacylglycerol phosphate, or phosphatidic acid. (d) The phosphatidic acid reacts with a third molecule of fatty acyl CoA to form a fatty acid ester at carbon-3 of glycerol, releasing CoA and phosphate. The product is the triacylglycerol.

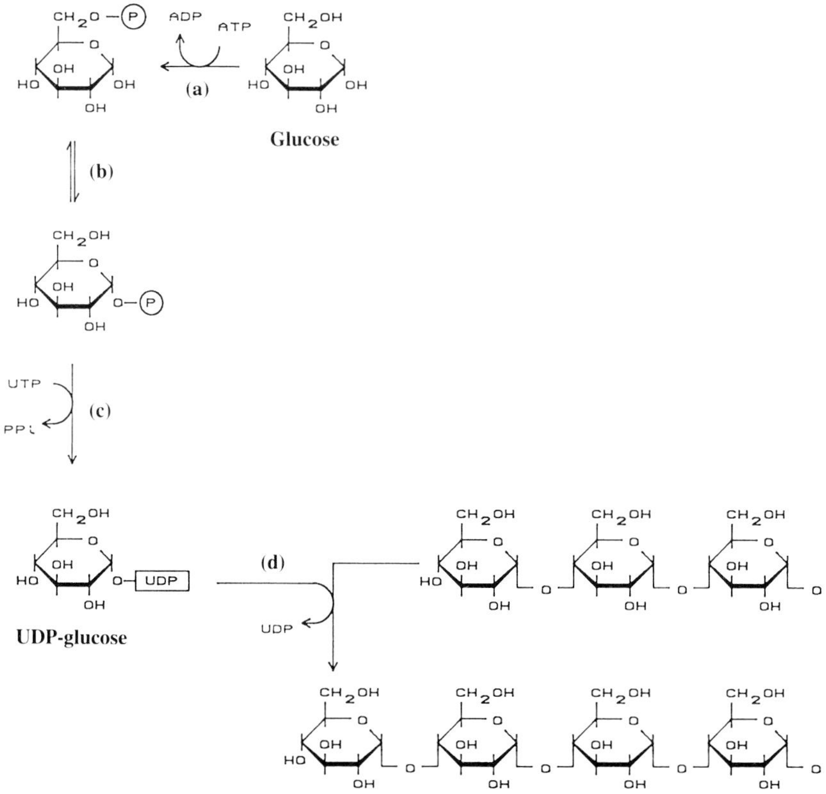

Figure 6.14 The synthesis of glycogen
(a) *Hexokinase*: glucose is phosphorylated to glucose-6-phosphate in a reaction in which ATP is the phosphate donor. This is the same as the first reaction of glycolysis (see Fig. 6.4). (b) *Glucose-6-phosphate isomerase*: glucose-6-phosphate is isomerized to glucose-1-phosphate. (c) *Uridyl transferase*: glucose-1-phosphate reacts with UTP, to form UDP-glucose, with the release of pyrophosphate. (d) *Glycogen synthase*: UDP-glucose reacts with carbon-4 of the glucose unit at the end of the growing glycogen chain, forming a glycoside bond and releasing UDP.

units one at a time from the many ends of the molecule. The reaction is a phosphorolysis – cleavage of the glycoside link between two glucose molecules by the introduction of phosphate. The product is glucose-1-phosphate, which is then converted to glucose-6-phosphate.

Gluconeogenesis: the synthesis of glucose Muscle and other tissues can use fatty acids and ketones as metabolic fuels in the fasting state, and muscle has considerable glycogen reserves, but the nervous system is reliant on a supply of glucose. It is only in prolonged starvation that the concentration of ketones (hydroxybutyrate and acetoacetate) in the blood rises high enough for the brain to be able to make use of them as a metabolic fuel. Therefore there is a need to maintain the blood concentration of glucose between about 3 and 5 mmol/l, even in the fasting state. If the plasma concentration of glucose falls below about 2 mmol/l there is a loss of consciousness – **hypoglycaemic coma**.

To a great extent, the plasma concentration of glucose can be maintained in short-term fasting by the use of liver glycogen as a source of free glucose, and by releasing free fatty acids from adipose tissues, and ketones from the liver, which are preferentially used by muscle, so sparing such glucose as is available for use by the brain (see Table 6.2).

Table 6.2 Changes of plasma concentrations of metabolic fuels in fasting and starvation.

	Fed	40h fasting	7 days starvation
Glucose (mmol/l)	5.5	3.6	3.5
Fatty acids (mmol/l)	0.3	1.15	1.19
Ketones (mmol/l)	0.01	2.9	4.5

However, there is only a relatively small amount of glycogen in the liver. Indeed, the total body pool of glycogen (that in both liver and muscle) would be exhausted within 24h of fasting if there were not another source of glucose. This is provided by the process of **gluconeogenesis** – the synthesis of glucose from non-carbohydrate precursors: amino acids from the breakdown of protein, and the glycerol of triacylglycerols.

It is important to note that although acetyl CoA, and hence fatty acids, can be synthesized from pyruvate (and therefore from carbohydrates), the decarboxylation of pyruvate to acetyl CoA cannot be reversed. Pyruvate cannot be formed from acetyl CoA. Since two molecules of carbon dioxide are formed for each two-carbon acetate unit metabolized in the citric acid cycle (see Fig. 6.8), there can be no net formation of oxaloacetate from acetate. *It is not possible to synthesize glucose from acetyl CoA. Therefore, fatty acids cannot serve as a precursor for glucose synthesis.*

The amino acids are metabolized by way of the same intermediates as arise in the metabolism of fatty acids and glucose. Those which give rise to intermediates of glucose metabolism, or provide a net increase in the amount of oxaloacetate in the citric acid cycle, can be used for the synthesis of glucose in the fasting state. During fasting, tissue protein is broken down, and the resultant amino acids are used either as metabolic fuels or as precursors for glucose synthesis.

The pathway of gluconeogenesis is essentially the reverse of the pathway of glycolysis, shown in Figure 6.4. However, at three steps there are separate enzymes involved in the breakdown of glucose (glycolysis) and gluconeogenesis. As discussed on p. 138, the reactions of pyruvate kinase (which converts phosphoenolpyruvate to pyruvate), phosphofructokinase and hexokinase cannot readily be reversed (i.e. they have equilibria which are strongly towards the formation of pyruvate, fructose bisphosphate and glucose-6-phosphate, respectively).

There are therefore separate enzymes, under distinct metabolic control, for the reverse of each of these reactions in gluconeogenesis:

(a) Pyruvate is converted to phosphoenolpyruvate for glucose synthesis by a two-step reaction, with the intermediate formation of oxaloacetate. As shown in Figure 6.15, pyruvate is carboxylated to oxaloacetate in an ATP-dependent reaction in which the vitamin biotin (see p. 271) is the coenzyme. This reaction can also be used to replenish oxaloacetate in the citric acid cycle when intermediates have been withdrawn for use in other pathways. Oxaloacetate then undergoes a phosphorylation reaction, in which it also loses carbon dioxide, to form phosphoenolpyruvate. The phosphate donor for this reaction is GTP.

(b) Fructose bisphosphate is hydrolysed to fructose-6-phosphate by a simple hydrolysis reaction catalysed by the enzyme fructose bisphosphatase.

(c) Glucose-6-phosphate is hydrolysed to free glucose and phosphate by the action of glucose-6-phosphatase. The glucose is then exported from the liver for use by the nervous system and other tissues. Glucose-1-phosphate arising from the phosphorolysis of liver glycogen can be converted readily to glucose-6-phosphate, and then hydrolysed to glucose for release into the bloodstream. Muscle glycogen cannot act as a source of blood glucose in the same way, since muscle cells lack glucose-6-phosphatase.

The other reactions shown in Figure 6.4 are readily reversible, and the overall direction of metabolism, either glycolysis or gluconeogenesis, will depend on the relative activities of the separate enzymes involved in the interconversions of pyruvate and phosphoenolpyruvate, and of fructose-6-phosphate and fructose bisphosphate.

The continuing requirement for gluconeogenesis from amino acids in fasting and starvation explains why there is often a considerable loss of muscle when people are fasted, even if they still have apparently adequate adipose tissue reserves. In people who have only small adipose tissue reserves, there will be more loss of muscle in starvation (see p. 172).

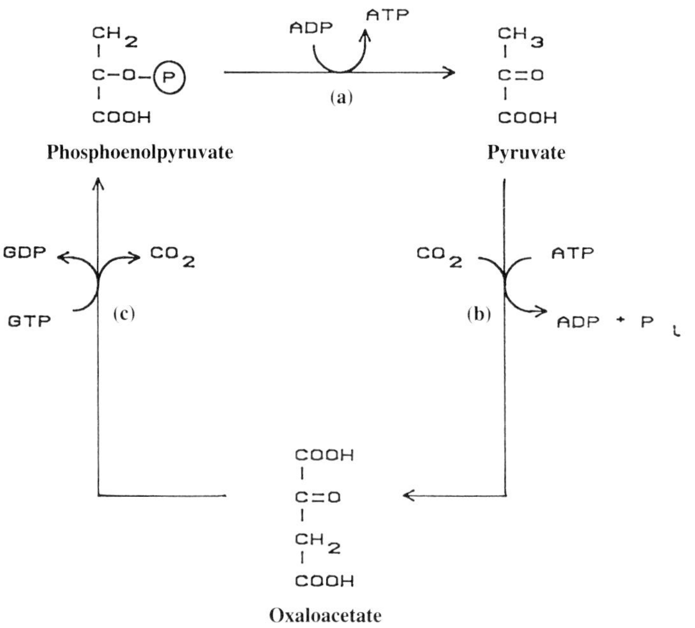

Figure 6.15 The reversal of the pyruvate kinase reaction in gluconeogenesis
a) *Pyruvate kinase*: the formation of pyruvate from phosphoenolpyruvate is essentially irreversible (see Fig. 6.5). Therefore, an alternative pathway must exist for the formation of phosphoenolpyruvate from pyruvate for gluconeogenesis. (b) *Pyruvate carboxylase*: pyruvate is carboxylated to oxaloacetate in a reaction in which ATP is hydrolysed to ADP and phosphate. (c) *Phosphoenolpyruvate carboxykinase*: oxaloacetate is phosphorylated in a reaction in which GTP is the phosphate donor, undergoing loss of carbon dioxide in the process, and forming phosphoenolpyruvate.

Control of the formation and utilization of tissue reserves of metabolic fuels

We would expect the availability of metabolic fuels in the fed state to lead towards the formation of glycogen and triglyceride reserves. Similarly, in the fasting state we would expect the utilization of metabolic fuels, without a continuing input from the gut, to result in the mobilization of triglyceride and glycogen reserves.

In addition, we can consider two types of control over the metabolic pathways concerned: control by intracellular metabolites and control by hormones secreted in response to changes in whole body metabolism. Hormonal control of metabolism is discussed in Chapter 10.

As well as the effects of the concentrations of their immediate substrates and products, some enzymes are sensitive to changes in the concentrations of other metabolites in the cell. Such regulatory factors include: the ratio of ATP:ADP; the ratio of NADH:NAD and the concentrations of a variety of compounds such as citrate and acetyl CoA, which can be considered to be the end-products of pathways. These compounds bind at a site other than the active site of the enzyme. They act by causing a conformational change in the enzyme protein, which affects the active site, and so either increases or decreases the activity of the enzyme.

As an example of this type of metabolic regulation, we can consider control over the reactions catalysed by phosphofructokinase and fructose-1,6-bisphosphatase in glycolysis and gluconeogenesis respectively (reaction c in Fig. 6.4). Factors which increase the activity of phosphofructokinase, and hence increase the formation of fructose bisphosphate (i.e. increase the rate of glycolysis) also act to decrease the activity of fructose bisphosphatase. Similarly, compounds which decrease the activity of phosphofructokinase increase the activity of fructose bisphosphatase. This ensures that only one of these two enzymes is active at any one time, and hence determines the overall direction of metabolism: glycolysis or gluconeogenesis.

Phosphofructokinase is inhibited by relatively high concentrations of ATP. We can consider ATP to be an end-product of glycolysis. Similarly, it is inhibited by a high concentration of hydrogen ions (H^+), as occurs when there is an accumulation of pyruvate and lactate, indicating a requirement for gluconeogenesis rather than continuing glycolysis. Citrate also inhibits phosphofructokinase. Again citrate can be considered to be an end-product of glycolysis when it accumulates in the cytosol for the synthesis of fatty acids (see p. 148).

Phosphofructokinase is activated by AMP and phosphate. AMP is formed from ADP when the tissue content of ATP is relatively depleted, and ADP is relatively high, as a result of the reaction:

$$2 \times ADP \rightleftharpoons ATP + AMP.$$

Thus, phosphofructokinase is inhibited when there is enough ATP being formed, and glycolysis can be slowed down, and it is activated when there is a need for additional ATP formation from ADP.

Energy balance

If the intake of metabolic fuels is equivalent to the energy expenditure of the body, we can say that the person is in energy balance. Overall his or her metabolism will show equal amounts of fed-state metabolism (during which nutrient reserves are accumulated as liver and muscle glycogen, adipose tissue triacylglycerols and labile protein stores), and fasting-state metabolism, during which these reserves are utilized. Averaged out over several days, there will be no change in body weight or body composition.

By contrast, if the intake of metabolic fuels is greater than is required to meet energy expenditure, the body will spend more time in the fed state than the fasting state; there will be more accumulation of nutrient reserves than utilization. The result of this is an increase in body size, and especially an increase in adipose tissue stores. If continued for long enough, this will result in overweight or obesity (see Ch. 7).

The opposite state of affairs is when the intake of metabolic fuels is lower than is required to meet energy expenditure. Now the body has to mobilize its nutrient reserves, and overall spends more time in the fasting state than in the fed state. The result of this is undernutrition, starvation and eventually death (see Ch. 8).

We know the metabolic energy yields of metabolic fuels (see Table 1.1 on p. 3). Therefore if we know a person's food intake, it is easy to calculate his or her energy intake, using food composition tables (see Appendix II).

Energy expenditure can be determined in three different ways:
(a) direct **calorimetry**;
(b) indirect calorimetry;
(c) double-labelled water techniques.

Direct calorimetry

We can measure energy expenditure quite simply by measuring a person's **heat output**. This requires a thermally insulated chamber, whose temperature can be controlled so as to maintain the subject's comfort, and in which it is possible to measure the amount of heat produced, for example by the increase in temperature of the water used to cool the chamber. **Calorimeters** of this sort are relatively small, so that it is only possible for measurements of direct heat production to be made for subjects performing a limited range of tasks.

Indirect calorimetry

We can estimate energy expenditure from the rate of consumption of oxygen and production of carbon dioxide. This is known as indirect calorimetry, since there is no direct measurement of the heat produced. We know from a series of studies in which heat production has been measured by direct calorimetry at the same time as oxygen consumption has been measured that there is an output or expenditure of 20kJ/litre of oxygen consumed, regardless of whether the fuel being metabolized is carbohydrate, fat or protein. This means that we can estimate energy expenditure by measuring the amount of oxygen consumed.

Measurement of oxygen consumption is quite simple using a respirometer. Such instruments are portable, so people can carry on more or less normal activities for several hours at a time, while their energy expenditure is being estimated.

Respiratory quotient If we measure both oxygen consumption and carbon dioxide production, we can gain more information. In the metabolism of starch, the same amount of carbon dioxide is produced as oxygen is consumed, i.e. the ratio of carbon dioxide produced/oxygen consumed = 1.0. This is because the overall reaction is

$$C_6H_{12}O_6 + 6O_2 \rightarrow 6CO_2 + 6H_2O.$$

By contrast, when fat is metabolized, more oxygen is required. Again, if we look at the chemistry involved, this is obvious, since in the oxidation of fatty acids to carbon dioxide and water we are considering mainly the oxidation of $-CH_2-$ units:

$$-CH_2 + 1\frac{1}{2}O_2 \rightarrow CO_2 + H_2O.$$

Allowing for the fact that in triacylglycerols we also have glycerol and three $-COOH$ groups, we find that for the metabolism of fat the ratio of carbon dioxide produced/oxygen consumed = 0.7.

The metabolism of proteins gives a ratio of carbon dioxide produced/oxygen consumed intermediate between that of carbohydrate and fat; this is because proteins contain relatively more oxygen per carbon atom than do fats, although less than carbohydrates. For protein metabolism the ratio of carbon dioxide produced/oxygen consumed is 0.8.

We can get a measurement of the amount of protein being metabolized in a quite different way, by measuring the excretion of **urea**. As discussed on p. 203, urea is the end-product of metabolism of the nitrogen of proteins and amino acids, so measuring how much is excreted in the urine gives information on how much protein is being oxidized.

We call the ratio of carbon dioxide produced/oxygen consumed the **respiratory quotient**. Together with measurement of the excretion of urea, it can be used to calculate of the relative amounts of fat, carbohydrate and protein being metabolized.

In the fasting state, when a relatively large amount of fat is being used as a fuel, the respiratory quotient is around 0.8; in response to a meal, when there is more carbohydrate being metabolized, the respiratory quotient rises to about 0.9.

Long-term measurement of energy expenditure – the double-labelled water method

Although indirect calorimetry has considerable advantages over direct calorimetry, it still only allows measurement of energy expenditure over a relatively short period of time, perhaps a few hours, or a day, at the very most. A recent development permits the estimation of total energy expenditure over a period of 1–2 weeks.

This method depends on the administration of a sample of water labelled with stable isotopes (see p. 30). Both the hydrogen and oxygen of the water are labelled, the hydrogen as deuterium (^{2}H) and the oxygen as ^{18}O. The rate at which the labelled water is lost from the body is found by measuring the amounts of these two isotopes in urine or saliva.

The deuterium (^{2}H) is lost from the body only as water. The labelled oxygen (^{18}O) is lost more rapidly. It can be lost as either water or carbon dioxide, because of the rapid equilibrium between carbon dioxide and bicarbonate:

$$H_2O + CO_2 \rightleftharpoons H^+ + HCO_3^-.$$

Since all three oxygen atoms in the bicarbonate ion are equivalent, label from $H_2{}^{18}O$ can end up in both water and carbon dioxide.

Measuring the difference between the rate of loss of the two labels from the body thus gives us an estimate of the total amount of carbon dioxide which has been produced. If we then estimate the respiratory quotient, from the proportions of fat, carbohydrate and protein in the diet, we can estimate the total amount of oxygen that has been consumed, and hence the **total energy expenditure** over the period of the study.

Energy expenditure depends on two factors:

(a) the requirement for maintenance of normal body structure and function and metabolic integrity – the **basal metabolic rate (Table 6.3)**; and

(b) the additional energy required for work and physical activity.

Basal metabolic rate (BMR) Basal metabolic rate can be measured by direct or indirect calorimetry. It is defined as the energy expenditure by the body when at rest, but not asleep, under controlled conditions of thermal neutrality, and neither immediately after a meal nor yet in the fasting state. It is the energy requirement for the maintenance of metabolic integrity, nerve and muscle tone, circulation and respiration, etc.

Calculating a person's energy expenditure

Obviously, measurements of energy expenditure of the type described above, whether by direct or indirect calorimetry or the dual-labelled water method, have been performed on only a very small number of people. We need some way in which we can estimate energy expenditure, and hence energy needs, without the need for individual laboratory investigations.

Table 6.3 Definitions in energy metabolism.

BMR	Basal metabolic rate	Energy expenditure in the post-absorptive state, under standardized conditions of thermal neutrality, awake but completely at rest
RMR	Resting metabolic rate	Energy expenditure at rest, but not under standardized conditions
PAR	Physical activity ratio	Energy cost of physical activities, as a ratio of BMR
PAL	Physical activity level	Sum of PAR × time spent for each activity over 24 h, as a ratio of BMR
DIT	Diet-induced thermogenesis	Increased energy expenditure associated with digestion and processing of foods, sometimes called the *specific dynamic action of foods*

A large number of measurements of basal metabolic rate have been made under carefully controlled conditions, and there is a series of equations which permit calculation of **average BMR** from age, sex and body weight. These equations are shown in Table 6.4.

Table 6.4 Equations for calculating average BMR from body weight (in kg).

Age (years)	Men	Women
10–17	$0.074 \times \text{wt} + 2.754$	$0.056 \times \text{wt} + 2.898$
18–29	$0.063 \times \text{wt} + 2.896$	$0.062 \times \text{wt} + 2.036$
30–59	$0.048 \times \text{wt} + 3.653$	$0.034 \times \text{wt} + 3.538$
60–74	$0.0499 \times \text{wt} + 2.93$	$0.0386 \times \text{wt} + 2.875$
over 75	$0.035 \times \text{wt} + 3.43$	$0.0410 \times \text{wt} + 2.61$

Physical activity   We can express the energy requirement for various activities as a multiple of BMR. Very gentle activities (sitting around and doing very little) use only about 1.1–1.2 × BMR. By contrast, vigorous exertion, such as climbing stairs, cross-country walking uphill, etc., may use 6–8 × BMR.

We call this multiple of BMR for different physical activities the **physical activity ratio (PAR)** – it is the ratio of the energy expended while performing the activity/that expended at rest (= BMR). Table 6.5 shows the range of PAR for a variety of different types of activity, and Table 6.6 shows the average PAR of different types of occupational work.

Obviously, the amount of time spent in different activities is at least as important as the intensity of those activities when we come to consider total daily energy expenditure. Therefore, if we want to estimate a sub-

Table 6.5 Physical activity ratios in different types of activity.

PAR 1.2 (range 1.0–1.4)
 lying, sitting or standing at rest
 e.g. watching TV, listening to radio, reading, writing, eating, playing cards and board games

PAR 1.6 (range 1.5–1.8)
 sitting: sewing, knitting, playing piano, driving
 standing: preparing vegetables, washing dishes, ironing, general office and laboratory work

PAR 2.1 (range 1.9–2.4)
 standing: mixed household chores, cooking, washing small clothes, playing snooker or bowls

PAR 2.8 (range 2.5–3.3)
 standing: dressing, undressing, showering, making beds, vacuum cleaning floors
 walking: 3–4km/h, playing cricket
 occupational: tailoring, shoemaking, electrical and machine tool industry, painting and decorating

PAR 3.7 (range 3.4–4.4)
 standing: mopping floors, gardening, cleaning windows, playing table tennis, sailing
 walking: 4–6km/h, playing golf
 occupational: motor vehicle repairs, carpentry and joinery, chemical industry, bricklaying

PAR 4.8 (range 4.5–5.9)
 standing: polishing furniture, chopping wood, heavy gardening, playing volley ball
 walking: 6–7km/h
 exercise: dancing, moderate swimming, gentle cycling, slow jogging
 occupational: labouring, hoeing, road construction, digging and shovelling, felling trees

PAR 6.9 (range 6.0–7.9)
 walking: uphill with load or cross-country, climbing stairs
 exercise: average jogging, cycling, energetic swiming, skiing, playing tennis or football

Table 6.6 Classification of types of occupational work by physical activity ratio.

Light work (PAR = 1.7)
 professional, clerical and technical workers, administrative and managerial staff, sales representatives, housewives

Moderate work (PAR = 2.2 for women, 2.7 for men)
 sales staff, domestic service, students, transport workers, joiners and roofing workers

Moderately heavy work (PAR = 2.3 for women, 3.0 for men)
 machine operators, labourers, agricultural workers, bricklaying and masonry

Heavy work (PAR = 2.8 for women, 3.8 for men)
 labourers, agricultural workers, bricklaying, masonry where there is little or no mechanization

Figures are the average PAR throughout the 8h working day, excluding leisure activities.

subject's **total energy expenditure**, we have to draw up an activity diary, where we note the time spent by the subject each day in different types of activity. When we have completed the energy diary, we can calculate the subject's overall average energy expenditure, relative to BMR. This is the subject's **physical activity level (PAL)** – the average of the physical activity ratio for the different types of activity indulged in, allowing for the time spent in each type of activity.

Calculations of total energy expenditure of this type give us a good estimate of peoples' energy requirements. Table 6.7 shows us the average energy expenditure (and hence requirements) for different groups of the population.

Table 6.7 Estimated average requirements for energy.

Age	Males (MJ/day)	Females (MJ/day)
1–3y	5.2	4.9
4–6y	7.2	6.5
7–10y	8.2	7.3
11–14y	9.3	7.9
15–18y	11.5	8.8
adults	10.6	8.0

Figures are based on average weights, and for adults assume PAL = 1.4 (UK Department of Health 1991).

CHAPTER SEVEN

Overweight and obesity

We have seen in Chapter 6 that if the intake of metabolic fuels (in other words the total intake of food) is greater than is required to meet energy expenditure, the result is storage of the excess, largely as triacylglycerols in adipose tissue.

It is normal and desirable to have some reserves of fat in the body. In an adult man about 16% of body weight is normally fat, increasing to 24% by age 65. For women, about 30% of body weight should normally be fat at age 25, increasing to about 36% by age 65. This is a biological difference between the sexes, and is based largely on the possible biological need of the woman for greater reserves of metabolic fuels for reproduction.

Men with less than about 10% of body weight as fat, and women with less than about 15%, are considered to be **underweight**, and to have inadequate reserves.

In this chapter we will consider the problems associated with excess body fat reserves, and ways in which people who are overweight or obese can be helped to lose excess body fat. A modest excess of body fat stores is known as **overweight**; a larger excess of body fat is a more serious problem, with increased risks to health. Here we use the term **obesity** rather than overweight.

Measurement of body fat

Various ways of measuring the fat content of a body have been used in research, including chemical analysis of the body (*post mortem*) and weighing people in air and in water. Neither of these is applicable in ordinary clinical practice, and other, less violent, research methods are also generally too cumbersome for routine use.

We can estimate the body content of fat fairly precisely by measuring the thickness of **sub-cutaneous deposits of fat**, using skin-fold callipers which exert a standard pressure. Obviously, we should aim to measure the thickness of subcutaneous fat deposits at as many sites on the body as possible. In practice we find that we can achieve a good estimate by taking the average of the thicknesses at four sites: the subscapular region, the iliac crest and over the biceps and triceps.

The reference ranges for average **skin-fold thickness** are:

men : 3–10mm

women : 10–22mm.

Values below the lower end of the range indicate depleted fat reserves, and hence undernutrition; values above the upper end of the range indicate excessive fat reserves, and hence overnutrition.

Body weight and body mass index

Obviously, we cannot just say that body weight should lie within a certain range; peoples' heights differ, and a tall person will have a greater body weight than a short person, even if both have exactly the same proportion of fat in the body. One answer is to define desirable ranges of weight for people of different height. The ranges of desirable body weight shown in Figure 7.1 are based on data collected by life insurance companies for ranges of body weight associated with optimum life expectancy.

Alternatively, we can calculate a simple numerical index using both height and weight, and use this to establish acceptable ranges. The most commonly used such index is the **Body mass index (BMI)**, sometimes also called Quetelet's index, after Quetelet, who first demonstrated its usefulness in nutritional studies.

Body mass index is calculated from the weight (in kilogram) divided by the square of the height (in metres):

$$BMI = weight (kg)/height^2 (m).$$

The reference or desirable ranges for BMI are:

men: 20.5–25.0

women: 18.7–23.8.

Values of BMI below the reference range indicate undernutrition; values above the reference range indicate overweight or obesity.

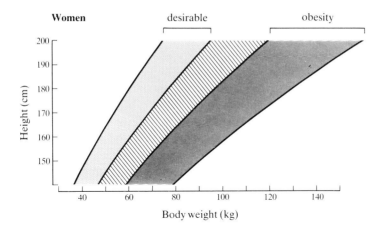

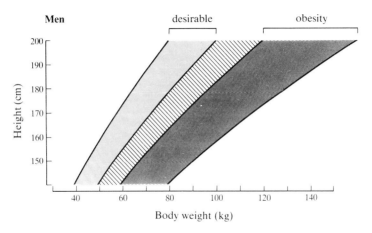

Figure 7.1 Desirable ranges of weight for height
The light shaded area shows the desirable range of weight for height, based on a body mass index between 18.7 and 23.8 for women (upper graph) or 20.5 and 25.0 for men (lower graph). Body weight to the right of the light shaded area is overweight, and in the dark shaded area (body mass index 30–40) obesity. Further to the right is severe obesity. Body weight to the left of the light shaded area is underweight.

The importance of overweight and obesity

Historically, a moderate degree of overweight was considered desirable. In a society where food was scarce, fatness demonstrated greater than average wealth and prosperity. This attitude persists in many developing countries today; food is scarce, and few people have enough to eat, let alone too much.

We can produce a good biological (evolutionary) argument in favour of a modest degree of overweight. A person who has reserves of fat is more likely to be able to survive a period of food deprivation or famine than a person with smaller fat reserves. So, at least in times past, fatter people may have been at an advantage. This is no longer so in developed countries. We no longer suffer from seasonal shortages of food, and widespread hunger is not been a problem in western Europe or North America, although, as discussed in Chapter 8, lack of food is still a major problem in many countries.

As food supplies have become more assured, we have changed our perceptions. Fatness is no longer regarded as a sign of wealth and prosperity. No longer are the overweight in society envied. Rather, they are likely to be mocked, reviled and made deeply unhappy by the unthinking comments and prejudices of their lean companions.

Because society at large considers obesity undesirable, and fashion emphasizes slimness, many overweight and obese people have major problems of a poor self-image, and low self-esteem. Obese people are certainly not helped by the all-too-common prejudice against them, the difficulty of buying clothes that will fit, and the fact that they are often regarded as a legitimate butt of crude and cruel humour. This may lead to a sense of isolation and withdrawal from society, and may frequently result in increased food consumption, for comfort; thus resulting in yet more weight gain, a further loss of self-esteem, further withdrawal, and more eating for compensation.

The psychological and social problems of the obese spill over to people of normal weight as well. There is continuous advertising pressure for "slimness", and newspapers and magazines are full of propaganda for slimness, and "diets" for weight reduction. This may be one of the factors in the development of major eating disorders such as anorexia nervosa and bulimia (see p. 181).

Health problems associated with overweight and obesity

There is a great deal of evidence, much of it coming originally from life insurance company data, that excessive body weight is associated with earlier death. Figure 7.2 shows how increasing body weight above the desirable range is associated with a steeply increasing risk of premature death. Underweight is also associated with increased mortality.

We can classify overweight according to its severity, as shown in Table 7.1. A modest excess of body weight (up to about 5 kg above desirable weight) gives no cause for concern. We can call this **plumpness**.

Overweight is indicated by a BMI between 25 and 30, and implies

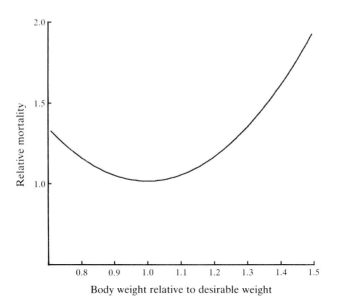

Figure 7.2 The effect of body weight on life expectancy
The graph shows the relationship between relative mortality and body weight relative to
desirable weight, which corresponds to a body mass index between 20 and 25. Relative
mortality is the ratio of the observed mortality for people of a given body weight/that for
people within the desirable range of body weight.

Table 7.1 The classification of oveweight and obesity.

	Body mass index	Excess weight (kg)	% of desirable weight
Plump	<25	<5	<110
Overweight	25–30	5–15	110–120
Obese	30–40	15–25	120–160
Severely obese	>40	>25	>160

between 5 and 15 kg excess weight, or about 110–120% of desirable
weight, for an adult. This may cause the person concerned some distress,
but there is little increased risk to life. The excess weight will exacerbate
problems due to varicose veins, arthritis and flat feet.

Obesity is indicated by a BMI between 30 and 40; some 15–25 kg in excess of desirable weight, or 120–160% of desirable weight. This is associated with increasing health problems and a significantly increased chance
of premature death. People who are 20–30% over desirable weight have
a 20–30% increased risk of premature death; people whose body weight
is 150% of desirable weight have a doubled risk of premature death.

Severe obesity represents a serious health problem. We are talking
about people with a BMI greater than 40, and carrying more than 25 kg
excess weight; in other words, they carry more than half as much weight

167

again as people whose weight is within the desirable range. The dangers to health and life are now very serious. Losing such a large amount of excess body weight can pose very severe problems, and will be a prolonged process.

It is important to realize that we define overweight and obesity in terms of what is desirable on the basis of life expectancy, not on the basis of the average weight of the population. Indeed, average weights are considerably higher than we would wish on health grounds. Department of Health studies show that in Britain we can classify some 45% of adult men, and 36% of adult women, as overweight (i.e. with a BMI greater than 25). More importantly, some 8% of men and 12% of women can be classified as obese, with a BMI greater than 30. This is an increasing proportion of the population. Between 1980 and 1987 the proportion of men with a BMI above 30 increased from 6% to 8% of the population; for women the increase is greater: from 8% in 1980 to 12% in 1987.

Table 7.2 Causes of premature death in obese people (figures show observed mortality from various causes, relative to the mortality in lean subjects from the same causes).

Cause of death	Men	Women
Cardiovascular disease	1.49	1.77
Diabetes mellitus	3.83	3.72
Liver cirrhosis	2.49	1.77
Appendicitis	2.23	1.95
Gallstones	2.06	2.34
Pneumonia	1.02	1.29
Cancer	0.97	1.00
Suicide	0.78	0.73

Table 7.2 shows the causes of **premature death** which are associated with obesity. The figures are expressed as the ratio of that condition as a cause of death in obese people/the expected rate in lean people.

While some of these figures show a simple relationship, in that obesity is a factor in the disease, others need a little explanation. The very high excess mortality from cirrhosis of the liver associated with obesity is due to the fact that excessive consumption of alcoholic beverages is a cause of both obesity and cirrhosis. It does not mean that obesity causes cirrhosis, nor that cirrhosis causes obesity.

Similarly, the excess mortality associated with appendicitis and gallstones is because surgery is very much more dangerous for obese people than for lean people. Indeed, because of this, it is common to try to reduce obese patients' weight to a more acceptable range before surgery, if it is possible to delay the surgery. Obviously, for emergency conditions such as gallstones and appendicitis, this is not possible. The surgery cannot be put off for several months until the patient has lost enough weight to reduce the risks of surgery.

Overall there is no increase in death from cancer associated with obesity; this is the result of grouping all types of cancer together. Obese people are more likely to develop cancer of the colon than lean people; obese men are more likely to develop cancer of the prostate, while obese women are more likely to develop cancer of the breast, uterus and ovary. The obese are less likely to develop cancer of the lung and some other tissues than lean people.

The causes of obesity

The cause of obesity is an intake of metabolic fuels greater than is required for energy expenditure, so that excess is stored, largely as fat in adipose tissue reserves. The simple answer to the problem of obesity is therefore just to redress the balance; reduce food intake and/or increase physical activity, and hence energy expenditure.

Most overweight and obese people are in energy balance, just as lean people are. Although the cause of excess body weight is an excessive intake of food compared with energy expenditure, as a person gains weight, so his or her energy expenditure increases. As discussed on p. 160, BMR depends very largely on body weight, because it is the energy requirement for maintenance of the body's metabolic functions, and the energy cost of these increases as the size of the body increases. Similarly, physical activity incurs a greater energy cost for a person whose body weight is high. You might like to try running up a flight of stairs with a 25 kg backpack, just to demonstrate this to yourself! *It is only during the development of obesity that energy intake is greater than expenditure.*

Part of the problem is the relatively low level of physical activity of many people in Western countries. The average PAL in Britain is only 1.4; in other words, physical activity accounts for only 40% more energy expenditure than BMR. At the same time, food is always readily available, with an ever-increasing array of attractive snack foods, which are easy to eat, and many of which are high in fat and sugar.

Sometimes we may find overweight and obese people whose problem can be attributed to a low rate of energy expenditure despite a reasonable level of physical activity. Although we can predict BMR fairly well from the formulae shown in Table 6.4 on p. 160, these are average figures. We can allow a range of 30% around this average to cope with individual variation. This means that some people will have a very low BMR, and hence a very low requirement for food. Despite eating very little compared with those around them, they may gain weight. Equally, we can expect to find people who have a relatively high BMR, who seem to be able to eat a large amount of food without gaining weight. This is normal biological variation.

We do not know how most people manage to balance their food intake with energy expenditure. Certainly we don't do it by sitting down with tables of food composition to calculate what we should eat to compensate for today's activities!

Changes in the concentrations of glucose, free fatty acids, amino acids and ketones in the bloodstream have all been suggested to act as signals to the appetite control centres in the hypothalamus, as have changes in the hormones associated with the control of nutrient metabolism. There is some evidence that the state of fullness or emptiness of the stomach may exert control over how much we eat.

Quite separately, some people seem to be able to modify their energy expenditure to match their food intake. Again we do not know how important this is, but many people become quite hot after meals, or when they are asleep. We believe that this is because in their brown adipose tissue they have some degree of uncoupling of electron transport from oxidative phosphorylation (see p. 126), and so are able to oxidize "surplus" fuel which would otherwise be stored as fat in adipose tissue. Such people tend to be lean. Other people seem to be much more energy efficient, and their body temperature may drop slightly while they are asleep. This means that they are using less metabolic fuel to maintain body temperature, and so are able to store more as adipose tissue. Such people tend to be overweight. (This response, lowering body temperature and metabolic rate to conserve food, is seen in a more extreme form in animals which hibernate. During their long winter sleep these animals have a very low rate of metabolism, and hence a low requirement for the fuel they have stored in adipose tissue reserves.)

Rarely, we come across people who have a very low metabolic rate for a medical reason; perhaps they have an underactive thyroid gland (the thyroid hormone controls the overall rate of metabolism). Here it is a matter of identifying the underlying medical problem, and treating that. Very rarely, we may come across people who have a physical defect of the appetite control centres in the brain, for example some tumours can cause damage to the satiety centre, so that the patient feels hunger, but not the sensation of satiety, and has no recognizable physiological cue to stop eating.

Part of the problem of obesity can be attributed to a **psychological**

failure of appetite control. At its simplest, this can be blamed on the variety of attractive foods available to us. We are tempted to eat more than we need, and it may take quite an effort of willpower to refuse a choice morsel. Even when we have had enough of one sort of food, the appearance of something different can tempt us to eat more. Experimental animals, which normally do not become obese, can be persuaded to eat too much, and to become obese, by providing them with a "cafeteria" array of attractive foods.

Studies comparing grossly obese people with lean people have shown that some of the obese do not seem to sense the normal cues to hunger and satiety. Rather, in many cases, it is the sight of food which prompts them to eat, regardless of whether they are "hungry" or not. If no food is visible, they will not feel hunger. Some obese people have a psychological dependence on eating and the actions of chewing and swallowing food, which is as severe a problem for them as is habituation or addiction to alcohol, tobacco or narcotics. There have been no such studies involving overweight or moderately obese people, so we do not know whether the apparent failure of appetite regulation is a general problem or whether it only affects the relatively small group of very obese people.

How obese people can be helped to lose weight

In considering the treatment of obesity, we have to think about two different aspects of the problem:

(a) the initial problem, which is to help the overweight or obese person to reduce his or her weight to within the desirable range, where life expectancy is maximum; and

(b) the long-term problem of helping the now lean person to maintain desirable body weight. This is largely a matter of education: increasing physical activity and changing eating habits – no simple problem, but the same guidelines for a good diet apply to the slimmed-down, formerly obese, person as to everyone else, as discussed in Chapter 2.

How fast can excess weight be lost?

The aim of any form of weight-reduction regime is to reduce the intake of food to below the level needed for energy expenditure. This will mean that in order to maintain basal metabolism and physical activity, body reserves of fat will have to be used.

We can calculate the theoretical maximum possible rate of weight loss quite easily. About two-thirds of the weight of adipose tissue is triacylglycerol. Since triacylglycerol is equivalent to 37 kJ/g, adipose tissue is equivalent to 25 kJ/g. If we consider someone whose physical activity level is such that he or she has an energy expenditure of 10 MJ/day, and we impose total starvation, we can calculate that there will be a daily loss of 400 g of adipose tissue – 2.8 kg/week. It is not possible to have a greater rate of weight loss than this, and this is calculated assuming that there is no intake of food at all.

Frequently, the first 1 or 2 weeks of a weight-reducing regime are associated with a very much greater loss of weight than this. Obviously, from the discussion above, this cannot be due to loss of fat. What is happening in the early stages of either total starvation or a severe restriction of intake is that there is a considerable utilization of **glycogen reserves** in liver and muscle. Glycogen is associated with very much more water than is fat, so a great deal of water is lost from the body. This does not continue for long, and after 1–2 weeks, when glycogen reserves are very much smaller, the rate of weight loss slows down to what we would expect from the energy deficit (i.e. the difference between energy expenditure and intake).

Although it is not sustained, the initial rapid rate of weight loss can be extremely encouraging for the obese person. The problem is to ensure that he or she realizes that it will not be sustained, and indeed cannot continue. This is something which should always be borne in mind when reading the claims of those who offer rapid rates of weight loss; we can calculate with reasonable precision the maximum possible rate of loss of adipose tissue, and anyone who claims to offer a greater rate than this for more than the first week or so is not being honest.

More or less **total starvation** has been used in a hospital setting for seriously obese patients, especially those who are to undergo elective surgery. Vitamins and minerals have to be supplied (see Ch. 11), as well as fluid, but apart from this an obese person can lose weight at about the predicted rate of 2.8 kg/week if starved completely.

There are two major problems with total starvation as a means of rapid weight loss:

(a) The problem of enforcement. It is very difficult to deprive someone of food and to prevent them finding more or less devious means of acquiring it; by begging or stealing from other patients, visitors and hospital volunteers, or even by walking down to the hospital shop or out-patients' cafeteria.

(b) A biochemical problem. We saw on p. 153 that the brain has to be provided with glucose even in the fasting state. Once glycogen reserves are exhausted (and this will occur within a relatively short time) there will be increasing **catabolism of tissue protein reserves** to provide substrates for gluconeogenesis. As much as half the weight lost in total starvation may be muscle and other tissues, not adipose tissue. This is not desirable; indeed, if we are preparing an obese patient for surgery, while we want a loss of adipose tissue, we most certainly do not want a loss of tissue protein. The stress of surgery causes a serious loss of protein in itself and we would not want to start this loss before surgery.

Total starvation has been more or less abandoned as a means of rapid weight loss, because there have been a few cases of sudden death, apparently due to loss of essential tissue proteins.

Very low-energy diets

Many of the problems associated with total starvation can be avoided by feeding a very low-energy intake, normally in a liquid formula preparation which provides adequate amounts of vitamins and minerals, together with some 1.0-1.5MJ/day, largely as protein. Such regimes have shown excellent results in the treatment of severe obesity. There is very much less loss of tissue protein than in total starvation, and with this small intake people feel less hungry than those who are starved completely.

If very low-energy diets are used together with a programme of exercise, the rate of weight loss can be 2–2.5 kg/week. Such diets should be regarded as a treatment of last resort, for people with a serious problem of obesity which does not respond to more conventional diet therapy. The manufacturers recommend that they should not be used for more than 3–4 weeks at a time without close medical supervision, because there is still a possible risk of loss of essential tissue proteins.

Conventional diets

For most people, the problem is not one of severe obesity, but a more modest excess body weight. Even for people who have a serious obesity problem, it is likely that less drastic measures than those discussed above will be beneficial. The aim is to reduce energy intake to below expenditure, and so ensure the utilization of adipose tissue reserves. To anyone who has not tried to lose weight, the answer would appear to be simple: just eat less. Obviously it is not so simple. As discussed above, we have a considerable, and increasing, problem of obesity in Western countries; and a vast array of diets, slimming regimes, special foods, appetite suppressants, etc.

The ideal approach to the problem of obesity and weight reduction

173

would be to provide people with the information they need to choose an appropriate diet for themselves. What we have to do is provide tables of the energy yield of different foods, and leave people to calculate for themselves what they should eat. This is not easy. It is not simply a matter of reducing energy intake, but of ensuring at the same time that intakes of protein, vitamins and minerals are adequate. The preparation of balanced diets, especially when the total energy intake is to be reduced, is a highly skilled job, and is one of the main functions of the dietitian. Furthermore, we have to consider the problem of long-term compliance of a seriously overweight or obese person with dietary restrictions.

Nevertheless, some degree of nutrition education can indeed help people to make informed choices of foods, and many people do manage to lose weight in just this way, both regaining a desirable body weight and altering their food and eating habits afterwards, to comply with what we would consider a prudent diet, as discussed in Chapter 2.

We can make it easier for people to lose weight by describing specific types of diet changes. A very simple way is to set up three lists of foods, based on food composition tables (see Appendix II):

(a) Energy-rich foods, which should be avoided. These are generally foods which are rich in fat and sugar, but provide little in the way of vitamins and minerals. Such foods include oils and fats, fried foods, fatter cuts of meat, cakes, biscuits, etc. and alcoholic beverages. They should be eaten with extreme caution, if at all.

(b) Foods which are relatively high in energy yield, but also good sources of protein, vitamins and minerals. They should be eaten with caution.

(c) Foods which are generally rich sources of vitamins and minerals, high in starch and non-starch polysaccharide, and low in fat and sugars. These can be eaten (within reason) as much as is wanted.

This advice is really no more than a more extreme version of the general advice for a healthy diet discussed in Chapter 2 – reduce the intake of fats and sugar, and increase consumption of fruits and vegetables.

At one time, there was a vogue for **low carbohydrate diets** for weight reduction. The idea was that fat and protein are more slowly digested and absorbed than carbohydrates. Therefore they have greater satiety value. At the same time, it was suggested that severe restriction of carbohydrate intake would limit the intake of other foods as well; one argument was that if you had no bread, you would have nothing on which to spread butter. Nowadays we would not recommend a low carbohydrate diet for weight reduction, since we are aiming to reduce the fat intake of the population as a whole, and this means that the proportion of metabolic fuel coming from carbohydrate must increase, rather than decrease. However, we would indeed recommend a reduction in the intake of non-milk extrinsic sugars (see p. 22).

"Diets" that probably won't work

We have seen above how the problem of weight reduction depends on reducing the intake of metabolic fuels (in other words the total amount of food eaten), but still ensuring that the intake of vitamins and minerals is adequate to meet requirements. Equally important is the problem of ensuring that the weight that has been lost is not replaced, in other words eating patterns must be changed after weight has been lost, to allow for the maintenance of body weight with a well balanced diet.

There is a bewildering array of different diet regimes on offer to help the overweight and obese to lose weight. Some of these are based on sound nutritional principles, as discussed above, and provide about half the person's energy requirement, together with adequate amounts of protein, vitamins and minerals. They permit a sustained weight loss of about 1–1.5 kg/week.

Other "diets" are neither scientifically formulated nor based on sound nutritional principles, and indeed frequently depend on pseudoscientific mumbo-jumbo to attempt to give them some validity. They frequently make exaggerated claims for the amount of weight that can be lost, and rarely provide a balanced diet. Publication of testimonials from "satisfied clients" cannot be considered to be evidence of efficacy, and publication in a book which is a best-seller, or in a magazine with wide circulation, cannot correct the underlying flaws in many of these "diets".

Some of the more outlandish diet regimes depend on such nonsensical principles as eating protein and carbohydrates at different meals, ignoring the fact that such "carbohydrate" foods as bread and potatoes provide a significant proportion of our protein intake as well (see p. 192). Others depend on a very limited range of foods. The most extreme have allowed the client to eat as many bananas (or some other food) as he or she wishes, but nothing else; others ascribe almost magical properties to certain fruits, again with a very limited range of other foods allowed.

The idea is that if you are permitted to eat as much as you like of only a very limited range of foods, you will end up eating very little; even if you liked bananas, they would soon pall. In practice, these "diets" do neither good nor harm. People get so bored that they give up before there can be any significant effect on body weight, or any adverse effects of a very unbalanced diet. This is all to the good, if people did stick to such diets for any length of time they might well encounter problems of protein, vitamin and mineral deficiency.

Aids to weight reduction

As well as diet regimes based on sound nutritional principles, there are other ways of helping the overweight person to lose weight: substitutes for sugar and fats, bulking agents to increase satiety and appetite suppressants. Low-fat foods are discussed on p. 18.

Sugar substitutes As discussed on p. 22, the average consumption of sugar is considerably higher than is considered desirable. There is a school of thought which blames the ready availability of sugar for much of the problem of overweight and obesity in Western countries. You might think it easy to say that an overweight person could reduce energy intake considerably simply by stopping taking sugar in tea and coffee, after all, a teaspoon of sugar is 5g of carbohydrate, and thus provides 80 kJ; in each of six cups of tea or coffee a day, two spoons of sugar would thus account for some 960 kJ – almost 10% of the average person's energy expenditure. Quite apart from this obvious sugar, which people can see they are adding to their intake, there is a great deal of sugar in beverages, for example a standard 330 ml can of lemonade provides 20 g of sugar.

Because many people like their tea and coffee sweetened, and to replace the sugar in lemonades, etc., we have a range of sugar substitutes. These are synthetic chemicals which are very much sweeter than sugar, but are not metabolized as metabolic fuels. Even those which can be metabolized (for example **aspartame**, which is an amino acid derivative) are taken in such small amounts that they make no significant contribution to intake.

Table 7.3 Some non-nutritive sweeteners listed in order of their sweetness relative to sucrose = 1.0.

	Relative sweetness
Thaumatin	3000–4000
Saccharine	300–550
Stevioside	300
Acesulphame K	200
Aspartame	180–200
Cyclamate	30–40

Note that not all of these sweeteners are permitted as food additives in all countries.

Table 7.3 shows the commonly used synthetic sweeteners (also known as non-nutritive sweeteners or intense sweeteners), together with approximately how sweet they are compared with sugar. All of these compounds have been extensively tested for safety; as a result of concerns about possible hazards, some are not permitted in some countries, although they are widely used elsewhere.

Bulking agents One of the signals to stop eating is the sensation of fullness – and one of the common complaints of people on energy-reduced diets is that they "feel empty". One solution to this problem is to recommend a "high-fibre" diet. As discussed on p. 24, a high intake of non-starch polysaccharides can make it difficult for a child to eat enough food to meet energy requirements. This is precisely what is required in a weight-reducing regime. A high intake of non-starch polysaccharides makes it easier to keep to a low-energy diet because such foods have high satiety value, but are generally low in fat.

It is generally desirable that the dietary sources of non-starch polysaccharides should be ordinary foods – fruits and vegetables, whole-grain cereal products, etc. – rather than "supplements". However, as an aid to weight reduction, several preparations of dietary fibre are available.

Some of these are more or less ordinary foods, but containing added non-starch polysaccharides of various kinds, which give texture to the food, and increase the feeling of fullness and satiety. Some of the special slimmers' soups, biscuits, etc. are of this type. They are formulated to provide about one-third of a day's requirement of protein, vitamins and minerals, but with a low energy yield. They are supposed to be taken in place of one meal each day, and to aid satiety they contain carboxymethyl-cellulose or another non-digested polysaccharide.

The alternative approach is to take tablets or a suspension of non-starch polysaccharide before a meal. This again creates a feeling of fullness, and so reduces the amount of food that will be eaten.

Appetite suppressants Some compounds act either to suppress the activity of the hunger centre in the hypothalamus, or to stimulate the satiety centre. Sometimes this is a highly undesirable side-effect of medicines used to treat various diseases. As an aid to weight reduction, especially in people who find it difficult to control their food intake, drugs which suppress appetite can be useful. Three compounds are in relatively widespread use as appetite suppressants: fenfluramine (and more recently the D-isomer, dexfenfluramine), diethylpropion and mazindol. Other compounds have been used in the past, including amphetamines and amphetamine derivatives, which carry a risk of addiction, and are controlled substances which cannot be prescribed except under special circumstances.

In general, the activity of appetite suppressants only lasts for a relatively short time, perhaps a few weeks, but this should be enough to encourage the overweight or obese person who has been having difficulty in losing weight. After this, some degree of tolerance or resistance to their action develops, and they have less effect the longer they are used. Needless to say, appetite suppressants will only be effective if they are taken before meals.

Help and support Especially for the severely obese person, weight loss is a lengthy and difficult experience. Friends and family can be supportive, but frequently specialist help and advice are needed. To a great extent, this is the rôle of the dietitian and other health-care professionals. In addition, there are several organizations, normally of formerly obese people, who can offer a mixture of professional nutritional and dietetic advice together with practical help and counselling. The main advantage of such groups is that they provide a social setting, rather than the formal setting of the dietitian's office in an out-patient clinic, and all the members have, or have been through, the same problems. Many people find the sharing of the problems and experiences of weight reduction extremely helpful.

CHAPTER EIGHT

Undernutrition

In this chapter we will be considering general malnutrition, sometimes also called protein–energy malnutrition, in other words the problems of an inadequate intake of food. Specific problems of protein deficiency are discussed on p. 193, and problems of individual vitamin and mineral deficiencies are discussed in Chapter 11.

We have already seen that if the intake of metabolic fuels is lower than is required for energy expenditure, the body's reserves of fat, carbohydrate (glycogen) and protein are used to meet energy needs. Especially in lean people, who have relatively small reserves of body fat, there is a relatively large loss of tissue protein when food intake is inadequate. As the deficiency continues, so there is an increasingly serious loss of tissue, until eventually essential tissue proteins are catabolized as metabolic fuels, a process which obviously cannot continue for long.

*The terms **protein–energy malnutrition** and **protein–energy deficiency** are incorrect*, although they are widely used. The problem is not one of protein deficiency, but rather of general inadequacy of food intake – a deficiency of metabolic fuels. Indeed, there may be a relative excess of protein, in that protein which might be used for tissue protein replacement, or for growth in children, is being used as a fuel because of the deficiency of total food intake.

This was demonstrated in a series of studies in India in the early 1980s. Children whose intake of protein was just adequate were given additional carbohydrate (in sugary drinks). They showed an increase in growth, and the deposition of new body protein. This was because originally their energy intake was inadequate, despite an adequate intake of protein. Increasing their intake of carbohydrate as a metabolic fuel spared dietary

179

protein for the synthesis of tissue proteins; initially they were "wasting" protein by using it as a fuel. The body's first requirement, at all times, is for an adequate source of metabolic fuels. Only when energy requirements have been met can dietary protein be used for tissue protein synthesis, and, as discussed on p. 217, protein synthesis also has a relatively high energy cost.

There are two extreme forms of protein–energy malnutrition: marasmus and kwashiorkor. **Marasmus** can occur in both adults and children, and as discussed on p. 181 will be seen in vulnerable groups of the population in developed countries as well as in developing countries. By contrast, **kwashiorkor** is a deficiency disease which only affects children, and has only been reported in developing countries. Marasmus is the predictable end-result of prolonged negative energy balance, while there are additional features involved in kwashiorkor which are not really fully understood.

Marasmus

The key feature of marasmus is extreme emaciation. The name is derived from the Greek for wasting away. Not only have the body's fat reserves been exhausted, but there is wastage of muscles as well. As the condition progresses, so there is loss of protein from the heart, liver and kidneys, although as far as possible essential tissue proteins are protected.

There is a general reduction in protein synthesis. As a result of this there is a considerable impairment of the immune response, so that under-nourished people are more at risk from infections than those who are adequately nourished. What we in the West consider to be relatively minor childhood illnesses can often prove fatal to undernourished children in developing countries. Measles is commonly cited as the cause of death, although it would be more correct to give the true cause of death as malnutrition; infection was simply the final straw.

One of the proteins secreted by the liver which is most severely affected by protein–energy malnutrition is the plasma retinol-binding protein, which transports vitamin A from liver stores to tissues where it is required (see p. 240). As the synthesis of retinol-binding protein is reduced, so there are increasing signs of vitamin A deficiency, although there may be adequate reserves of the vitamin in the liver. The problem is that without adequate synthesis of the binding protein, these liver reserves cannot be transported to the tissues where they are required. It is quite common for signs of vitamin A deficiency to be associated with protein–energy mal-nutrition, but supplements of vitamin A have no effect, since the problem is in the transport and utilization of the vitamin. Nevertheless, as discussed on p. 240, dietary deficiency of vitamin A is also a serious problem in many developing countries.

A more serious effect of protein–energy malnutrition is impairment of the regeneration of the intestinal mucosa. Intestinal mucosal cells turn over rapidly. The process from cell replication in the crypts to shedding of cells into the intestinal lumen at the tip of the villus takes about 48 hours. Normally there are some 20–40 villi/mm^2 of intestinal mucosa, each projecting some 0.5–1.5 mm into the lumen. This gives a total of some 300 m^2 of absorptive surface in the small intestine. In protein–energy malnutrition the villi are very much shorter than usual, and in severe cases the intestinal mucosa is almost flat. This results in a very considerable reduction in the surface area of the intestinal mucosa, and hence a considerable reduction in the area over which such nutrients as are available from the diet can be absorbed. As a result, diarrhoea is commonly a feature of protein–energy malnutrition. Thus, not only does the undernourished person have an inadequate intake of food, but the absorption of what is available is impaired, so making the problem worse.

Causes of marasmus, and vulnerable groups of the population

In developing countries, the causes of marasmus are either a chronic shortage of food or the more acute problem of famine, where there will be very little food available at all. All too frequently, famine comes on top of a long-term shortage of food, so its effects are all the more rapid and serious. A simple lack of food is unlikely to be a problem in developed countries, although obviously the most socially and economically disadvantaged in the community are at risk of hunger and perhaps even protein–energy undernutrition in extreme cases.

Three different factors may cause marasmus in developed countries: disorders of appetite and eating behaviour, impairment of the absorption of nutrients and increased metabolic rate.

Disorders of appetite: anorexia nervosa and bulimia It was noted above (see p. 166) that there is considerable pressure on people in Western countries to be slim; we are bombarded with more or less well-informed or ill-informed articles about the evils of obesity in magazines, newspapers, and on radio and television. While obesity is indeed a serious health problem, one side-effect of the propaganda is to put considerable pressure on some people to reduce their body weight, even though they are within the acceptable and healthy weight range. In some cases this pressure may be a factor in the development of anorexia nervosa – a major psychological disturbance of appetite and eating behaviour. Those most at risk are adolescent girls, although similar disturbances of eating behaviour can occur in older women, and (rarely) in adolescent boys and men.

The key feature of anorexia nervosa is a refusal to eat, with the obvious result of very considerable weight loss. Despite all evidence and arguments to the contrary, the anorectic subject is convinced that she is overweight, and restricts her eating very severely. Dieting becomes the primary focus of her life. She has a preoccupation with, and often a considerable knowledge of, food, and frequently has a variety of stylized compulsive behaviour patterns associated with food. As a part of her pathological obsession with thinness, the anorectic subject frequently takes a great deal of strenuous exercise, often exercising to exhaustion in solitude. She will go to extreme lengths to avoid eating, and frequently when forced to eat will induce vomiting soon afterwards. Many anorectics also make excessive use of laxatives.

Surprisingly, many anorectic people are adept at hiding their condition, and it is not unknown for the problem to remain unnoticed, even in a family setting. Food is played with, but little or none is actually eaten; excuses are frequently made to leave the table in the middle of the meal, perhaps on the pretext of going into the kitchen to prepare the next course.

Some anorectic subjects also exhibit a further disturbance of eating behaviour – **bulimia** or **binge eating**. After a period of eating little or nothing, they suddenly eat an extremely large amount of food (40 MJ or more in a single meal, compared with an average daily requirement of 8–12 MJ), frequently followed by deliberate induction of vomiting and heavy doses of laxatives. This is followed by a further prolonged period of anorexia.

Bulimia also occurs in the absence of anorexia nervosa: a person of normal weight will consume a very large amount of food (commonly 40–80 MJ over a period of a few hours), again followed by induction of vomiting and excessive use of laxatives. In severe cases such binges may occur five or six times a week.

Anorexia nervosa is a psychological problem, rather than a simple nutritional one, and requires sensitive specialist treatment. It is not simply a matter of "persuading" the patient to eat. One theory is that the root cause of the problem, at least in adolescent girls, is a reaction to the physical changes of puberty. By refusing food, the girl believes that she can delay or prevent these changes. To a considerable extent this is so. Breast development slows down or ceases as the energy balance becomes more negative, and as body weight falls below about 45 kg, menstruation also ceases. Obviously, the considerable pressure for slimness from the media and her peers, and the continual discussion of "diets", places an additional stress on the anorectic subject.

According to some estimates, almost 2% of adolescent girls go through at least a short phase of anorexia. In most cases it is self-limiting, and normal eating patterns are re-established as the emotional crises of adolescence resolve themselves. Others may require specialist counselling and treatment, and in an unfortunate few the problems of eating behaviour persist into adult life.

Malabsorption Any clinical condition which impairs the absorption of nutrients from the intestinal tract will lead to undernutrition, although in this case the intake is apparently adequate. The problem is one of digestion and/or absorption of the food.

Obviously, major intestinal surgery will result in a reduction in the amount of intestine available for the digestion and absorption of nutrients. Here we are at least aware of the problem in advance, and can take precautionary measures. These generally involve a period of intravenous feeding, to supplement normal food intake, and careful counselling by a dietitian, so as to ensure adequate nutrient intake despite the problems.

A variety of infectious diseases can cause malabsorption and diarrhoea. In many cases this lasts only a few days, and so has no long-term consequences. However, intestinal parasites can cause long-lasting diarrhoea and damage to the intestinal mucosa, leading to malnutrition if the infection remains untreated for too long.

Food intolerances and allergies Allergic reactions to foods may cause a wide variety of signs and symptoms, including dermatitis, eczema and urticaria, asthma, allergic rhinitis, muscle pain, rheumatoid arthritis and migraine, as well as having effects on the gastrointestinal tract. All of these will be likely to impair the sufferer's appetite, and hence may contribute to undernutrition. There can be serious damage to the intestinal mucosa, leading to severe malabsorption, and hence malnutrition despite an apparently adequate intake of food. One of the best understood such conditions is coeliac disease.

Coeliac disease is an allergy to one specific protein in wheat – the gliadin fraction of wheat gluten. The result is a considerable loss of intestinal mucosa, and flattening of the intestinal villi, so that the appearance of the intestine is similar to that seen in marasmus. This reduction in the absorptive surface of the intestine leads to persistent diarrhoea and a failure to absorb nutrients. The result is undernutrition; although the intake of food is apparently adequate, there is inadequate digestion and absorption of nutrients. Severe emaciation can occur in patients with untreated coeliac disease.

Once the diagnosis is established, and the immediate problems of undernutrition have been dealt with, treatment is relatively simple – avoidance of all wheat and rye-based products. In practice, this is less easy than it sounds; apart from the obvious foods, like bread and pasta, wheat flour is used in a great many food products. There is therefore a need for counselling from a dietitian, and careful reading of labels for lists of ingredients. Some products have the symbol of the Coeliac Society on the label, to show that they are known to be free from gluten, and therefore safe for patients to eat.

Other intolerances or allergic reactions to foods can also lead to similar persistent diarrhoea, loss of intestinal mucosa and hence malnutrition. The problem of disaccharide intolerance was discussed on p. 133. In general, once the offending food has been identified, the patient's condition has stabilized and body weight has been restored, continuing treatment is relatively easy, although avoidance of some common foods may provide significant problems.

It is the identification of the offending food which provides the greatest problem, and frequently calls for lengthy investigations, maintaining the patient on a very limited range of foods, then gradually introducing additional foods, until the offending item is identified.

Patients with food intolerances or allergies are generally extremely ill after they have eaten the offending food, and this may persist for several days. Even after the offending foods have been identified, and the patient's condition has been stabilized, there may be continuing problems of appetite and eating behaviour.

Metabolic causes of malnutrition Any disease which involves a prolonged increase in the BMR, or prolonged fever, will increase energy expenditure, and can thus lead to severe weight loss and the development of marasmus despite an apparently normal intake of food. This is a problem among people with human immunodeficiency virus (HIV) infection and the acquired immune deficiency syndrome (AIDS), as well as several other chronic infections, and in people who have an overactive thyroid gland (hyperthyroidism).

The thyroid hormones are involved in controlling BMR, and excess secretion leads to considerable additional heat production, and hence negative energy balance. A hyperthyroid patient may well have a BMR 50–100% above normal; under such conditions a normal intake of food will be grossly inadequate to meet requirements. Here the answer is to treat the overactivity of the thyroid gland, and so reduce the patient's metabolic rate to normal, so that energy balance can be restored, and weight regained.

Cancer cachexia Patients with advanced cancer are frequently undernourished. Physically they show all the signs of marasmus, but there is more loss of body protein than occurs in starvation. The condition is called **cachexia** (from the Greek for "in a poor condition").

There are two aspects to the problem:

(a) The patients are extremely sick, and their appetite may be impaired because of this. Also, both cancer itself and many of the drugs used in chemotherapy can cause nausea, loss of appetite and alteration of the senses of taste and smell, so that foods which were appetizing are now either unappetizing or even repulsive.

(b) One of the reactions of the body to cancer is the secretion of **cachexin (tumour necrosis factor)**. This has a beneficial effect, in that it causes slowing of the development of the tumour, but it also increases the metabolic rate, and so causes a negative energy balance. One of the main actions of cachexin is to increase the rate of breakdown of muscle protein; this means that there is greater loss of protein, and earlier, in cachexia than in marasmus or starvation.

There has been considerable success with nutritional support of patients. In addition to such food as they are able to eat, their nutritional status is enhanced by providing nutrients by intravenous or intragastric tubes.

Kwashiorkor

Kwashiorkor was first described in Ghana, in west Africa, in 1932. The name is the Ga name for the disease which afflicts the first child when the second is born, and it is therefore weaned. In addition to the wasting of muscle tissue, loss of intestinal mucosa and decreased immune responses seen in marasmus, children with kwashiorkor show several characteristic features which distinguish this disease:

(a) fluid retention and hence severe oedema, associated with a decreased concentration of plasma proteins; the puffiness of the limbs, due to the oedema, masks the severe wasting of arm and leg muscles;

(b) enlargement of the liver – this is due to the accumulation of abnormally large amounts of fat in the liver, to the extent that instead of its normal reddish-brown colour, the liver is pale yellow when examined at post-mortem or during surgery. The metabolic basis for this fatty infiltration of the liver is not known. It is the enlargement of the liver which causes the paradoxical "pot-bellied" appearance of children with kwashiorkor; together with the oedema, they appear, from a distance, to be plump, yet they are starving;

(c) characteristic changes in the texture and colour of the hair – this is most noticeable in African children; instead of tightly curled black hair, children with kwashiorkor have sparse, wispy hair, which is less curled than normal, and poorly pigmented – it is often reddish or even grey;

(d) a sooty, sunburn-like skin rash;

(e) a characteristic expression of deep misery.

Kwashiorkor traditionally affects children aged between 3 and 5 years. In many societies a child continues to suckle until about this age, when the next child is born. As a result, the toddler is abruptly weaned, frequently onto very unsuitable food. In some societies, children are weaned onto a dilute gruel made from whatever is the local cereal; in others the child may be fed on the water in which rice has been boiled – it may look like milk, but has little nutritional value. Sometimes the child is given little or no special treatment, but has to compete with the rest of the family for its share from the stew-pot. A small child has little chance of getting an adequate meal under such conditions, especially if there is not much food for the whole family anyway.

The underlying cause of kwashiorkor is thus an inadequate intake of food, as is the case for marasmus. However, it is frequently a result of ignorance of suitable weaning foods, rather than just a lack of food. Many clinics in developing countries run education programmes to prevent kwashiorkor by teaching mothers about more suitable ways of weaning their children.

We cannot account satisfactorily for the development of kwashiorkor, rather than marasmus. At one time it was believed that it was due to a lack of protein, with a more or less adequate intake of energy. We now know that this is not correct. As discussed on p. 193, protein deficiency results in reduction of growth. Furthermore, many of the signs of kwashiorkor, and especially the oedema, begin to improve early in treatment, when the child is still receiving a low-protein diet (see below).

We do know that *infections frequently precipitate kwashiorkor* in children whose nutritional status is inadequate, even if they are not yet showing signs of malnutrition. Indeed, paediatricians in developing countries have come to expect an outbreak of kwashiorkor a few months after an outbreak of measles.

The most likely cause of kwashiorkor is that superimposed on general food deficiency there is a deficiency of the "anti-oxidant nutrients" such as zinc, copper, carotene and vitamins C and E. These nutrients are involved in overcoming the toxic effects of oxygen radicals, both those generated during normal metabolism and those produced by cells of the immune system as a part of the process of killing bacteria. Thus, in deficient children, the added oxidant stress of an infection may well trigger the sequence of events which leads to the development of kwashiorkor.

Rehabilitation of malnourished children

It is obvious from the description of the problems of marasmus and kwashiorkor that the intestinal tract of the malnourished patient is in a very poor state. This means that the patient is not able to deal at all adequately with a rich diet, or a large amount of food. Rather, treatment begins with small, frequent feeding of liquids: a dilute sugar solution for the first few days, followed by diluted milk, and then full-strength milk. This may be achieved by use of a nasogastric tube, so that the dilute solution can be provided at a slow and constant rate throughout the day and night. Where such luxuries are not available, the malnourished infant is fed from a teaspoon, a few drops at a time, more or less continually.

Once the patient has begun to develop a more normal intestinal mucosa (when the diarrhoea ceases), ordinary foods can gradually be introduced. Recovery is normally rapid in children, and they soon begin to grow at a normal rate.

CHAPTER NINE

Protein nutrition and metabolism

The need for protein in the diet was demonstrated early in the 19th century, when it was shown that animals which were fed only on fats, carbohydrates and mineral salts were unable to maintain their body weight, and showed severe wasting of muscle and other tissues. It was known that proteins contain nitrogen (mainly in the in the amino groups of their constituent amino acids, see p. 88), and methods of measuring total amounts of nitrogenous compounds in foods and excreta were soon developed. Although nucleic acids also contain nitrogen (see p. 95), protein is the major dietary source of nitrogenous compounds, and measurement of total nitrogen intake gives a good estimate of protein intake.

Nitrogen balance and protein requirements

Early studies showed that there is normally a balance or equilibrium between the intake of nitrogenous compounds in food and the output of nitrogenous compounds from the body. This output is largely in the urine and faeces, but significant amounts may also be lost from the body in sweat and shed skin cells, and in longer-term experiments even the growth of hair and nails must be taken into account. Obviously, any loss of blood or tissue will also involve a loss of protein.

Although the intake of nitrogenous compounds is mainly as protein, the output is not. Most of the nitrogenous output from the body is urea (see p. 203), although small amounts of other products of amino acid metabolism are also excreted, as shown in Table 9.1.

Table 9.1 The average daily excretion of nitrogenous compounds in the urine.

Urea	10–35 g (150–600 mol)	depends on the intake of protein
Ammonium	340–1200 mg (20–70 mmol)	depends on the state of acid-base balance
Amino acids	1.3–3.2 g	⅓ as free amino acids ⅓ as small peptides ⅓ as conjugates
Protein	< 60 mg	significant proteinuria indicates kidney damage
Uric acid	250–750 mg 1.5–4.5 mmol	
Creatinine	♂ 1.8 g (16 mmol) ♀ 1.2 g (10 mmol)	depends on muscle mass
creatine	< 50 mg (< 400 μmol)	significant exretion of creatine indicates muscle catabolism

Under normal conditions, an adult in good health loses the same amount of nitrogen from the body each day as is taken in from the diet. This is called **nitrogen balance** or **nitrogen equilibrium**.

If we try to determine the state of nitrogen balance in a child, we find that there is a difference between intake and excretion. A growing child puts out less nitrogen than the dietary intake. There is an increase in the amount of protein in the child's body as it grows. When there is an overall retention of nitrogen in the body (i.e. when the output of nitrogenous compounds is less than the intake), we say that the subject is in **positive nitrogen balance**, gaining total body nitrogen from the diet.

We can also see the opposite, a net loss of nitrogen from the body: the output is greater than the intake. This is called **negative nitrogen balance**, and means that there is an overall loss of protein from the body. Negative nitrogen balance is never normal; it always reflects either a pathological condition or dietary inadequacy.

Dynamic equilibrium

The proteins of the body are continually being broken down and replaced. Some, and especially enzymes which have a rôle in controlling metabolic pathways, may turn over within a matter of minutes or hours; others last for longer before they are broken down, perhaps days or weeks. Some proteins only turn over very slowly; for example, the connective tissue protein, collagen, is broken down and replaced so slowly that it is almost

189

impossible to measure the rate – perhaps half of the body's collagen is replaced in a year.

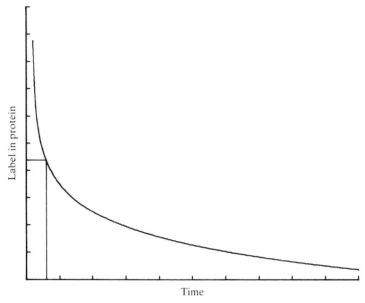

Time

Figure 9.1 The loss of label from a protein, showing metabolic turnover
An isotopically labelled amino acid was given at time 0. The label is incorporated into newly synthesized proteins, then lost as proteins are broken down and replaced.

We call this continual breakdown and replacement **dynamic equilibrium**. Superficially, there is no change in the body protein. In an adult there is no detectable change in the amount of protein in the body, or the relative amounts of different proteins, from one month to the next. Nevertheless, if we give a test dose of an isotopically labelled amino acid, we can follow the process of turnover. As shown in Figure 9.1, the label rapidly becomes incorporated into newly synthesized proteins, then is gradually lost with time as the proteins are broken down. The rate at which the label is lost from any one protein depends on the rate at which that protein is broken down and replaced.

The process of protein breakdown is enzymic hydrolysis to release free amino acids, as occurs in the intestinal tract in digestion. What we do not yet understand is how individual proteins are targeted for breakdown, and why some last so much longer than others. The processes involved in protein synthesis are discussed on p. 204

Protein requirements

The continuous breakdown of tissue proteins creates the requirement for protein in the diet. Although some of the amino acids released by breakdown of tissue proteins can be re-used, most are metabolized, by pathways which are discussed on p. 198 yielding a variety of intermediates which can be used as metabolic fuels, and urea, which is excreted. This means that there is a need for dietary protein to replace the lost tissue proteins, even in an adult who is not growing. In addition, relatively large amounts of protein are lost from the body in mucus, enzymes and other proteins which are secreted into the gastrointestinal tract and are not completely digested and reabsorbed.

An adult who is fed a diet which is otherwise adequate, but devoid of protein, continues to excrete nitrogenous compounds, the end-products of amino acid metabolism, in the urine. The average daily amount excreted is equivalent to breakdown of 0.5g of body protein/kg body weight: about 33g of tissue protein broken down each day in a 65 kg person. We call this the **obligatory nitrogen loss**, it reflects the tissue protein which is broken down and must be replaced by dietary intake.

Measurements of nitrogen balance are used to determine protein requirements. If the intake is inadequate to replace the protein that has been broken down, then there is negative nitrogen balance – a greater output of nitrogen from the body than the dietary intake. Once the intake is adequate to meet requirements, nitrogen balance is restored. The proteins that have been broken down can be replaced, and any surplus intake of protein can be used as a metabolic fuel.

From studies of nitrogen balance, we have a good estimate of protein requirements. For adults the *average daily requirement is 0.6 g of protein/ g body weight*, or 39 g/day for a 65 kg person. From this, allowing for individual variation, the **reference nutrient intake** (RNI, see p. 231) for protein is 0.75 g/kg body weight, or 49 g/day for a 65 kg person.

Average intakes of protein in developed countries are considerably greater than the requirement – of the order of 80–100 g/day. There is thus little likelihood of people in developed countries suffering from protein deficiency. Indeed, it is unlikely that adults will suffer from protein deficiency at all, if they are eating enough food to meet their energy requirements.

We can express protein requirements as the percentage of total energy intake which must be met from protein. The energy yield of protein is 17 kJ/g; using the average energy expenditure discussed on p. 162, the average adult's requirement for protein is 6.25% of energy intake (and the RNI is 7.8% of energy intake). In Western countries protein provides on average 15% of the energy intake.

Table 9.2 Protein content of various cereals, as percentage of energy yield.

	Energy (kJ/100g)	Protein (g/100g)	(kJ/100g)	% energy
Wheat, wholemeal	1350	13.2	224	16.6
Wheat, white flour	1430	11.3	192	13.4
Spaghetti	1610	13.6	231	14.3
Maize	520	4.1	70	13.5
Oatmeal	1700	12.4	211	12.4
Semolina	1490	10.7	182	12.2
Rye	1430	8.2	139	9.8
Potato	370	2.1	36	9.6
Barley	1540	7.9	134	8.7
Rice	1540	6.5	111	7.2
Yam	560	2.0	34	6.1
Cassava	460	0.9	15	3.3

Table 9.2 shows the protein content of some cereals and other "starchy" foods, as a percentage of the energy they provide. It is obvious that almost all of these provide enough protein, if enough is eaten to meet energy needs. Only cassava, yam and possibly rice provide insufficient protein (as a percentage of energy) to meet adult requirements. The shortfall in protein provided by a diet based on yam or rice would be made up by *small* amounts of other foods which are good sources of protein, such as those shown in Table 9.3. With diets based largely on cassava there is a more serious problem in meeting protein requirements.

Table 9.3 Sources of protein in the average diet; the figures show the average percentage of total protein intake obtained from different types of food.

Meat and meat products	36
Cereal products	23
(bread	(14)
Milk and milk products	17
Fruit and vegetables	10
Fish	6
Eggs	4

Table 9.3 shows the proportion of the protein which comes from different sources on average in Western countries. We are accustomed to regard

meat, fish, eggs and dairy produce as "protein foods" and bread and potatoes as "starchy foods". However, it is obvious from this table that cereal products (mainly bread and pasta) account for a significant proportion of average protein intake. Fish accounts for only a relatively small proportion of the protein on average because not many people eat much fish. On average, potatoes provide as much of our protein intake as fish. Although potatoes are relatively low in protein, they are widely eaten in relatively large amounts.

We can also see from Tables 9.2 and 9.3 that it is unlikely that vegetarians will be short of protein. Even people who eat meat or fish daily get half of their protein from vegetable sources; and anyway the average diet provides twice as much protein as is required. If the meat or fish is replaced with increased amounts of vegetables and nuts, then it is obvious that vegetarians are able to maintain a more than adequate intake of protein.

Protein deficiency in children   Since children are growing, and increasing the total amount of protein in the body, they have a proportionally greater requirement for protein than adults. A child should be in positive nitrogen balance while he or she is growing. Even so, the need for protein for growth is relatively small compared with the requirement to replace proteins which are turning over. Table 9.4 shows the protein requirements of children at different ages. As for adults, children in Western countries receive more protein than is needed to meet their requirements.

Table 9.4 Reference nutrient intakes for protein (UK Department of Health 1991).

Age (years)	Males (g/day)	Females (g/day)
1–3	15	15
4–6	20	20
7–10	28	28
11–14	42	41
15–18	55	45
19–50	56	45
over 50	53	47

If a child is receiving a protein-deficient diet (which may occur in developing countries, although it is most unlikely in Western countries), the result is a slowing of the rate of growth. A protein-deficient child will grow more slowly than one receiving an adequate intake of protein. This is **stunting of growth**. An important consequence of stunting is that the child's requirement for protein now falls. If the restriction is severe enough, then growth ceases more or less completely, and the requirement is now only for replacement of protein which is turning over. This is the same as for an adult: an average requirement of 0.6g/kg body weight and an RNI of 0.75g/kg body weight.

A deficiency specifically of protein, with an adequate intake of metabolic fuels, results in slower growth and stunting. The protein–energy deficiency diseases, marasmus and kwashiorkor (see Ch. 8) result from a general lack of food (and hence metabolic fuels), not a specific deficiency of protein.

Protein requirements in convalescence Patients can lose significant amounts of body protein as a result of physiological responses to surgical and other trauma, and even prolonged inactivity. One of the body's reactions to a major trauma, such as a burn, a broken limb or surgery, is an increase in the rate of breakdown of tissue proteins. This seems to be a means of mobilizing amino acids ready for increased protein synthesis to repair damaged tissue and the synthesis of specific trauma-response proteins, but a great deal is wasted, and there is an increase in the loss of nitrogenous compounds in the urine in response to trauma. Together with the loss of blood associated with injury, total losses of body protein may be as much as 1 kg. Even prolonged bed rest results in a considerable loss of protein, because there is atrophy of muscles which are not used. Muscle protein is catabolized as normal, but without the stimulus of exercise it is not completely replaced.

This loss of protein has to be made good as a part of the process of convalescence, and therefore we would expect patients who are convalescing to be in positive nitrogen balance. However, this does not mean that a convalescent patient requires a diet which is richer in protein than usual. We have seen that the average requirement for maintenance of protein turnover is 0.6 g of protein/kg body weight, yet the average intake is twice this. In other words, a normal diet will provide plenty of "spare" protein to permit replacement of the losses due to illness and hospitalization.

Essential amino acids Early studies of nitrogen balance showed that not all proteins are the same. Greater amounts of some proteins than others are needed for the maintenance of nitrogen balance. This is because different proteins contain different amounts of the various amino acids (see p. 86). The body's requirement is not just for protein, but for the amino acids which make up proteins, in the correct proportions to replace the body proteins that are being broken down.

We can feed people with mixtures of amino acids, rather than whole proteins, and so find the requirements for each amino acid in turn. If we do this, we find that the amino acids can be divided into two groups: some are absolutely required in the diet, while others can be omitted without causing any problems, as long as the total amount of protein (or amino acids) in the diet is adequate.

Table 9.5 Essential and non-essential amino acids.

Dietary essential (indispensable) amino acids
   lysine, methionine, threonine
   leucine, isoleucine, valine
   phenylalanine, tryptophan
   [histidine, arginine]

In addition
   tyrosine is synthesized from phenylalanine
   cysteine is synthesized from methionine

Non-essential amino acids
   glycine, alanine, serine, proline
   glutamate, glutamine, aspartate, asparagine

The amino acids that can be omitted from the diet are called the dispensable, or **non-essential amino acids** (see Table 9.5). The reason that they do not have to be provided in the diet is that they can be synthesized readily in the body, from a variety of common metabolic intermediates, as long as there is enough total protein in the diet.

Eight amino acids (shown in Table 9.5) cannot be synthesized in the body at all, but must be provided preformed in the diet. These are called the indispensable or **essential amino acids**. If one of these is lacking or provided in inadequate amount, then, regardless of the total intake of protein or amino acids, it will not be possible to maintain nitrogen balance, since there will not be a source of the amino acid for replacement protein synthesis.

There is a ninth essential amino acid, histidine. Although histidine can be synthesized in the body, the amount that can be made is not adequate to meet requirements if none at all is provided in the diet. Thus, while it is rarely, if ever, a cause for nutritional concern, histidine must be regarded as an essential amino acid, since the body's capacity to synthesize it is not adequate to meet requirements.

For infants and young children we have to consider a tenth essential amino acid, arginine. Although adults can synthesize adequate amounts of arginine to meet their requirements, the capacity for arginine synthesis is low in infants, and is not adequate to meet the requirements for growth.

Two amino acids occupy an intermediate position, in that they can be synthesized in the body, but only from an essential amino acid. They are cysteine, which is formed from methionine, and tyrosine, which is formed from phenylalanine. Adequate amounts of cysteine and tyrosine can be formed only if there is an adequate intake of the precursor essential amino acids, methionine and phenylalanine. The amount of cysteine and tyrosine which is provided in the diet will affect the requirement for the precursor amino acids. If the intake of cysteine is relatively high, then less methionine will be used for the formation of cysteine, and more can be used as methionine. Similarly, an adequate dietary intake of tyrosine reduces the requirement for phenylalanine, since less will have to be used for the synthesis of tyrosine.

Protein quality We can now refine our estimates of protein requirements. The average requirement is 0.6g of protein/kg body weight. However, the requirement is actually for the appropriate amount of each of the essential amino acids, plus an adequate total amount of the non-essential amino acids, in any proportions, since they can be formed in the body quite freely as long as there is an adequate total intake of amino acids.

We can compare the amounts of the essential amino acids in various proteins with the amounts that are required, as a means of assessing **protein quality** or **nutritional value**. If a protein provides at least as much of each of the essential amino acids as is required, then it will be completely usable for tissue protein synthesis. Such a protein has a **protein score** of 1.0.

If a protein provides less of one of the essential amino acids than the requirement for that amino acid, then it is not completely usable for tissue protein synthesis, and will have a protein score of less than 1.0. Thus, a protein which provided only half of the required amount of lysine (but more than half the requirement of the other amino acids) would only be able to meet half of the requirement for tissue protein synthesis before the available lysine was exhausted. Such a protein would have a protein score of 0.5.

The **limiting amino acid** of a protein is the essential amino acid which is present in the lowest amount relative to the requirement for that amino acid. The protein score is determined by the proportion of the requirement for the limiting amino acid which is met by that protein.

The limiting amino acid in cereal proteins is lysine, while in animal and most other vegetable proteins the limiting amino acid is methionine. (Correctly the sum of methionine plus cysteine, since, as discussed above, cysteine is synthesized from methionine, and the presence of cysteine reduces the requirement for methionine.)

The protein score, which we have used above to discuss protein nutritional value or quality, is based on chemical analysis of the essential amino acids present in the protein, compared with the amounts that are required. Other methods of assessing protein quality are biological assays based on the ability of minimally adequate amounts of the protein to support growth or the maintenance of nitrogen balance. You may come across protein nutritional value expressed in terms of "biological value", "net protein utilization" or "protein efficiency ratio". These are the results of various biological assay methods for determining protein quality.

If a protein has a low nutritional value, it means that in order to meet our requirement for the limiting essential amino acid, we have to eat more of that protein than would be the case for a protein with a higher nutritional value. *As the quality of the protein falls, so the amount needed to maintain nitrogen balance increases.*

Complementation We do not get our protein from only a single source. We eat a variety of different proteins. Even the most deprived communities in the poorest developing countries have five or more different sources of protein in their diet. The importance of this is that different proteins are limited by different amino acids, and have a relative excess of other essential amino acids.

The result of mixing different proteins in a diet is to give an unexpected increase in the nutritional value of the mixture. For example, wheat protein provides only 62% of the requirement for lysine, and thus has a protein score of 0.62. However, it provides more than enough methionine plus cysteine to meet requirements. Pea protein provides only 49% of the requirement for methionine plus cysteine, and thus has a protein score of 0.49. However, it provides more than the requirement of lysine. A mixture of equal parts of wheat and pea proteins is limited by methionine plus cysteine, but provides 77% of the requirement. In other words the mixture has a protein score of 0.77. This is as high as the protein score of meat. A mixture of proteins has a considerably higher nutritional quality than you would expect from the average of the scores for the two proteins.

This complementation between different proteins, which might individually be of low quality, to give mixtures of high nutritional value is reflected in whole diets. The average Western diet, made up of the mixture of protein sources shown in Table 9.3, has a protein score of 0.73. The poorest diets in developing countries, with a more restricted range of foods available, and very little milk, meat or fish, have a protein score of 0.6. We have to consider the mixture of protein sources that make up the diet as a whole, rather than being concerned with the apparent quality of single protein sources.

Since people eat mixtures of different types of protein, it doesn't make

197

sense to try to divide individual proteins into "first class" and "second class" categories. Most diets have very nearly the same protein quality, regardless of the individual protein sources.

The metabolism of amino acids

The need for a dietary intake of protein is to replace the amino acids lost as a result of the turnover of tissue proteins. Therefore we have to consider the metabolic fate of those amino acids, as well as any amino acids from the diet which are not required for protein synthesis. Overall, for an adult in nitrogen balance, the total amount of amino acids being metabolized will be equal to the total intake of amino acids in dietary proteins.

We can consider the metabolism of amino acids in two parts: the metabolism of the amino nitrogen, which gives rise to nitrogenous compounds in the urine, and the metabolism of the carbon skeletons as metabolic fuels. Many amino acids are also required for the synthesis of a variety of different metabolic products in the body, including the purines and pyrimidines of nucleic acids (see p. 93), hormones, neurotransmitters, etc. In general, the requirement for these purposes is small compared with the requirements for the maintenance of nitrogen balance, and we will not consider these pathways here.

The initial step in the metabolism of amino acids is the removal of the amino group ($-NH_2$), leaving the carbon skeleton of the amino acid. Chemically, these carbon skeletons are **oxo-acids** (sometimes also called **keto-acids**). An oxo-acid has a $C=O$ group in place of the $HC-NH_2$ group of an amino acid.

Some amino acids can be directly oxidized to their corresponding oxo-acids, releasing ammonia: the process of **deamination** (see Fig. 9.2). There is a general amino acid oxidase which catalyses this reaction, but it has a low activity. Two amino acids are deaminated by specific enzymes:

(a) **glycine** is deaminated to its oxo-acid, glyoxylic acid, and ammonium ions by glycine oxidase;
(b) **glutamic acid** is deaminated to oxoglutarate and ammonium ions by glutamate dehydrogenase.

Other amino acids are not deaminated directly, but undergo the process of **transamination**. The amino group of the amino acid is transferred onto the enzyme, leaving the oxo-acid. In the second half of the reaction, the enzyme transfers the amino group onto an acceptor, which is a different oxo-acid, so forming the amino acid corresponding to that oxo-acid. This reaction is shown in Figure 9.3.

(a) **Amino acid oxidase**

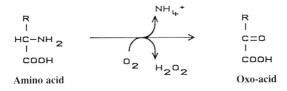

Amino acid   Oxo-acid

(b) **Glycine oxidase**

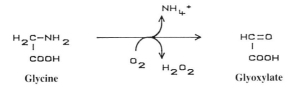

Glycine   Glyoxylate

(c) **Glutamate dehydrogenase**

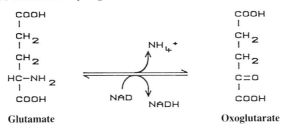

Glutamate   Oxoglutarate

Figure 9.2 The deamination of amino acids
(a) *Amino acid oxidase* acts on more or less all amino acids, but has low activity. The reaction is an oxidation, utilizing oxygen, and forming hydrogen peroxide. (b) *Glycine oxidase* acts in the same way as amino acid oxidase, but is specific for glycine, forming the oxo-acid glyoxylate. (c) *Glutamate dehydrogenase* catalyses the release of the amino group of glutamate as ammonium, forming oxoglutarate, linked to the reduction of NAD to NADH.

If the acceptor oxo-acid is oxoglutarate, then glutamate is formed, and glutamate can be oxidized readily back to oxoglutarate, with the release of ammonia. Similarly, if the acceptor oxo-acid is glyoxylate, then the product is glycine. Again, glycine can be oxidized back to glyoxylate and ammonia. Thus, by means of a variety of transaminases, and using the

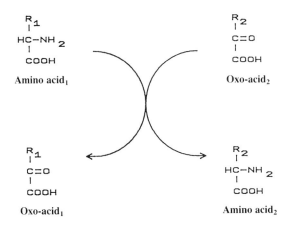

Figure 9.3 The reaction of transamination
(a) An amino acid reacts with the enzyme, transferring its amino group onto the enzyme, and thus forming the oxo-acid corresponding to that amino acid. (b) An oxo-acid reacts with the amino form of the enzyme; the amino group is transferred onto the oxo-acid, forming the corresponding amino acid, and restoring the enzyme to its original state, so that it can react with another amino acid. Many of the oxo-acids corresponding to amino acids are common metabolic intermediates. The oxo-acids of four amino acids are especially important:

Amino acid	*Oxo-acid*
glycine	glyoxylate
alanine	pyruvate
aspartate	oxaloacetate
glutamate	oxoglutarate

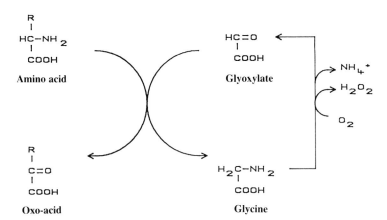

Figure 9.4 Transamination linked to glycine oxidase
Many transaminases, acting on a variety of amino acids, are linked to glyoxylate as the oxo-acid substrate, forming glycine. Glycine can then be deaminated by the action of glycine oxidase, releasing ammonium (NH_4^+) and reforming glyoxylate, which is then able to react with another molecule of amino acid.

200

reactions of glutamate dehydrogenase or glycine oxidase, all of the amino acids can be converted to their oxo-acids and ammonia (Figs 9.4, 9.5).

The oxo-acids produced by transamination or deamination of the amino acids are metabolized as metabolic fuels. Many of them either comprise intermediates of metabolic pathways already discussed in Chapter 6, or can readily be converted into such intermediates. In this way, the carbon skeletons of the amino acids join the same metabolic pathways as carbohydrates and fatty acids.

The process of transamination can also be used for the synthesis of any amino acid for which there is a source of the corresponding oxo-acid. The oxo-acids of the non-essential amino acids are intermediates in the metabolism of carbohydrates (and fatty acids), or can easily be formed from these intermediates. Thus there is a ready source of the carbon skeletons for the synthesis of these amino acids. This explains why, as long as the total intake of amino acids from dietary protein is adequate, the individual non-essential amino acids are not important; they can be made from metabolic intermediates by transamination from other amino acids. By contrast, the oxo-acids of the essential amino acids can only be formed from the amino acids in the first place, and therefore these amino acids cannot be synthesized in the body.

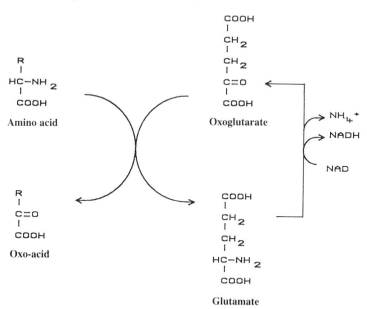

Figure 9.5 Transamination linked to glutamate dehydrogenase
Many transaminases, acting on a variety of amino acids, are linked to oxoglutarate as the oxo-acid substrate, forming glutamate. Glutamate can then be deaminated by the action of glutamate dehydrogenase, releasing ammonium (NH_4^+) and reforming oxoglutarate, which is then able to react with another molecule of amino acid.

201

The metabolism of ammonia

The deamination of amino acids (and several other reactions in the body) results in the formation of ammonium ions. Ammonia is very toxic. The normal plasma concentration is less than $50\,\mu mol/l$. An increase to only 80–$100\,\mu mol/l$ results in disturbance of consciousness, and in patients whose blood ammonia rises above about $200\,\mu mol/l$ ammonia intoxication leads to brain damage and may be fatal.

At any time, the total amount of ammonia to be transported around the body, and eventually excreted, is greatly in excess of the toxic level. However, as it is formed, ammonia is metabolized, mainly by the formation of glutamate from oxoglutarate, and then **glutamine** from glutamate, in a reaction catalysed by **glutamine synthetase**, as shown in Figure 9.6. Glutamine is transported in the bloodstream, to the liver and kidneys.

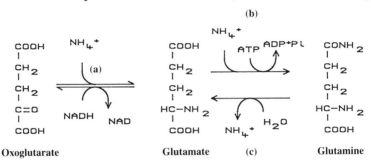

Figure 9.6 The removal of ammonium: the reactions of glutamate dehydrogenase and glutamine synthetase

(a) *Glutamate dehydrogenase*: the equilibrium of glutamate dehydrogenase is such that the direction of reaction depends on the relative concentrations of glutamate, oxoglutarate and, most importantly, ammonium. (b) *Glutamine synthetase*: in tissues other than the liver and kidney, glutamine is synthesized from glutamate and ammonium in a reaction in which ATP is hydrolysed to ADP and phosphate. (c) *Glutaminase*: in the liver and kidneys, glutamine is hydrolysed to glutamate and ammonium.

In the kidneys, some glutamine is converted back to glutamate (which remains in the body) and ammonia, which is excreted in the urine to neutralize excess acid excretion. This reaction is a simple hydrolysis, as shown in the lower half of Figure 9.6.

In the liver, glutamine is also hydrolysed to glutamate and ammonia. Here the ammonia is metabolized further, to form **urea**, which is then transported to the kidneys for excretion. The pathway for urea synthesis is shown in Figure 9.7. It is a cyclic pathway. The key compound is ornithine, which acts as a carrier on which the molecule of urea is built up. At the end of the reaction sequence, urea is released by the hydrolysis of arginine, yielding ornithine to begin the cycle again.

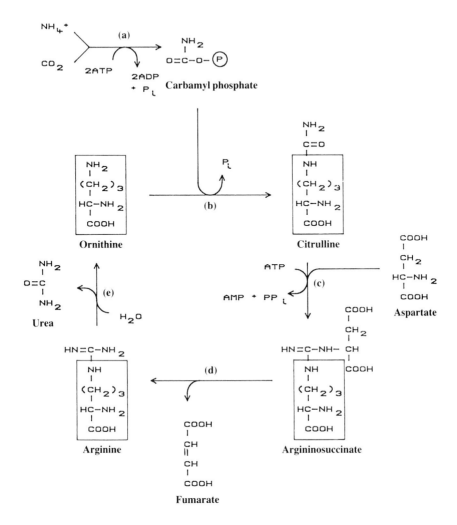

Figure 9.7 The synthesis of urea
One of the two nitrogen atoms of urea comes from ammonium and the other from aspartate. The pathway of urea synthesis is cyclic; the growing urea molecule is built up on the side-chain amino group of the amino acid ornithine, eventually forming arginine. Arginine is then hydrolysed to release urea and ornithine, which is available to undergo another cycle of reactions. The structure of ornithine is shown in the boxes in the diagram; it is unchanged during the cycle. (a) *Carbamyl phosphate synthetase*: carbamyl phosphate is formed from ammonium and carbon dioxide, in a reaction in which ATP is the phosphate donor. A second molecule of ATP is hydrolysed to ADP and phosphate in this reaction. (b) *Ornithine carbamyl transferase*: the carbamyl part of carbamyl phosphate is transferred onto the side-chain amino group of ornithine, forming citrulline and releasing phosphate. (c) *Argininosuccinate synthetase*: citrulline and aspartate undergo a condensation reaction linked to the hydrolysis of ATP to AMP and pyrophosphate (which is hydrolysed to 2 mol of phosphate), forming argininosuccinate. (d) *Argininosuccinase*:

The urea synthesis cycle is also the pathway for the synthesis of the amino acid **arginine**. Ornithine can be synthesized readily from glutamate, and then undergoes the reactions shown in Figure 9.7 to form arginine when the dietary intake is not enough to meet the requirements for protein synthesis.

It was noted on p. 195 that arginine is an essential amino acid for infants – they cannot synthesize as much of it as is necessary to meet the requirement for growth. The limitation on their ability to synthesize arginine is due to a limited capacity of the urea synthesis cycle. This has important implications for infant feeding. A limited capacity for urea synthesis means a limited capacity for ammonia metabolism, and hence a limited capacity to metabolize excess protein. *Infants fed on too high an intake of protein are at risk of ammonia intoxication.*

This becomes important when we consider the use of cows' milk as a substitute for human milk. Both types of milk have the same energy yield, but cows' milk contains 3.3g of protein/100 ml, while human milk contains 1.3 g of protein/100 ml. In order to avoid problems of ammonia intoxication, cows' milk must be diluted so as not to provide too much protein. However, if it is simply diluted with water, the infant will be starved of metabolic fuels. Human milk contains almost twice as much carbohydrate as cows' milk; infant formula based on cows' milk is diluted to reduce the concentration of protein, and has carbohydrate (usually lactose) added to maintain the intake of metabolic fuels.

Protein synthesis

We have already seen on p. 95 that DNA in the nucleus of cells contains the information needed for the synthesis of all the various proteins that are needed for the normal functioning of the body. What we now have to consider is how this information is used in the synthesis of specific proteins. The process can be divided into two phases:

(a) transcription of specific regions of DNA to form messenger RNA;
(b) translation of the message carried by mRNA into protein.

---

the bond between the amino group of the aspartate part of argininosuccinate and the carbon skeleton is cleaved, releasing fumarate and leaving arginine. Fumarate can enter the citric acid cycle and undergo oxidation to oxaloacetate (see Fig. 6.8 on p. 142). Oxaloacetate can then act as an amino acceptor in a variety of transamination reactions, so "collecting" amino groups from a variety of amino acids to reform aspartate for reaction (c). (e) *Arginase*: arginine is hydrolysed, releasing urea, which is excreted, and reforming ornithine, which is available to undergo a further cycle of reactions.

Transcription

In the transcription of DNA to form mRNA a part of the desired region of DNA is uncoiled, and the two strands of the double helix are separated. A **complementary copy** of one DNA strand is then made, in the same way as happens in DNA replication in cell division (see p. 100), except that in this case it is ribonucleotides which form the growing strand, rather than deoxyribonucleotides. This process is shown in Figure 9.8.

There are three main differences between the replication of DNA and transcription:

(a) only one of the two strands of DNA is transcribed to form messenger RNA, whereas in DNA replication both strands are copied at the same time;

(b) in replication, the whole of the DNA is copied; in transcription only specific regions, (individual genes, corresponding to the individual proteins) are copied;

(c) only one copy of the DNA is made in the process of replication, while in transcription multiple copies of the gene are made.

It was noted on p. 100 that only about 10% of the total DNA in a cell actually codes for proteins. The remainder consists of apparently redundant regions called introns, regions which act as "spacers" between genes, a variety of regions associated with the control of replication and regions which control the process of transcription.

The **transcription control sites** include start and stop messages, and promoter and enhancer sequences. The main promoter region for any gene is about 25 bases before (upstream of) the beginning of the gene to be transcribed. It is the signal that what follows is a gene to be transcribed.

Enhancer regions may be found further upstream of the message, downstream or sometimes even in the middle of the message. An enhancer may be several thousand base-pairs away from the gene it controls. The function of enhancer regions is to increase the rate at which the gene is transcribed.

It may not seem very useful to have enhancer sequences away from, and even after, the gene to be controlled if you regard DNA simply as a linear sequence of bases. However, when we consider the way in which DNA is coiled around proteins in the nucleus, it is obvious that regions which are quite far apart in the linear sequence can come to be close together when we look at the surface of the DNA–protein complexes. Thus, the information content of DNA depends not only on the linear sequence of bases, but also on the way in which that linear sequence is coiled around proteins, bringing distant regions close together, and even allowing regions which occur later in the linear sequence to be "seen" earlier on.

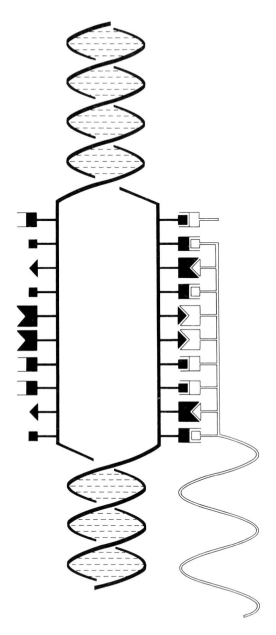

Figure 9.8 The transcription of DNA to form messenger RNA
A small region of the double helix of DNA is unwound and a copy of one strand is made.
Each base in the strand of DNA being copied forms hydrogen bonds to its complementary
nucleotide triphosphate, then the 3′-5′phosphate links are formed between the ribose
units, with the elimination of pyrophosphate. As the process is completed, so the growing
chain of RNA leaves the DNA strand to which it was attached, and the DNA double helix
reforms.

206

The first step in the transcription of a gene is to uncoil that region of DNA from its associated proteins, so as to allow the various enzymes involved in transcription to gain access to the DNA. In some circumstances this process can be seen under the microscope. Regions of DNA which are being transcribed appear as "puffs" or fluffy areas, quite distinct from the condensed chromatin of inactive DNA coiled around proteins. The DNA is uncoiled from its associated proteins, and a short region of the double helix is opened at a time.

The enzyme RNA polymerase moves along the DNA strand which is to be transcribed, and matches complementary ribonucleotide triphosphates one at a time to the bases in the DNA. Cytosine in DNA is matched by guanosine triphosphate, guanine by cytidine triphosphate and thymine by adenosine triphosphate. However, adenine in DNA is matched by uridine triphosphate – RNA contains uracil rather than thymine as in DNA.

As each base is put into place, so a phosphate bond is formed by reaction between the new nucleoside and the growing RNA chain. This proceeds faster than the similar process in DNA replication, at a rate of about 40 nucleotides/second. Although it is obviously important that the mRNA should be a good copy of the DNA, occasional mistakes would be less important than in DNA replication, so there is no need for the slow meticulous proof-reading that occurs in DNA replication (see p. 100). The message in DNA must be preserved as near perfectly correct as possible, since this is the master copy of the message for the cell. By contrast, messenger RNA has a short life, turning over within a few hours, and an occasional faulty copy would not have major consequences.

At the end of the gene being transcribed, there is a specific **termination region** in the DNA. This causes cessation of the activity of RNA polymerase and release of the RNA to undergo further processing. RNA polymerase can then begin the synthesis of another copy of the same or another region of DNA. At any time there are many molecules of RNA polymerase moving along any one gene, so that multiple copies of the message are made at the same time.

There are three steps in the **processing of the RNA** formed by RNA polymerase before it can be exported from the nucleus as messenger RNA:

(a) The 5' end of the RNA is blocked by the formation of the unusual base 7-methylguanosine. This is called the "cap", and has an important rôle in the initiation of protein synthesis (see p. 211). The 5' end of the RNA is the first to be synthesized, and the cap is added before transcription has been completed.

(b) A tail is added to the 3' end of the RNA, after the termination codon. This tail is a sequence of between 20 and 250 adenosine residues, and therefore is called the poly-A tail. The poly-A tail of messenger RNA has been extremely useful to molecular biologists, providing a simple way of separating mRNA from the other forms of RNA in the cell. We do not know the function of the poly-A tail *in vivo*. Experimental systems can be manipulated to produce tailless mRNA; it is transported from the nucleus to the cytosol like normal mRNA, and is translated equally well.

(c) The DNA sequence which is the gene coding for any single protein consists of code sequences for the beginning and end of each message, as you would expect. However, between these two markers, not all the information is required for the synthesis of protein. There are regions of DNA in the middle of genes which seem to carry no useful information, although some of them are enhancer regions. They are called **introns**, because they are introduced in the middle of genes. Before the newly transcribed RNA can be translated it has to undergo "editing" to remove these extraneous sequences of DNA and splice the coding sequences together to give a simple translatable message. This is messenger RNA (mRNA), which is then transported out of the nucleus into the cytosol to be used for protein synthesis.

Translation

The process of protein synthesis consists of translating the message carried by the sequence of bases on mRNA into amino acids, and then forming peptide bonds between the amino acids to form a protein. This occurs on the ribosome, and requires a variety of enzymes, as well as specific transfer RNA (tRNA) molecules for each amino acid.

The genetic code   The bases of mRNA are read three at a time. These "words" are called **codons** – the units in which the genetic code is read. There are 64 possible combinations of three out of four different bases, and so with only four bases it would be possible to code for more than the 20 amino acids which are involved in protein synthesis.

The genetic code is shown in Tables 9.6 and 9.7. Three codons (UAA, UAG and UGA) do not code for amino acids at all, but act as **stop signals** to show the end of the message to be translated and so terminate protein synthesis. The remaining 61 codons all code for amino acids. In many cases only the first two bases of the codon have to be read to identify the amino acid; the third base can be either purine (either A or G, it doesn't matter) or either pyrimidine (C or U, again it doesn't matter). In some cases, it makes no difference which base in the third position (A, G, C or U). As discussed on p. 288, this redundancy in the genetic code, where a change in one base may well have no effect on the amino acid which is coded for, provides protection against mutations.

Table 9.6 The genetic code. This table shows the various codons for each amino acid; the bases are for mRNA, in DNA T would replace U.

Amino acid		Codon(s)
Alanine	Ala	GCU GCC GCA GCG
Arginine	Arg	CGU CGC CGA CGG AGA AGG
Asparagine	Asn	AAU AAC
Aspartic acid	Asp	GAU GAC
Cysteine	Cys	UGU UGC
Glutamic acid	Glu	GAA GAG
Glutamine	Gln	CAA CAG
Glycine	Gly	GGU GGC GGA GGG
Histidine	His	CAU CAC
Isoleucine	Ile	AUU AUC AUA
Leucine	Leu	UUA UUG CUU CUC CUA CUG
Lysine	Lys	AAA AAG
Methionine	Met	AUG
Phenylalanine	Phe	UUU UUC
Proline	Pro	CCU CCC CCA CCG
Serine	Ser	UCU UCC UCA UCG AGU AGC
Threonine	Thr	ACU ACC ACA ACG
Tryptophan	Trp	UGG
Tyrosine	Tyr	UAU UAC
Valine	Val	GUU GUC GUA GUG
	STOP	UAA UAG UGA

Transfer RNA (tRNA) The key to translating the message carried by the codons on mRNA into amino acids is transfer RNA (tRNA). There are 56 different types (species) of tRNA in the cell. They all have the same general structure, as shown in Figure 9.9, RNA twisted into a clover-leaf shape, and consisting of some 70–90 nucleotides. About half the bases in tRNA are paired by hydrogen bonding; this is important for the maintenance of the shape of the molecule.

The different species of tRNA have many regions in common with each other, and all have a -CCA tail at the 3' end, which reacts with the amino acid. The most important region of differences between the different species of tRNA is the **anticodon** – a sequence of three bases at the "bottom" of the clover-leaf. The bases in the anticodon are complementary to the bases of the codons of mRNA, and each species of tRNA binds specifically to one codon, or, in some cases, two closely related codons for the same amino acid.

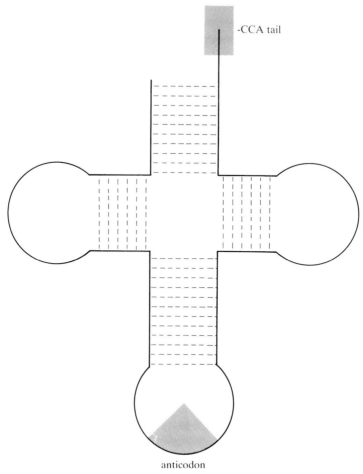

-CCA tail

anticodon

Figure 9.9 Transfer RNA
There are 56 different types of tRNA in the cell; all have the same general structure, a clover-leaf shape which is maintained by hydrogen bonds. At the base of the clover-leaf is the anticodon; at the other end is the -CCA tail to which the amino acid will be bound.

Amino acids bind to "**activating enzymes**" (aminoacyl-tRNA synthetases), which recognize both the amino acid and the appropriate tRNA molecule. The first step is reaction between the amino acid and ATP, to form aminoacyl-AMP, releasing pyrophosphate. The aminoacyl-AMP then reacts with the -CCA tail of tRNA to form amino acyl-tRNA, releasing AMP.

The specificity of these activating enzymes is obviously critically important to the process of translation. Each enzyme recognizes only one amino acid, but will bind and react with all the various tRNA species which carry an anticodon for that amino acid. Mistakes are extremely rare. The easiest possible mistake would be the attachment of valine to the tRNA for isoleucine, or vice versa, because of the close similarity between the structures of these two amino acids (see p. 87). However, it is only about once in every 3,000 times that this mistake occurs. This is very much lower than would be expected. Aminoacyl-tRNA synthetases have a second active site which checks that the correct amino acid has been attached to the tRNA, and, if not, hydrolyses the newly formed bond, releasing tRNA and the amino acid.

Table 9.7 The genetic code. This table shows the bases in mRNA; in DNA T would replace U.

First position	Second position				Third position
	U	C	A	G	
U	Phe	Ser	Tyr	Cys	U
U	Phe	Ser	Tyr	Cys	C
U	Leu	Ser	STOP	STOP	A
U	Leu	Ser	STOP	Trp	G
C	Leu	Pro	His	Arg	U
C	Leu	Pro	His	Arg	C
C	Leu	Pro	Gln	Arg	A
C	Leu	Pro	Gln	Arg	C
A	Ile	Thr	Asn	Ser	U
A	Ile	Thr	Asn	Ser	C
A	Ile	Thr	Lys	Arg	A
A	Met	Thr	Lys	Arg	G
G	Val	Ala	Asp	Gly	U
G	Val	Ala	Asp	Gly	C
G	Val	Ala	Glu	Gly	A
G	Val	Ala	Glu	Gly	G

Protein synthesis on the ribosome The subcellular organelle concerned with protein synthesis is the ribosome. This consists of two subunits, composed of RNA with a variety of associated proteins. The ribosome permits the binding of the anticodon region of aminoacyl-tRNA to the codon on mRNA, and aligns the amino acids for formation of peptide bonds. As shown in Figure 9.10, the ribosome binds to mRNA, and has two tRNA binding sites. One, the P site, contains the growing peptide chain, attached to tRNA, while the other, the A site, binds the next aminoacyl-tRNA to be incorporated into the peptide chain.

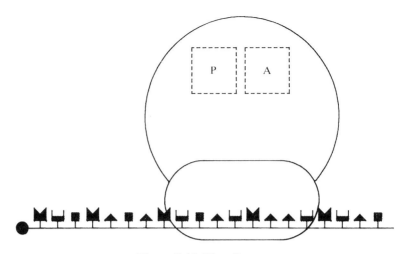

Figure 9.10 The ribosome

The first codon of mRNA (the **initiation codon**) is always AUG, the codon for methionine. This means that the amino terminal of all newly synthesized proteins is methionine, although this may well be removed in post-translational modification of the protein (see p. 215).

A special initiator methionine-tRNA forms a complex with the small ribosomal subunit, then together with a variety of initiation factors (enzymes and other proteins) binds to the initiator codon of mRNA, and finally to a large ribosomal subunit, to form the complete ribosome, as shown in Figure 9.11a. The 5' cap of mRNA is important for this process, since it shows where the initiator codon is. AUG is the only codon for methionine, and anywhere else in mRNA, it binds the normal methionine-tRNA. It is only immediately next to the cap that AUG binds the initiator methionine-tRNA.

After the ribosome has been assembled, with the initiator tRNA bound at the P site and occupying the AUG initiator codon, the next aminoacyl-tRNA binds to the A site of the ribosome, with its anticodon bound to the next codon in the sequence. This is shown in Figure 9.11b.

The methionine is released from the initiator tRNA at the P site, and forms a peptide bond to the amino group of the aminoacyl-tRNA at the A site of the ribosome. The initiator tRNA is then released from the P site, and the growing peptide chain, attached to its tRNA, moves from the A site to the P site. Since the peptide chain is attached to tRNA, which occupies a codon on the mRNA, this means that as the peptide chain moves from the A site to the P site, so the whole assembly moves one codon along the mRNA. This is shown in Figure 9.11c.

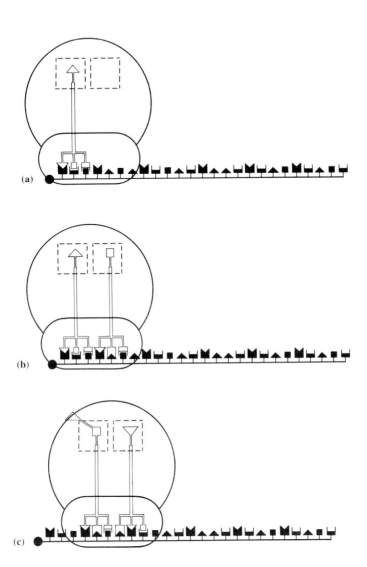

Figure 9.11 The synthesis of proteins on the ribosome
(a) Initiator tRNA-methionine binds to the P site of the ribosome, with its anticodon hydrogen bonded to the first codon of the mRNA. (b) The next tRNA with its amino acid attached binds to the next codon on the mRNA, and occupies the A site of the ribosome. (c) The amino acid attached to tRNA at the A site displaces the initiator tRNA from the methionine, forming a peptide bond and releasing initiator-tRNA. In the process, the tRNA moves from the A site of the ribosome to the P site. Immediately, the next codon forms hydrogen bonds to its tRNA with the appropriate amino acid attached. *(Continued overleaf.)*

213

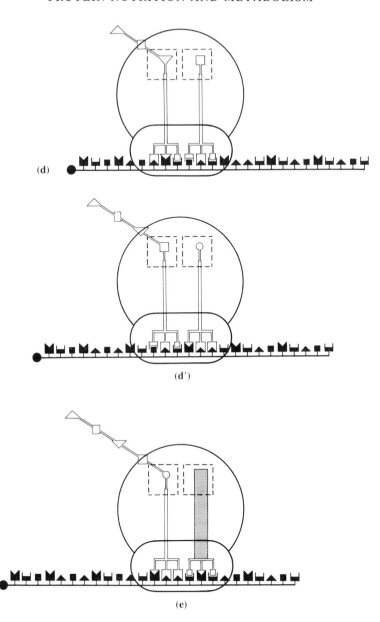

Figure 9.11 (continued) The synthesis of proteins on the ribosome

(d) Each amino acid attached to tRNA at the A site of the ribosome displaces the growing peptide chain from tRNA at the P site, forming a new peptide bond, and moving onto the P site. (e) When there is a stop codon under the A site of the ribosome, this interacts with a termination factor, which blocks the A site, and causes hydrolysis of the bond linking the growing peptide chain to tRNA at the P site. This releases the newly synthesized protein, and causes the two subunits of the ribosome to separate, ready to come together again at the initiator site of mRNA.

214

occupies the A site, covering its codon. The growing peptide chain is transferred from the tRNA at the P site, forming a peptide bond to the amino acid at the A site. Again the free tRNA at the P site is released, and the growing peptide, attached to tRNA, moves from the A site to the P site, moving one codon along the mRNA as it does so. This is shown in Figure 9.11d, and is repeated until the codon under the A site is a stop codon.

The **stop codons** (UAA, UAG and UGA) are not read by tRNA, but by protein release factors. These occupy the A site of the ribosome, as shown in Figure 9.11e, and hydrolyse the peptide-tRNA bond. This releases the finished protein from the ribosome. As the protein leaves, so the two subunits of the ribosome separate, and leave the mRNA; they are now available to bind another initiator tRNA and begin the process of translation over again.

Termination, and release of the protein from the ribosome requires the presence of a stop codon and the protein release factors. However, protein synthesis can also come to a halt if there is not enough of one of the amino acids bound to tRNA. In this case, the growing peptide chain is not released from the ribosome, but remains, in arrested development, until the required aminoacyl-tRNA is available. This means that if the intake of one of the essential amino acids is inadequate, then once supplies are exhausted, protein synthesis will come to a halt.

Just as several molecules of RNA polymerase can transcribe the same gene at the same time (see p. 207), so several ribosomes translate the same molecule of mRNA at the same time. As the ribosomes travel along the ribosome, so each has a longer growing peptide chain than the one before. Such assemblies of ribosomes on a molecule of mRNA are called **polysomes**.

Post-translational modification of proteins Just as the RNA produced by transcription has to undergo editing and further processing before it is translatable mRNA, so the initial products of translation frequently undergo modification before they are mature active proteins.

Proteins which are to be exported from the cell are synthesized with a hydrophobic signal sequence of amino acids at the amino terminal to direct them through the membrane of the endoplasmic reticulum. This is removed early in the process of post-translational modification. Many other proteins have regions removed from the amino or carboxyl terminal during post-translational modification.

Many proteins contain carbohydrates and lipids, covalently bound to amino acid side-chains. Others contain covalently bound cofactors and prosthetic groups, such as vitamins and their derivatives, metal ions or haem. Again the attachment of these non-amino-acid parts of the protein is part of the process of post-translational modification to form the active protein.

Some proteins contain unusual amino acids, for which there is no codon, and no tRNA. These are formed by modification of the protein after translation is complete. Such amino acids include:

(a) **methyl histidine** in the contractile proteins of muscle;
(b) **hydroxyproline** and **hydroxylysine** in the connective tissue proteins; the formation of hydroxyproline and hydroxylysine requires vitamin C as a cofactor, explaining why wound healing, which requires new synthesis of connective tissue, is impaired in vitamin C deficiency (see p. 273);
(c) γ-**carboxyglutamate** in several of the blood-clotting proteins; the formation of γ-carboxyglutamate requires vitamin K, and this explains the rôle of vitamin K in blood clotting (see p. 252).

Antibiotics Many of the antibiotics in common use act by inhibiting the synthesis of protein by bacteria, and so (gradually) killing the organisms which cause disease. Fortunately, there are differences between the ribosomes and enzymes of protein synthesis of bacteria and higher organisms (including man). To be useful clinically, an antibiotic must inhibit the bacterial protein synthesis system while having little or no effect on the human system. Antibiotics which inhibit protein synthesis in man as well as in bacteria may be useful tools for research, but they have no clinical use. They would kill the patient as well as the disease-causing organism!

Tetracyclines bind to bacterial ribosomes, and so prevent the binding of aminoacyl-tRNA to the A site. **Streptomycin** binds to the small subunit of the bacterial ribosome and distorts its shape. This leads to abnormal codon–anticodon interactions, and hence to misreading and garbled translation. The resultant nonsense peptides are useless to the bacteria. **Erythromycin** inhibits the bacterial enzyme which is responsible for the translocation of the peptide-tRNA from the A site to the P site of the ribosome. **Chloramphenicol** inhibits the bacterial transpeptidase, which catalyses the formation of the peptide bond between the peptide chain attached to tRNA in the P site and the next amino acid to be added, in the A site.

Biosynthetic human proteins

One of the major advances in the treatment of some diseases over the past few years has been the development of the ability to synthesize human hormones and other proteins. The principle of the method is that the

216

human gene for the desired protein is inserted into the DNA of a bacterium, yeast or mammalian cell in culture, and the host cell is persuaded to transcribe and translate the new gene, so producing a protein which is identical to the normal human protein.

For many proteins, it is relatively easy to isolate the mRNA from human tissue or cells in culture. This mRNA is used to synthesize a complementary copy, as DNA – the process is the reverse of the process of transcription described on p. 205, and indeed the enzyme used is called **reverse transcriptase**. It uses an RNA template to synthesize a strand of DNA, using deoxyribonucleotides, in the same way as RNA polymerase forms mRNA by copying the DNA template. The single strand of DNA can then be used to form its own complementary strand, as occurs normally in DNA replication. We now have a double-stranded length of DNA, carrying the desired gene. Under appropriate conditions, it is possible to insert this newly synthesized DNA into the DNA of a host cell, together with a suitable promoter region, and possibly also enhancer regions. If all has gone well, the new strain of the host cell can be cultured, and will contain and express the gene for a human protein.

As a result of the development of such techniques of genetic engineering and biotechnology, we can now treat people with diabetes using **human insulin**, rather than insulin extracted from the pancreas of pigs or cows (which differs slightly in structure from human insulin, and gradually results in the development of antibodies in people using it over many years).

We also have an ample supply of **human growth hormone** for the treatment of children of extremely short stature, whereas until the advent of biosynthetic human growth hormone there was only enough of the hormone available from cadavers to treat the most serious cases.

We can now produce **blood-clotting factors** for the treatment of patients with haemophilia and other disorders of blood clotting, without relying on donated blood and the associated risks of infection with HIV or hepatitis.

The same techniques can be used to prepare pure viral and bacterial proteins for use in immunization, avoiding the risks associated with the use of attenuated strains of disease-causing organisms.

The energy cost of protein synthesis

The body's first requirement is for a source of metabolic fuels, and if the total intake of food is inadequate to meet energy expenditure, then protein will be used as a fuel rather than for replacement of tissue proteins (see p. 179). We also have to consider the metabolic energy required for protein synthesis; a considerable proportion of the basal metabolic rate (see p. 160) is concerned with the energy cost of protein synthesis.

The synthesis of mRNA requires the nucleoside triphosphates; RNA polymerase releases pyrophosphate, which is then broken down to free phosphate. This means that for each base incorporated into mRNA there is a net cost equivalent to the hydrolysis of 2mol of ATP to ADP and phosphate. This includes those bases which are incorporated into non-coding regions of the precursor of mRNA (5'- and 3'-tail regions and introns) which are subsequently excised and broken down to release free nucleotides during the post-transcriptional modification to yield mRNA.

There are many copies of the mRNA for each different protein being synthesized in the cell, and, as noted above, mRNA has a rapid turnover. For proteins which vary in response to hormone stimulation (see p. 226), the mRNA may have a half-life of only minutes, while even for proteins which are synthesized in more or less constant amount the mRNA has a half-life of hours – 30 h would be a long half-life for an mRNA molecule.

The process of translation is also energy expensive:

(a) Formation of the aminoacyl-tRNA requires the formation of amino-acyl-AMP, with the release of pyrophosphate, which again breaks down to yield phosphate. Hence, for each amino acid attached to tRNA there is a cost equivalent to 2mol of ATP hydrolysed to ADP and phosphate.

(b) The binding of each aminoacyl-tRNA to then A site of the ribosome involves the hydrolysis of GTP to GDP and phosphate, which is equivalent to the hydrolysis of ATP to ADP and phosphate.

This gives a cost equivalent to the hydrolysis of 3mol of ATP to ADP and phosphate for each amino acid incorporated into protein; this includes those amino acids incorporated into regions of the protein which are removed during post-translational modification.

There is also a requirement for both GTP and ATP for the initiation of protein synthesis and the assembly of the ribosome on mRNA, and again a requirement for GTP in the binding and action of the protein release factor at the stop codon.

CHAPTER TEN

The hormonal control of metabolism

We saw on p. 109 how changes in the concentrations of metabolites in a cell can regulate key steps in metabolic pathways, and thus control the fate of substrates and metabolites. This is a mechanism for moment-by-moment regulation of metabolism, within each cell separately.

There is also regulation and integration of metabolism on a whole-body basis, to ensure co-ordination between metabolic pathways in different tissues and organs. This is achieved by the actions of hormones.

Hormones are synthesized and secreted by the endocrine glands, in response to various stimuli. The stimulus to change the amount of a hormone secreted may be a change in the concentration of a key metabolite in the bloodstream, nervous stimulation of the endocrine gland or the action of another hormone.

After their release, hormones circulate throughout the body, and therefore are potentially able to act on all cells in the body. However, a hormone can only act on cells which have **receptors** for that hormone. Cells which do not have receptors are unaffected by changes in the concentration of the hormone in the bloodstream. Hormones are slowly metabolized to inactive forms; sometimes this happens in the liver, sometimes inside the cells which have responded to hormone action.

Hormones control metabolism in one of two main ways:
(a) by altering the activity of enzymes in the cell, by means of reversible chemical modification of the enzyme protein;
(b) by changing the amount of enzyme protein in the cell, changing the rate at which individual genes are expressed.

Changes in the amount of enzyme in the cell can be considered to be a mechanism of long-term regulation, since the effects last for some time,

219

while changes in enzyme activity by modification of the protein are short-term regulation, since they can be reversed rapidly.

Hormonal control of the formation and utilization of metabolic fuel reserves

As an example of the way in which hormones regulate and integrate metabolism, we can consider the actions of various hormones in the control of the formation and utilization of tissue reserves of metabolic fuels. Hormones which increase the synthesis of tissue reserves act in the fed state, while in the fasting state other hormones act to increase the mobilization and utilization of tissue reserves.

Insulin

Insulin is secreted by the ß-cells of the pancreas in response to an increase in the concentration of glucose in the bloodstream. Its action is to increase the formation of tissue reserves of metabolic fuels. Insulin has five main actions:

(a) stimulation of the uptake of glucose into muscle and adipose tissue;
(b) stimulation of the formation of glycogen from glucose in muscle and liver;
(c) increased formation of fatty acids and triacylglycerols from glucose in liver and adipose tissue;
(d) stimulation of the uptake of amino acids into muscle, increasing the rate of muscle protein synthesis;
(e) inhibition of the hydrolysis of triacylglycerols in adipose tissue, and hence inhibition of the release of fatty acids.

Glucagon

Glucagon is secreted by the α-cells of the pancreas when the blood concentration of glucose falls, i.e. the opposite of the conditions under which insulin is secreted. High circulating concentrations of glucose, which stimulate insulin secretion, inhibit the secretion of glucagon.

Glucagon is the main hormone of the fasting state, and its actions are to increase the mobilization of tissue reserves of metabolic fuels. Glucagon has three main actions:

(a) inhibition of the synthesis of glycogen and stimulation of the activity of glycogen phosphorylase, so increasing the breakdown of glycogen; this results in the release of glucose from the liver;

(b) inhibition of the formation of fatty acids and triacylglycerols in liver and adipose tissue and stimulation of lipase in adipose tissue, resulting in the release of fatty acids;

(c) stimulation of gluconeogenesis from pyruvate and other substrates derived from amino acids.

Adrenaline

Adrenaline (sometimes called epinephrine) is secreted by the adrenal glands, especially in response to fright or fear. Its actions are to achieve rapid mobilization of tissue reserves of metabolic fuels for fighting or escape. Adrenaline has two main actions:

(a) activation of glycogen phosphorylase in muscle and liver; in muscle this provides additional glucose-6-phosphate for rapid muscle activity;

(b) activation of lipase in adipose tissue, resulting in the release of fatty acids as an additional metabolic fuel.

Growth hormone

Growth hormone is secreted by the hypothalamus. In addition to its actions to stimulate growth, it increases the activity of lipase in adipose tissue, so increasing the release of fatty acids from adipose tissue triacylglycerol reserves.

Cortisol

The glucocorticoid hormone cortisol is secreted by the adrenal cortex. Increased secretion results in a decrease in new protein synthesis, and hence an increase in the net breakdown of proteins and increased gluconeogenesis.

This action of cortisol is indirect; it has no direct effect on any of the enzymes of protein synthesis or gluconeogenesis. Rather, the effect of cortisol secretion is increased synthesis of two enzymes in the liver, tryptophan oxygenase and tyrosine transaminase, which are key steps in the catabolism of these two amino acids. As a result of increased activity of these two enzymes, there is depletion of the body pool of free tryptophan, tyrosine and phenylalanine. This results in a reduction in the rate of protein synthesis throughout the body. However, the breakdown of tissue proteins continues at the normal rate. Therefore there is an accumulation of amino acids which cannot be used for protein synthesis because of the relative deficit of tryptophan, tyrosine and phenylalanine. These are metabolized in the liver, either as metabolic fuels, or, if possible, as substrates for gluconeogenesis.

Changes in enzyme activity as a result of modification of the enzyme protein

Change in the activity of existing enzyme protein is a rapid control mechanism; the effects can be switched on or off within seconds. It is the mechanism of the responses to hormones such as insulin, glucagon, adrenaline and growth hormone. Neurotransmitters and some growth factors act by way of the same type of mechanism.

The key to understanding this type of metabolic regulation is the fact that a simple chemical modification of one or more reactive groups on the surface of some enzymes results in conformational changes which increase or decrease the activity of the enzyme very considerably. Commonly, the chemical modification is either the phosphorylation of the hydroxyl group of serine or tyrosine (catalysed by an enzyme known as a **protein kinase**), or the reverse reaction – dephosphorylation of phosphoserine or phosphotyrosine, catalysed by **protein phosphatase**. Some enzymes are activated by phosphorylation; others are inactivated.

The action of hormones is thus to activate or inhibit the enzymes which catalyse the phosphorylation and dephosphorylation of regulatory enzymes. This is achieved indirectly, by the production of a **second messenger** inside the cell. The sequence of events is as follows:

1. The hormone binds to a **receptor** on the outer surface of the cell membrane. The receptor is a relatively large protein, which spans the cell membrane. Binding of the hormone at the outer surface causes a conformational change, which carries through the membrane to the protein at the inner surface. Directly or indirectly, this results in activation of an enzyme inside the cell.
2. The activated enzyme catalyses a reaction which results in the release into the cell of the second messenger.
3. The second messenger binds to one or more enzymes in the cell. This either increases or decreases their activity.
4. The activated enzymes catalyse the phosphorylation or dephosphorylation of further enzymes, thus altering their activity. Sometimes the

enzymes whose activity is altered in this way are the enzymes catalysing the key metabolic steps which are to be regulated. More commonly, they are intermediate enzymes which in turn activate or inactivate the final target enzymes by phosphorylation or dephosphorylation.

The effect of this cascade of actions is a considerable amplification of the signal from the hormone:

(a) For as long as the hormone remains bound to the cell surface receptor, the enzyme at the inner surface of the cell membrane will continue to synthesize and release the second messenger. This means that many molecules of second messenger will be formed in response to the binding of a single molecule of hormone.

(b) For as long as the second messenger is being produced, it will activate (or inhibit) the enzymes it affects. This means that each molecule of second messenger can have a considerable effect on the amount of the product of the affected enzyme which can be formed.

(c) Once an enzyme has been activated by phosphorylation (or dephosphorylation), it can catalyse the conversion of many molecules of substrate. It will remain activated until the process is reversed, normally in response to another hormone.

Adenyl cyclase and the formation of cyclic AMP as a second messenger

The cell surface receptors for hormones such as glucagon and adrenaline activate the enzyme adenyl cyclase, which catalyses the formation of cyclic AMP (cAMP) from ATP:

$$ATP \rightarrow cAMP + pyrophosphate.$$

In turn, cAMP activates enzymes which modify the activity of protein kinases and phosphatases.

The receptors are complex multi-subunit proteins. One subunit binds GDP at the inner face of the membrane in the resting state. Binding of the hormone causes a conformational change in the whole protein complex, resulting in the release of GDP and binding of GTP.

The subunit with GTP bound then leaves the receptor–protein complex, and binds to adenyl cyclase, activating it, so that it forms cAMP from ATP. Cyclic AMP then activates protein kinases and phosphatases which phosphorylate or dephosphorylate other proteins, altering their activity.

Cyclic AMP is hydrolysed to AMP by phosphodiesterase, so that stimulation or inhibition of the enzymes only lasts for as long as cAMP continues to be formed.

The receptor subunit with GTP bound slowly catalyses the hydrolysis of its GTP to GDP and phosphate. When this happens, it dissociates from adenyl cyclase. This causes the adenyl cyclase to lose activity, and the formation of cyclic AMP ceases. The protein subunit with GDP bound returns to bind to the inner surface of the receptor. If hormone stimulation continues, it will again lose its GDP, bind GTP and activate adenyl cyclase once again.

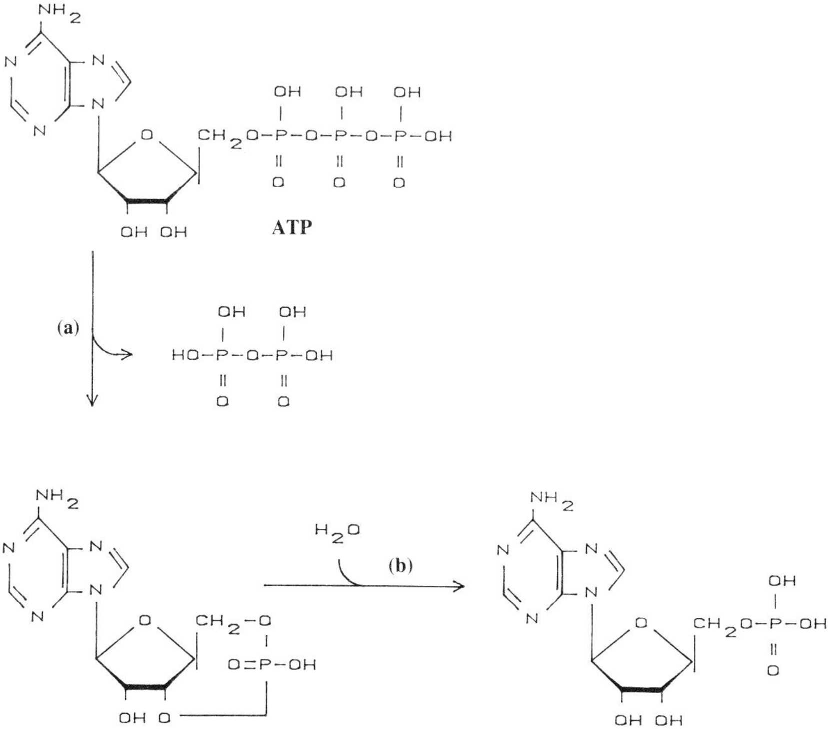

Figure 10.1 The formation and hydrolysis of cyclic AMP as a second messenger in hormone action

(a) *Adenyl cyclase*: cAMP is formed from ATP in a reaction in which pyrophosphate is eliminated. The pyrophosphate is then hydrolysed to 2 mol of phosphate. Adenyl cyclase is an intracellular membrane-associated enzyme which is activated, directly or indirectly, by the binding of the hormone or other agonist to the cell-surface receptor. (b) *Phosphodiesterase*: cAMP is hydrolysed by phosphodiesterase, to yield AMP, which does not affect the activity of enzymes whose activity is modified by cAMP. AMP can be rephosphorylated to ATP.

*Phospholipase and the formation of
inositol triphosphate as a second messenger*

Some responses to hormones and other modifiers of cell metabolism occur by way of a different type of second messenger response, the phosphatidyl

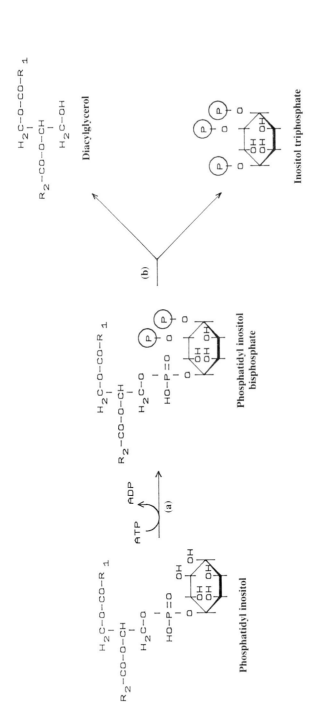

Figure 10.2 The formation of inositol triphosphate and diacylglycerol as second messengers in hormone action
(a) *Phosphatidyl inositol kinase*: phosphatidyl inositol in membranes undergoes two phosphorylations in which ATP is the phosphate donor, forming phosphatidyl inositol bisphosphate. (b) *Hormone-sensitive phospholipase*: binding of the hormone to the cell-surface receptor results in activation of membrane-associated phospholipase which hydrolyses phosphatidyl inositol bisphosphate to yield inositol triphosphate and diacylglycerol.

inositol cascade.

One of the phospholipids in cell membranes is phosphatidyl inositol, and much of this is phosphorylated to phosphatidyl inositol bisphosphate (see Fig. 10.2 and p. 82). Binding of the hormone to the cell-surface receptor causes a conformational change which activates a phospholipase. This acts specifically on phosphatidyl inositol bisphosphate, resulting in the release into the cell of two second messengers: inositol triphosphate and diacylglycerol.

Inositol triphosphate increases the concentration of calcium ions in the cytoplasm, by releasing calcium from stores in the endoplasmic reticulum. This calcium is bound by a specific calcium-binding protein, **calmodulin**. Calmodulin with calcium bound to it affects the activity of several enzymes, including some of the protein kinases which phosphorylate key regulatory enzymes.

The **diacylglycerol** released by the action of phospholipase increases the sensitivity of these protein kinases to activation by calcium bound to calmodulin.

Inositol triphosphate gradually undergoes either dephosphorylation or further phosphorylation to inactive products, and diacylglycerol undergoes hydrolysis to glycerol and free fatty acids. At the same time, the concentration of calcium in the cytosol is reduced by pumping calcium ions back into the endoplasmic reticulum.

Changes in the amount of enzyme in the cell

There is a continual turnover of proteins in the cell, and not all proteins are broken down and replaced at the same rate. Some are relatively stable, while others, and especially enzymes which are important in metabolic regulation, have short half-lives, of the order of minutes or a few hours. This rapid turnover means that it is possible to control metabolic pathways by changing the rate at which a key enzyme is synthesized, and hence the total amount of that enzyme in the tissue.

An increase in the rate of synthesis of an enzyme or other protein by a hormone or other compound is called **induction**. The reverse, a decrease in the rate of synthesis of the enzyme by a metabolite, is called **repression**. Many key enzymes in metabolic pathways are induced by their substrates, and similarly many are repressed by high concentrations of the end-products of the pathways they control.

Enzyme induction is the mechanism of action of the steroid hormones such as cortisol, the sex steroids (androgens, oestrogens and progesterone), vitamins A and D (see pp. 236 and 242), thyroid hormone, and a variety of growth factors. Unlike the rapidly acting hormones discussed above, which bind to cell-surface receptors, these hormones enter the cell and bind to receptor proteins in the nucleus. The hormone–receptor complex then binds to an enhancer site on DNA (see p. 205). This increases the rate of transcription of the gene (or a family of related genes).

There is amplification of the hormone signal. One molecule of hormone–receptor complex bound to the enhancer site will enhance transcription of that gene for as long as it remains bound, so producing many molecules of messenger RNA. Each molecule of messenger RNA can then be translated many times over, producing many molecules of the enzyme.

Both the binding of the hormone–receptor complex to the enhancer site and the binding of the hormone to the receptor are equilibrium reactions, and there is metabolism of the hormone to an inactive form in the cell. This means that as the secretion of the hormone ceases, so there is a reduction in the concentration in the bloodstream, and a reduction in the concentration available to bind to receptors in the nucleus. Thus, as the concentration of hormone falls, so transcription of the gene also falls. The amounts of both the messenger RNA and the enzyme then fall gradually back to the original level.

This type of metabolic regulation is obviously slower and longer-lasting than changing the activity of an existing molecule of enzyme protein. It takes some time for there to be a noticeable increase in the amount of enzyme in the cell. After the end of hormone stimulation, the fall in enzyme activity is relatively slow, since it depends on the rate at which the enzyme (and its messenger RNA) are broken down.

The control of gene expression by steroid hormones is not generally an "on/off" affair. Rather, the hormone causes an increase in the expression of a gene which is anyway being transcribed, albeit at a low rate. Similarly, the secretion of steroid hormones is not a strictly "on/off" affair, rather a matter of changes in the amount being secreted.

CHAPTER ELEVEN

Micronutrients: the vitamins and minerals

In addition to an adequate source of metabolic fuels (carbohydrates, fats and proteins) and protein (and the essential amino acids) for protein synthesis, we have a requirement for very much smaller amounts of other nutrients: the vitamins, minerals and essential fatty acids.

Vitamins are organic compounds which are required for the maintenance of normal health and metabolic integrity. They cannot be synthesized in the body, but must be provided in the diet. They are required in very small amounts, of the order of μg or mg/day, and thus can be distinguished from the essential fatty acids (see p. 81) and the essential amino acids (see p. 195), which are required in larger amounts, several g/day.

The essential minerals are those inorganic elements which have a physiological function in the body. Obviously, since they are elements, they must be provided in the diet, because elements cannot be interconverted. The amounts required vary from g/day for sodium and calcium, through mg/day (e.g. iron) to μg/day for the trace elements (so called because they are required in such small amounts).

The vitamins

As can be seen from Table 11.1, the vitamins are named in a curious way. This is a historical accident, and results from the way in which they

228

Table 11.1 The vitamins.

Vitamin		Principal metabolic functions	Deficiency disease
A	retinol	visual pigments in the retina; cell differentiation	night blindness; xerophthalmia; keratinization of skin
	ß-carotene	ß-carotene is an antioxidant	
D	calciferol	maintenance of calcium balance; enhances intestinal absorption of Ca^{2+} and mobilizes bone mineral	rickets = poor mineralization of bone; osteomalacia = bone demineralization
E	tocopherols tocotrienols	antioxidant, especially in membranes	extremely rare – serious neurological dysfunction
K	phylloquinone menaquinones	coenzyme in formation of carboxyglutamate in enzymes of blood clotting and bone matrix	impaired blood clotting, haemorrhagic disease
B_1	thiamin	coenzyme in pyruvate and 2-oxoglutarate dehydrogenases, and transketolase; poorly defined function in nerve conduction	peripheral nerve damage (beriberi) or CNS lesions (Wernicke–Korsakoff syndrome); acidosis
B_2	riboflavin	coenzyme in oxidation and reduction reactions; prosthetic group of flavoproteins	lesions of corner of mouth, lips and tongue; seborrhoeic dermatitis
niacin	nicotinic acid nicotinamide	coenzyme in oxidation and reduction reactions, functional part of NAD and NADP	pellagra – photosensitive dermatitis, depressive psychosis, fatal
B_6	pyridoxine pyridoxal pyridoxamine	coenzyme in transamination and decarboxylation of amino acids and glycogen phosphorylase; role in steroid hormone action	disorders of amino acid metabolism, convulsions
	folic acid	coenzyme in transfer of one-carbon fragments	megaloblastic anaemia
B_{12}	cobalamin	coenzyme in transfer of one-carbon fragments and metabolism of folic acid	pernicious anaemia = megaloblastic anaemia with degeneration of the spinal cord
	pantothenic acid	functional part of CoA and acyl carrier protein	peripheral nerve damage (burning-foot syndrome)
	biotin	coenzyme in carboxylation reactions in gluconeogenesis and fatty acid synthesis	impaired fat and carbohydrate metabolism, dermatitis
C	ascorbic acid	coenzyme in hydroxylation of proline and lysine in collagen synthesis; anti-oxidant; enhances absorption of iron	scurvy – impaired wound healing, loss of dental cement, subcutaneous haemorrhage

were discovered. Studies at the beginning of the 20th century showed that there was something in milk that was essential, in very small amounts, for the growth of mice fed on a diet consisting of purified fat, carbohydrate, protein and mineral salts.

These early studies showed that two factors were essential: one was found in the cream and the other in the watery part of milk. Logically, they were called Factor A (fat-soluble, in the cream) and Factor B (water-soluble, in the watery part of the milk). Factor B was identified as being chemically an amine, and in 1913 the name "vitamin" was coined for these "vital amines".

Further studies showed that "Vitamin B" was a mixture of compounds, with different actions in the body, and so they were given numbers as well: vitamin B_1, vitamin B_2, and so on. There are gaps in the numerical order of the B vitamins. When what might have been called vitamin B_3 was discovered, it was found to be a chemical compound that was already known, nicotinic acid. It was therefore not given a number. Other gaps are because compounds which were assumed to be vitamins, and were given numbers, such as B_4, B_5, etc., were later shown either not to be vitamins, or to be vitamins which had already been described by other workers, and given other names.

Vitamins C, D and E were named in the order of their discovery. The name "vitamin F" was used at one time for what we now call the essential fatty acids (see p. 81); "vitamin G" was later found to be what was already known as vitamin B_2. Biotin is still sometimes called vitamin H. Vitamin K was discovered by Henrik Dam, in Denmark, as a result of studies of disorders of blood coagulation, and he named it for its function "*koagulation*" in Danish, hence vitamin K.

We now know the chemistry of all the vitamins, and therefore we can give them proper names, as shown in Table 11.1. Where only one chemical compound has the biological activity of the vitamin, this is quite easy. Thus, vitamin B_1 is thiamin, vitamin B_2 is riboflavin, etc.

With several of the vitamins, several chemically related compounds found in foods can be interconverted in the body, and all show the same biological activity. We call such chemically related compounds **vitamers**, and we use a general name (a **generic descriptor**) to mean all compounds which display the same biological activity. Thus, niacin is the generic descriptor for two compounds, nicotinic acid and nicotinamide, which have the same biological activity. Vitamin B_6 is used to describe the six compounds which have vitamin B_6 activity.

The definition of essentiality

Correctly, for a compound to be classified as a vitamin, it should be a dietary essential. In other words, it is something that must be provided in the diet, and cannot be synthesized in the body. By this strict definition, two vitamins should not really be included, since they can be made in the body. **Vitamin D** is made in the skin in sunlight (see p. 242), and should really be regarded as a steroid hormone rather than a vitamin. It is only when sunlight exposure is inadequate that a dietary source is required. Similarly, **niacin** can be formed from the essential amino acid tryptophan. Indeed, synthesis from tryptophan is probably more important than a dietary intake of preformed niacin. Nevertheless, both vitamin D and niacin were discovered as a result of investigations of deficiency diseases, and they are always considered as vitamins.

Deficiency of a vitamin causes a specific disease, which is cured by restoring the vitamin to the diet. This is important, it is not enough just to show that the compound has effects when added to the diet. After all, aspirin will cure a headache, but this does not mean that headache is an aspirin deficiency disease, nor that aspirin is a dietary essential!

We now know the metabolic functions of all the vitamins. Therefore, before we would accept a new substance as a possible vitamin, we would require not only evidence that deprivation caused a specific deficiency disease which could be cured only with that compound, but also at least some idea of its metabolic function. Here we are specifically excluding pharmacological actions; we are looking for essential metabolic functions. We are confident that all the compounds listed in Table 11.1 are dietary essentials and therefore vitamins (with the anomaly of vitamin D and niacin referred to above).

The determination of requirements

Before we can estimate requirements for a vitamin, mineral or any other nutrient, we have to consider what we mean by adequacy; in other words, we have to answer the question "Requirement for what purpose?"

We have to distinguish between requirements for the maintenance of normal health and metabolic integrity, and possible pharmacological or drug-like actions at higher levels of intake. Here we are concerned with requirements to maintain normal health, and not possible actions of higher amounts of nutrients in treating diseases.

The maintenance of normal health and metabolic integrity is difficult to define. Certainly, we cannot consider the absence of clinical deficiency disease as a criterion of any more than minimal adequacy.

We use a variety of different **criteria of adequacy**: maintenance of normal metabolic responses; saturation of enzymes with their vitamin-derived cofactors; urinary excretion of metabolites of the vitamin; concentration in the plasma or red blood cells. Several of these may be used in studies of requirements for any one vitamin, in which groups of volunteers are maintained on deficient diets until specific changes develop, then the intake required to correct the abnormalities is found by restoring varying amounts of the vitamin to the diet. We can also measure the rate at which the body content of the vitamin turns over (for example using isotopically labelled vitamin); the requirement is then the amount which is required to replace what is lost each day. Problems arise in interpreting the results, and therefore defining requirements, when different markers of adequacy respond to different levels of intake.

Individuals do not all have the same requirement for vitamins and other nutrients, even when expressed relative to body size or energy expenditure. Figure 11.1 shows the results of determining the requirements of 1,000 subjects for a vitamin (it is theoretical; even taking all the studies of vitamin requirements that have ever been performed, we probably do not have results on 1,000 people). There is a wide spread of individual requirements, although most people have requirements around the middle of the range the average, or statistical mean, requirement.

If we analyze the results statistically, we can determine not only the average requirement, but also the **standard deviation (SD)** of the results; a measure of the spread of the results around the mean. For results such as those shown in Figure 11.1, a statistically normal distribution, *95% of the population have a requirement within the range -2SD to +2SD around the mean*.

An intake equal to the average requirement will be *more than enough* to meet the requirements of 50% of the population. An intake equal to the average plus 2SD will be more than enough to meet the requirements of 97.5% of the population. By contrast, an intake equal to the average minus 2SD will only be adequate to meet the requirements of 2.5% of the population.

We take the range of ±2SD around the average requirement (the requirement of 95% of the population) as a **reference range**, against which we can compare the adequacy of diets. We can then define three levels of intake:

(a) The **Lower Reference Nutrient Intake (LRNI)** or lowest threshold intake, below which it is unlikely that most peoples' requirements can be met. This is either the level of intake below which we know from experimental studies that metabolic integrity cannot be maintained, or, where such experimental evidence is not available, 2SD below the average requirement.

232

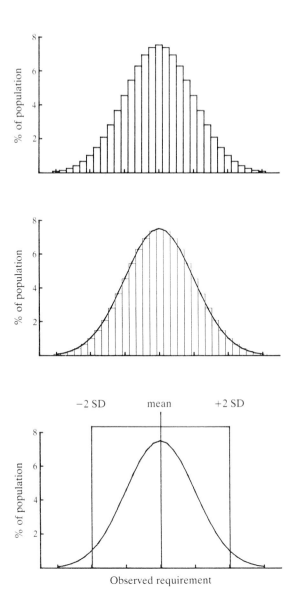

Figure 11.1 The determination of Reference Nutrient Intakes
(a) If we determined the requirements of 1,000 people for any given nutrient, we would find that they had different individual requirements; we plot a histogram of the percentage of the subjects whose requirements lie within each range. (b) We can join up the midpoints of each bar of the histogram to produce a smooth curve. This is the statistically normal distribution curve, with equal numbers of people having requirements above and below the average or mean. (c) A range of $2\times$ standard deviation around the mean includes 95% of the population.

If we take a value $2\times$ standard deviation *above* the mean requirement, we have more than met the requirements of 97.5% of the population. This is the Reference Nutrient Intake; it is greater than the requirements of essentially everyone in the population. If we take a value $2\times$ standard deviation *below* the mean requirement, we have failed to meet the requirements of 97.5% of the population. This is the Lower Reference Nutrient Intake, below which it is most unlikely that adequate nutrient will be supplied.

(b) The **average requirement**. This is just what it seems to be the average of the requirements of the individuals who have been studied.

(c) The **Reference Nutrient Intake (RNI)**. This is 2SD above the average requirement, and hence is *more than adequate to meet the requirements of 97.5% of the population*. This is the level of intake which is sometimes called the Recommended Daily Amount (RDA), Recommended Daily Intake (RDI) or Population Reference Intake (PRI).

Until 1991 the British Department of Health tables of nutrient requirements used the term RDA. The United States, and many other countries, still use the term. However, it is misleading:

(a) We do not have to have an intake of any nutrient every day; on average over a period of time we have to meet our requirements, but it does not matter if intake varies quite widely from day to day.

(b) More importantly, the RNI or RDA is *not a recommended intake for an individual*, but a reference standard against which to compare intakes of a population or group of people, and a target for catering in hospitals and other institutions, to ensure that intakes are more than adequate to meet individual requirements. It is obvious from the discussion above that very few people have a requirement as high as the RNI.

Tables 11.2 and 11.3 show the RNIs for vitamins and minerals.

Pharmacological actions of vitamins, and problems of toxicity

Reference nutrient intakes of vitamins and minerals are established on the basis of being more than adequate to meet requirements for the maintenance of normal health and metabolic integrity. Some of the vitamins have different actions in larger amounts, generally considerably higher than could be obtained from foods. Some of these actions may be useful in the treatment of diseases other than deficiency diseases. Here we are talking about pharmacological or drug-like actions of compounds which, by chance, are vitamins in smaller amounts.

It is a curious quirk of the law that compounds which are nutrients can generally be sold over the counter without any need for proof of efficacy in the treatment of the conditions for which they are recommended. By contrast, a compound which is not a nutrient must undergo rigorous testing for safety and efficacy before it can be granted a Product Licence for sale as a medicine. This means that many of the claims made for vitamins at (non-nutritionally) high levels of intake are untested. Without evidence of efficacy and safety, it is difficult to justify the sale or consumption of vitamin and mineral supplements which provide more than about the RNI.

Table 11.2 Reference nutrient intakes for vitamins
(UK Department of Health 1991).

	A	B$_1$	B$_2$	niacin	B$_6$	B$_{12}$	folate	C
	(μg)	(mg)	(mg)	(mg)	(mg)	(μg)	(μg)	(mg)
0–3 months	350	0.2	0.4	3	0.2	0.3	50	25
4–6 months	350	0.2	0.4	3	0.2	0.3	50	25
7–12 months	350	0.2	0.4	4	0.3	0.4	50	25
10 monthly	350	0.3	0.4	5	0.4	0.4	50	25
1–3yr	400	0.5	0.6	8	0.7	0.5	70	30
4–6yr	500	0.7	0.8	11	0.9	0.8	100	30
7–10yr	500	0.7	1.0	12	1.0	1.0	150	30
Males								
11–14yr	600	0.9	1.2	15	1.2	1.2	200	35
15–18yr	700	1.1	1.3	18	1.5	1.5	200	40
19–50yr	700	1.0	1.3	17	1.4	1.5	200	40
over 50yr	700	0.9	1.3	16	1.4	1.5	200	40
Females								
11–14yr	600	0.7	1.1	12	1.0	1.2	200	35
15–18yr	600	0.8	1.1	14	1.2	1.5	200	40
19–50yr	600	0.8	1.1	13	1.2	1.5	200	40
over 50yr	600	0.8	1.1	12	1.2	1.5	200	40
pregnant	700	0.9	1.4	14	1.2	1.5	300	50
lactating								
0–4months	950	1.0	1.6	16	1.2	2.0	260	70
over 4months	950	1.0	1.6	16	1.2	2.0	260	70

Simply because a compound is a dietary essential in small amounts does not mean that high intakes are safe. Several of the vitamins are known to be toxic in excess. In general this is at very high levels of intake, as would be obtained from supplements, not the amounts which are found in foods. There is an exception here in the case of vitamin A; as discussed on p. 241, liver may contain unexpectedly high levels of vitamin A, and pregnant women are specifically recommended not to eat liver because of the possible teratogenic effects of vitamin A in excess. Where we have information about undesirable effects of high intakes of vitamins and minerals, these are discussed in the following pages.

The absence of any information does not mean that a vitamin is safe in unlimited amounts, simply that we have no information yet. Vitamin B$_6$

Table 11.3 Reference nutrient intakes for minerals (UK Department of Health 1991).

	Ca	P	Mg	Na	K	Cl	Fe	Zn	Cu	Se	I
	(mg)	(mg)	(mg)	(mg)	(mg)	(mg)	(mg)	(mg)	(mg)	(μg)	(μg)
0–3 months	525	400	55	210	800	320	1.7	4.0	0.2	10	50
4–6 months	525	400	60	280	850	400	4.3	4.0	0.3	13	60
7–9 months	525	400	75	320	700	500	7.8	5.0	0.3	10	60
10 monthly	525	400	80	350	700	500	7.8	5.0	0.3	10	60
1–3yr	350	270	85	500	800	800	6.9	5.0	0.4	15	70
4–6yr	450	350	120	700	1100	1100	6.1	6.5	0.6	20	100
7–10yr	550	450	200	1200	2000	1800	8.7	7.0	0.7	30	110
Males											
11–14yr	1000	775	280	1600	3100	250	11.3	9.0	0.8	45	130
15–18yr	1000	775	300	1600	3500	2500	11.3	9.5	1.0	70	140
19–50yr	700	550	300	1600	3500	2500	8.7	9.5	1.2	75	140
over 50yr	700	550	300	1600	3500	2500	8.7	9.5	1.2	75	140
Females											
11–14yr	800	625	280	1600	3100	2500	14.8	9.0	0.8	45	130
15–18yr	800	625	300	1600	3500	2500	14.8	7.0	1.0	60	140
19–50yr	700	550	270	1600	3500	2500	14.8	7.0	1.2	60	140
over 50yr	700	550	270	1600	3500	2500	8.7	7.0	1.2	60	140
pregnant	700	550	270	1600	3500	2500	14.8	7.0	1.2	60	140
lactating											
0–4 months	1250	990	320	1600	3500	2500	14.8	13.0	1.5	75	140
over 4 months	1250	990	320	1600	3500	2500	14.8	8.5	1.5	75	140

(see p. 260) was generally regarded as quite safe until about 10 years ago, when side-effects of very high intakes became apparent; until then no-one had taken such high intakes, and therefore they had not been tested.

Vitamin A

Two groups of compounds have vitamin A activity: retinol (preformed vitamin A), which is found only in animal foods, and a variety of carotenes which are found in yellow, red and green vegetables (see Figure 11.2). The main sources of preformed vitamin A are meat (and especially liver), milk and milk products, and eggs. Vitamin A is added to margarine to achieve the same level as is found in butter.

Many, but not all, of the carotenes can be metabolized in the intestinal

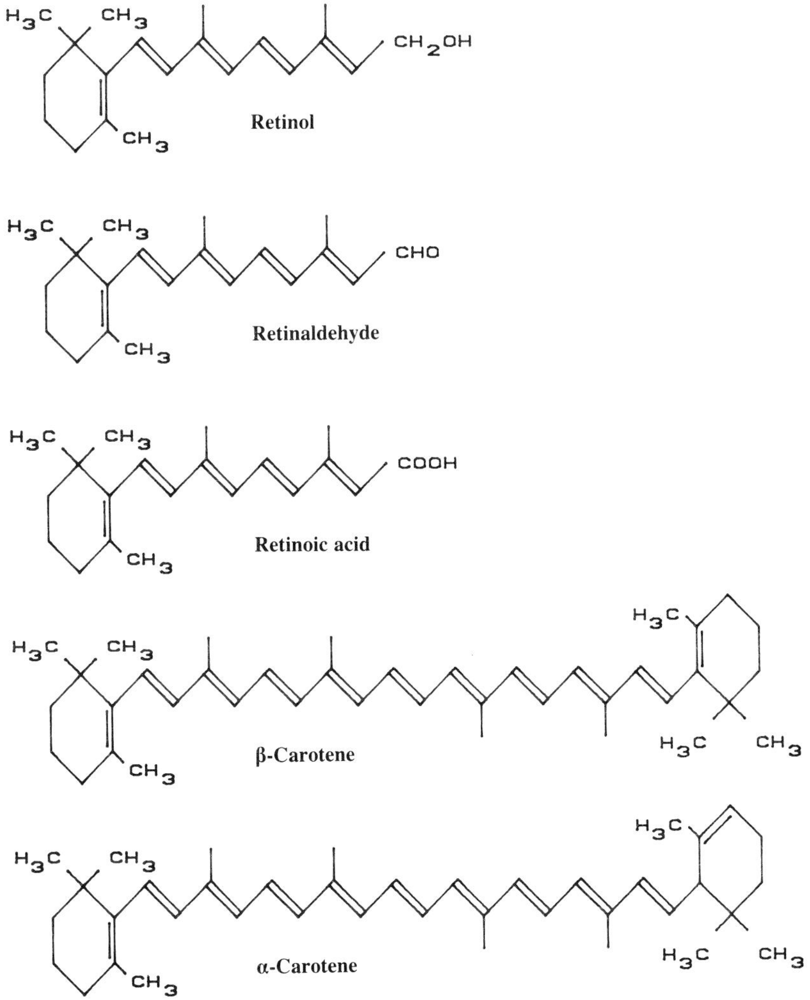

Figure 11.2 Vitamin A vitamers
Retinol, retinaldehyde and retinoic acid are sometimes referred to as preformed vitamin A; carotenes that can be cleaved to yield retinaldehyde are referred to as pro-vitamin A carotenoids.

mucosa to give rise to retinol. These are known as pro-vitamin A carotenoids. The most important of the carotenes with vitamin A activity is ß-carotene. Although it would appear from its structure, shown in Figure 11.2, that one molecule of ß-carotene would give rise to two molecules of retinol, this is not so in practice, since a considerable amount is absorbed as carotene. Nutritionally, $6\,\mu g$ of ß-carotene is equivalent to $1\,\mu g$ of preformed retinol. For other carotenes with vitamin A activity, $12\,\mu g$ is equivalent to 1 μg of preformed retinol.

We express the total amount of vitamin A in foods as μg **retinol equivalents**. This is calculated by adding:

μg preformed vitamin A

+ 1/6 x μg ß-carotene

+ 1/12 x μg other provitamin A carotenoids.

You will sometimes see vitamin A expressed in **international units (iu)**, although the international unit is now obsolete. Before pure vitamin A was available for chemical analysis, the vitamin A content of foods was determined by biological assays, and the results expressed in standardized experimental units (iu):

$$1\text{iu} = 0.3\,\mu\text{g retinol}$$
$$1\,\mu\text{g of retinol} = 3.33\text{iu}.$$

Metabolic functions

The best known, and best defined, function of vitamin A is in vision. The sequence of events is shown in Figure 11.3. Retinol undergoes a conformational change to the *cis*-isomer, which is then oxidized to *cis*-retinaldehyde. This then binds to the protein opsin, forming the pigment **rhodopsin**. When rhodopsin is exposed to light, it undergoes a conformational change which results in the release of the retinaldehyde, which undergoes isomerization to the all-*trans*-form.

The altered form of opsin interacts with other proteins, activating a second messenger system which results in the transmission of a nervous impulse. *Trans*-retinaldehyde is oxidized to retinol, then slowly converted to *cis*-retinaldehyde for the formation of rhodopsin. Under conditions where there is little retinol or retinaldehyde in the eye (i.e. in deficiency), vision is impaired (see below).

Although this is the best understood function of vitamin A, its main function in the body is in the control of **cell differentiation** and turnover. Both retinol and retinoic acid are active in the promotion of growth, development and tissue differentiation; they have different actions in different tissues. Like the steroid hormones (see p. 226) and vitamin D (see p. 244), retinol and retinoic acid bind to intracellular receptors, and regulate the transcription of genes. A large number of genes are sensitive to control by retinol and retinoic acid in different tissues, and at different stages in development.

Carotene Quite apart from their rôle as precursors of vitamin A, carotenes may be important in their own right. As discussed on p. 249, free-radical damage to tissues can have a variety of serious effects, including

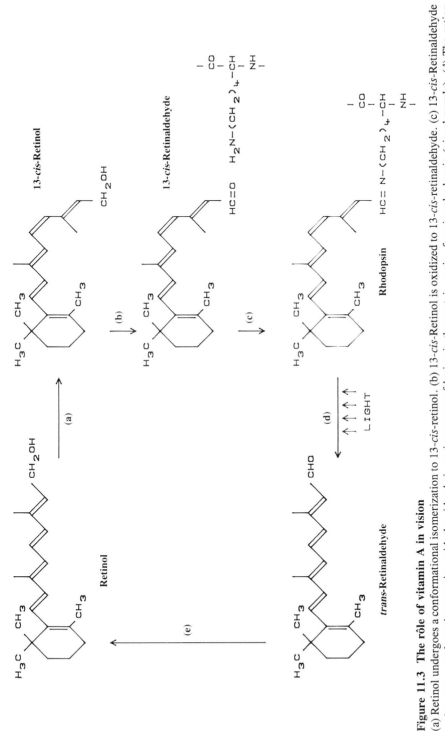

Figure 11.3 The rôle of vitamin A in vision

(a) Retinol undergoes a conformational isomerization to 13-*cis*-retinol. (b) 13-*cis*-Retinol is oxidized to 13-*cis*-retinaldehyde. (c) 13-*cis*-Retinaldehyde undergoes a condensation reaction with the side-chain amino group of lysine in the protein opsin, forming rhodopsin (visual purple). (d) The action of light on rhodopsin causes isomerization of 13-*cis*-retinaldehyde to *trans*-retinaldehyde, and cleavage of the bond between retinaldehyde and opsin. The conformational change in opsin is responsible for the initiation of nerve transmission to the brain. (e) Retinaldehyde is reduced back to retinol.

damage to DNA, which may result in the development of cancer. Carotene is one of a group of micronutrients collectively known as the **antioxidant nutrients**, because they can prevent oxidative damage to cells. Carotenes can react with radicals to form relatively stable, unreactive, radicals because the unpaired electron can be delocalized through the conjugated double-bond system of carotene.

There is epidemiological evidence that high intakes of carotene are associated with a lower risk of developing some forms of cancer, or at least that some forms of cancer are associated with low intakes of fruits and vegetables rich in carotene, and low plasma and tissue concentrations of carotene. There is little evidence yet as to whether supplements of carotene above that obtained from a normal mixed diet provide protection against cancer or other diseases, and no evidence on which to base reference intakes of carotene other than as a precursor of retinol.

Deficiency

The earliest signs of vitamin A deficiency are connected with vision. Initially, there is a loss of sensitivity to green light; this is followed by impairment of the ability to adapt to dim light, followed by inability to see at all in dim light: **night blindness**. More prolonged or severe deficiency leads to the condition called **xerophthalmia**: keratinization of the cornea, followed by ulceration. This is the most important preventable cause of blindness in the world. At the same time there are changes in the skin, again with considerable excessive formation of keratinized tissue.

As discussed on p. 180, signs of vitamin A deficiency also occur in protein–energy malnutrition, regardless of whether or not the intake of vitamin A is adequate. This is due to impairment of the synthesis of the **plasma retinol-binding protein** which is required to transport retinol from liver reserves to its sites of action. Hence functional vitamin A deficiency can occur secondary to protein–energy malnutrition.

Requirements

Vitamin A requirements are based on the intakes required to maintain a concentration of $20\,\mu g$ retinol/g in the liver. This concentration is adequate to maintain normal plasma concentrations of the vitamin, and people with this level of liver reserves can be maintained on a vitamin A-free diet for many months before they develop any detectable signs of deficiency. As the concentration of retinol in the liver increases above about $20\,\mu g/g$, so there is an increased rate of metabolism and excretion of the vitamin. The average requirement to maintain a concentration of $20 \mu g/g$ of liver is $6.7 \mu g$ retinol equivalents/kg body weight.

Toxicity

Although there is an increase in the rate of metabolism and excretion of retinol as the concentration in the liver rises above $20 \mu g/g$, there is only a limited capacity to metabolize the vitamin. Excessively high intakes lead to undesirable accumulation in the liver and other tissues, and can cause liver and bone damage, hair loss, vomiting and headaches. While large single doses can be acutely toxic, the main concern is with the chronic toxicity of habitually high intakes. Children are more sensitive to vitamin A intoxication than adults.

Although it is required for normal limb development, vitamin A can be teratogenic in excess. Pregnant women are recommended to consume no more than $3,300 \mu g/day$. Indeed, because of the high vitamin A content of some liver on sale, pregnant women have been advised to avoid eating liver and liver products.

The recommended upper limits of habitual intake of retinol are shown in Table 11.4. These apply only to preformed retinol. Excessive intake of carotene is not known to have any adverse effects, apart from giving an orange-yellow colour to the skin.

Table 11.4 Recommended upper limits of habitual intakes of preformed retinol.

	Upper limit of intake ($\mu g/day$)	RNI ($\mu g/day$)
Infants	900	350
1–3 years	1800	400
4–6 years	3000	500
6–12 years	4500	500
13–20 years	6000	600–700
Adult men	9000	700
Adult women	7500	600
Pregnant women	3300	700

Vitamin D

The normal dietary form of vitamin D is cholecalciferol. This is also the compound which is formed in the skin in sunlight. Some foods are enriched or fortified with the synthetic compound ergocalciferol. Ergocalciferol undergoes the same metabolism as cholecalciferol, and has the same biological activity.

Like vitamin A, vitamin D was measured in international units of biological activity before the pure compound was isolated. Although the iu is now obsolete, you will sometimes find it used:

1iu = 25 ng of cholecalciferol

1 μg of cholecalciferol = 40 iu.

Synthesis of vitamin D in the skin

As shown in Figure 11.4, the steroid 7-dehydrocholesterol (which is an intermediate in the synthesis of cholesterol), can undergo a non-enzymic reaction in the dermis on exposure to ultraviolet light, yielding first of all a compound called previtamin D. This slowly undergoes a further reaction (over a period of many hours) to form cholecalciferol, which is absorbed into the bloodstream.

Although, as discussed below, excessive dietary vitamin D is toxic, excessive exposure to sunlight does not lead to vitamin D poisoning. There is a limited capacity to form the precursor, 7-dehydrocholesterol, in the skin, and a limited capacity to take up cholecalciferol from the skin. Furthermore, prolonged exposure of previtamin D to ultraviolet light results in further reactions to yield biologically inactive compounds.

There are very few rich dietary sources of vitamin D: oily fish such as herring and mackerel, eggs, butter and margarine. In temperate climates there is a marked seasonal variation in the plasma concentration of vitamin D; it is highest at the end of summer, and lowest at the end of winter. Although there may be bright sunlight in winter, even in the south of England there is very little ultraviolet radiation of the appropriate wavelength for cholecalciferol synthesis when the sun is low in the sky. By contrast, in summer, when the sun is more or less overhead, there is a considerable amount of ultraviolet light even on a slightly cloudy day, and enough can penetrate thin clothes to result in significant formation of vitamin D.

In northerly climates, and especially in polluted industrial cities with little sunlight, people may well not be exposed to enough ultraviolet light to meet their vitamin D needs, and they will be reliant on the few dietary sources of the vitamin.

242

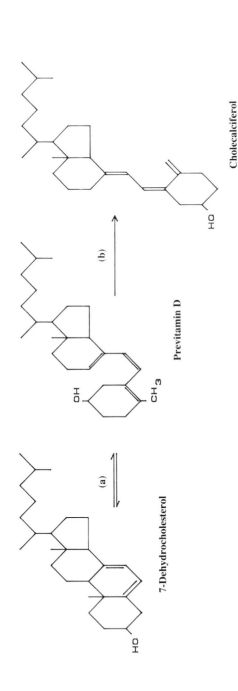

7-Dehydrocholesterol

(a)

Previtamin D

(b)

Cholecalciferol

Figure 11.4 The synthesis of vitamin D from 7-dehydrocholesterol
(a) 7-Dehydrocholesterol in the skin undergoes a reversible cleavage reaction on exposure to ultra-violet light, resulting in the formation of previtamin D. (b) Previtamin D undergoes a slow isomerization reaction to form cholecalciferol (vitamin D) which is then absorbed into the bloodstream.

The metabolism of vitamin D

Cholecalciferol, either synthesized in the skin or taken in from foods, is metabolized as shown in Figure 11.5. In the liver it is hydroxylated to form calcidiol, then in the kidney this is converted to either calcitriol, which is the active hormone, or to 24-hydroxycalcidiol, which has no biological activity, but is metabolized further, then excreted in the bile.

The metabolic rôle of vitamin D is in the control of **calcium homeostasis**. In turn, the activities of the two enzymes which metabolize calcidiol to either (active) calcitriol or (inactive) 24-hydroxycalcidiol are controlled by the state of calcium balance. As serum calcium falls, **parathyroid hormone** is secreted from the parathyroid gland. Parathyroid hormone both stimulates the enzyme which forms calcitriol and inhibits the enzyme which forms 24-hydroxycalcidiol. Thus, as serum calcium falls, so there is increased formation of the active metabolite of vitamin D, which acts to raise serum calcium.

Metabolic functions of vitamin D

Calcitriol acts like a steroid hormone (see p. 226). It enters cells of the intestinal mucosa and binds to a nuclear receptor protein. The calcitriol-receptor complex then binds to the enhancer site of the gene coding for a calcium-binding protein, increasing its transcription and so increasing the amount of calcium-binding protein in the cell. This increases the capacity of the intestinal mucosa to absorb calcium from the diet, and raises the plasma concentration of calcium.

Calcitriol also stimulates the mobilization of calcium from the bones, in order to maintain an adequate plasma concentration for nerve and muscle action. However, it also acts to stimulate the laying down of new bone to replace that lost.

Deficiency: rickets and osteomalacia

Historically, rickets is a disease of toddlers, especially in northern industrial cities. The bones are undermineralized, as a result of poor absorption of calcium in the absence of adequate amounts of calcitriol. When the child begins to walk, the long bones of the legs are deformed, leading to bow-legs or knock knees. More seriously, rickets can also lead to collapse of the rib-cage, and deformities of the bones of the pelvis. Similar problems may also occur in adolescents who are deficient in vitamin D during the adolescent growth spurt, when there is again a high demand for calci-

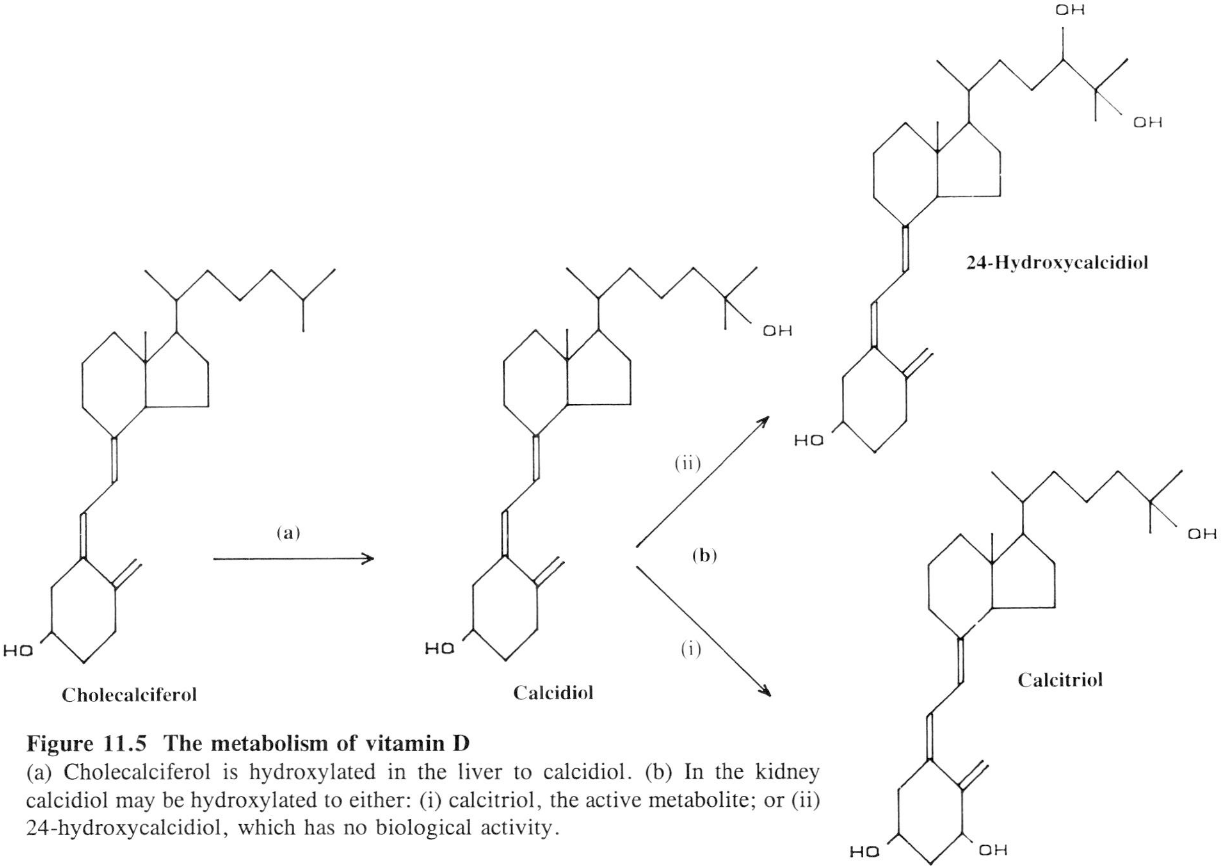

Cholecalciferol

(a)

Calcidiol

(ii)

(b)

(i)

24-Hydroxycalcidiol

Calcitriol

Figure 11.5 The metabolism of vitamin D

(a) Cholecalciferol is hydroxylated in the liver to calcidiol. (b) In the kidney calcidiol may be hydroxylated to either: (i) calcitriol, the active metabolite; or (ii) 24-hydroxycalcidiol, which has no biological activity.

um for new bone formation.

Osteomalacia is the adult equivalent of rickets. It results from the demineralization of bone, rather than the failure to mineralize it in the first place, as is the case with rickets. Women who have little exposure to sunlight are especially at risk from osteomalacia after several pregnancies, because of the strain which pregnancy places on their marginal reserve of calcium. Osteomalacia also occurs fairly commonly in the elderly. Here again the problem may be inadequate exposure to sunlight, but there is also evidence that the capacity to form 7-dehydrocholesterol in the skin decreases with advancing age, so that the elderly are more reliant on the few dietary sources of vitamin D.

Rickets and osteomalacia are an important problem of public health and nutrition among Asians living in northern Europe. Three factors combine to put this group of people at particular risk:

(a) As noted above, there are few dietary sources of vitamin D, and strict vegetarians will receive little or no preformed vitamin D in the diet.

(b) A diet based on unleavened wholemeal bread (chapattis) contains a large amount of phytate, which seriously reduces the absorption of calcium (see p. 282). Calcium deficiency may be a factor in the aetiology of rickets and osteomalacia independent of vitamin D status.

(c) Traditional modesty means that in general Asian people, and especially women and girls, are less exposed to sunlight, and expose less of their bodies, than do other groups of the population. In any case, there is considerably less ultraviolet radiation in northern Europe than in India or east Africa. It is unlikely that skin pigmentation is a factor here, since rickets and osteomalacia are not a significant problem among African and Afro-Caribbean people in northern Europe.

The other degenerative bone disease of the elderly is **osteoporosis**. This is not associated with vitamin D deficiency (although it may occur together with osteomalacia in some people). The underlying cause of osteoporosis is the loss of oestrogens (in women) and androgens (in men) with increasing age; the sex steroids are important in controlling the normal metabolism of bone. Supplements of vitamin D do not affect the development and progression of osteoporosis.

Requirements

It is difficult to determine requirements for vitamin D, since the major source is synthesis in the skin. For this reason, there are no RNIs for children over 4 years of age, or for adults aged under 65.

For the elderly, the RNI is $10\,\mu$g/day, a level of intake which maintains a plasma concentration of calcidiol above 20 nmol/l, the lower end of the reference range in younger people who have adequate sunlight exposure. This will almost certainly require either fortification of foods with the vitamin or the use of vitamin D supplements the average intake of vitamin D from the few foods which are rich sources is less than 4 μg/day.

Toxicity

During the 1940s and 1950s, rickets was more or less totally eradicated in Britain. This was the result of the enrichment of a large number of infant foods with vitamin D. However, a small number of infants suffered from vitamin D poisoning, the most serious effect of which is an elevated plasma concentration of calcium. This can lead to contraction of blood vessels, and hence dangerously high blood pressure. It can also lead to calcinosis: the calcification of soft tissues, including the kidney, heart, lungs and blood vessel walls.

Some infants are sensitive to intakes of vitamin D as low as 50 μg/day (compared with an RNI of 8.5 μg for infants). In order to avoid the serious problem of vitamin D poisoning in these susceptible infants, the extent to which infant foods are fortified with vitamin D has been reduced considerably. Unfortunately, this means that a small proportion, who have relatively high requirements, are now at risk of developing rickets. The problem is to identify those who have high requirements, and provide them with supplements.

The toxic threshold in adults is not known, but all those patients suffering from vitamin D intoxication who have been investigated were taking more than 250 μg of vitamin D/day.

Vitamin E

Vitamin E is the generic descriptor for two families of compounds, the **tocopherols** and the tocotrienols (see Fig. 11.6). The different vitamers have different biological potency. The most active is α-tocopherol, and it is usual to express vitamin E intake in terms of **mg α-tocopherol equivalents**. This is calculated by adding:

mg α-tocopherol
+ 0.5 x mg ß-tocopherol
+ 0.1 x mg γ-tocopherol
+ 0.3 x mg α-tocotrienol.

The other vitamers either occur in negligible amounts in foods or have negligible vitamin activity.

Although it is obsolete, the international unit of vitamin E activity is still sometimes used:

1iu = 0.67mg α-tocopherol equivalent

1mg α-tocopherol = 1.49iu.

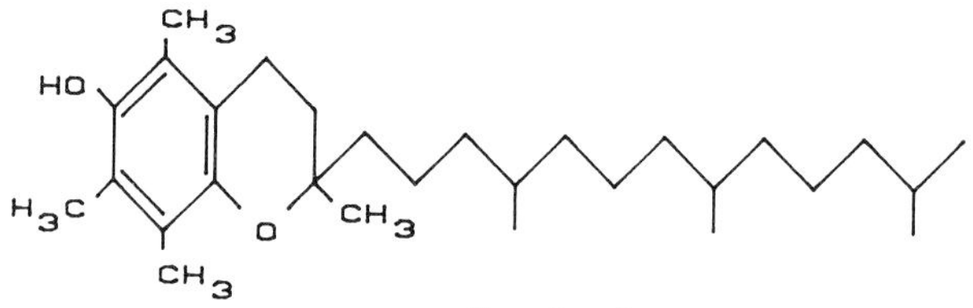

α-Tocopherol

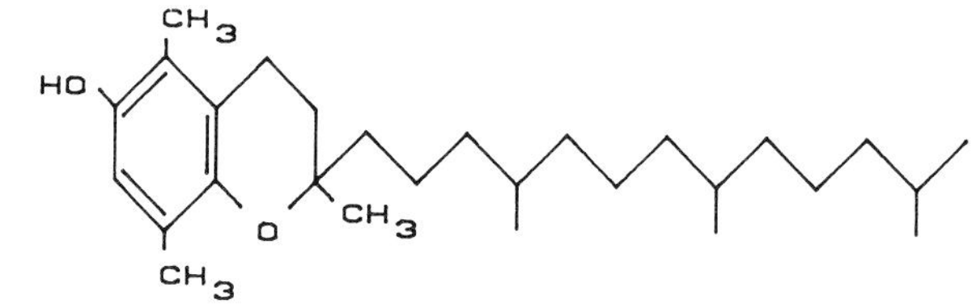

β-Tocopherol

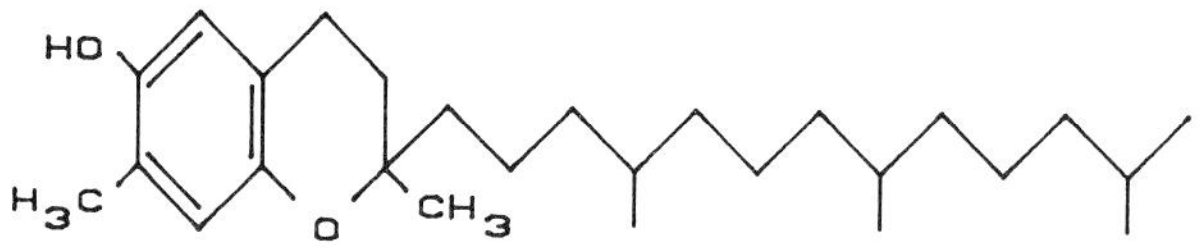

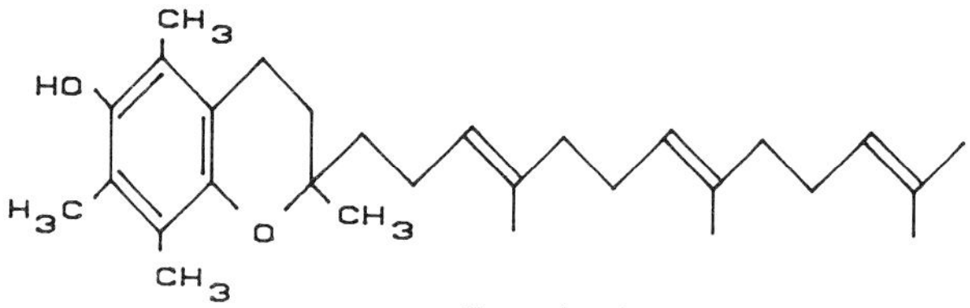

γ-Tocopherol

α-Tocotrienol

Figure 11.6 The major forms of vitamin E

The different vitamin E vitamers have different biological activity. The most potent is α-tocopherol.

Relative potency
(α-tocopherol = 1.0)

ß-tocopherol	0.49
γ-tocopherol	0.10
α-tocotrienol	0.29

Synthetic α-tocopherol does not have the same biological potency as the naturally occurring compound. This is because the side-chain of tocopherol has three centres of asymmetry and when it is synthesized chemically the result is a mixture of the various isomers. In the naturally occurring compound all three centres of asymmetry have the *R*-configuration (see p. 67). Therefore naturally occurring α-tocopherol is sometimes called all-*R*, or *RRR*-α-tocopherol.

Metabolic functions and deficiency

The function of vitamin E is as a **radical-trapping antioxidant**, especially in cell membranes. It is especially important in limiting oxidative radical damage to polyunsaturated fatty acids. As discussed on p. 67, free radicals are chemically highly reactive, because they have an unpaired electron. They interact with other compounds, creating a new radical in turn.

The most important radicals in terms of causing damage to cells are oxygen radicals. They are formed as a part of the normal oxidative metabolism of the cell, including the oxidation of reduced flavoproteins (see p. 119). In addition, oxygen radicals are produced by activated lymphocytes and macrophages as a part of their cytotoxic action, and also in the metabolism of a variety of chemicals that we are exposed to through environmental pollution and sometimes as medication.

Radiation (e.g. from X-rays and radioactive isotopes) also leads to the formation of radicals. The formation of radicals is responsible for the beneficial effects of radiotherapy in killing tumour cells, but also for the undesirable effects (carcinogenesis and mutagenesis) of environmental and occupational exposure to radiation.

The main biological damage caused by oxygen radicals is to polyunsaturated fatty acids in cell membranes (see p. 83). Polyunsaturated fatty acids can be oxidized to lipid peroxides, which are highly reactive radicals and can go on to attack further molecules of polyunsaturated fatty acid. This sets up a chain reaction, causing irreparable damage to the cell membrane. The products of the breakdown of lipid peroxides are also reactive compounds, and can interact with proteins and nucleic acids. Damage to DNA can result in inappropriate base-pairing during replication; if this occurs in the germ cells (ova or spermatozoa) the result is a **mutation**; in other cells the damage to DNA may lead to the development of cancer.

We have already seen that carotene acts to trap free radicals before they can cause tissue damage. Vitamin E has a similar action, trapping free radicals formed by oxidative attack on polyunsaturated fatty acids before they can establish a chain reaction in the membrane. The radical formed from vitamin E is relatively unreactive, and quenches the chain reaction.

The vitamin E radical is inactivated, and the active vitamin reformed, by reaction with vitamin C, as shown in Figure 11.7.

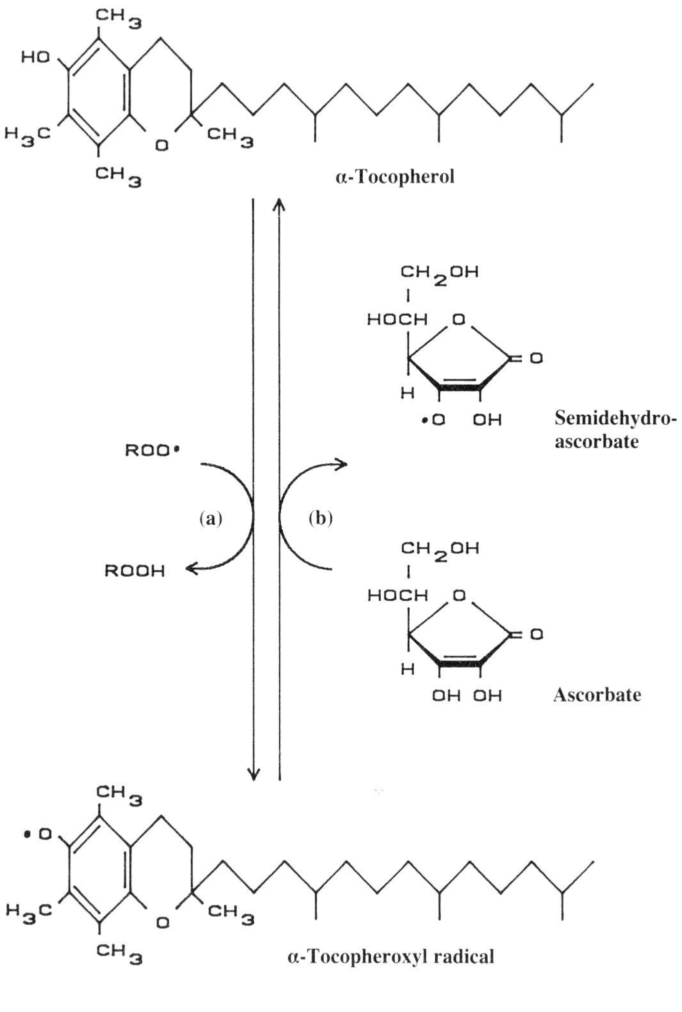

Figure 11.7 The rôle of vitamin E as a chain-breaking antioxidant
(a) α-Tocopherol in membranes can react with lipid hydroperoxide radicals, formed by the action of oxygen radicals on unsaturated fatty acids, to yield stable non-radical products. In the process, the relatively stable tocopheroxyl radical is formed. (b) The tocopheroxyl radical can be reduced back to α-tocopherol by reaction with ascorbic acid (vitamin C) in the plasma or extracellular fluid. This results in the formation of the stable semidehydro-ascorbate radical, which can be reduced back to ascorbate (see Fig. 11.19).

250

Dietary deficiency of vitamin E in human beings is unknown, although patients with severe fat malabsorption, cystic fibrosis, some forms of chronic liver disease and (very rare) congenital lack of plasma ß-lipoprotein, suffer deficiency because they are unable to absorb the vitamin or transport it around the body. They suffer from severe damage to nerve and muscle membranes.

Premature infants are at risk of vitamin E deficiency, since they are often born with inadequate reserves of the vitamin. The red blood cell membranes of deficient infants are abnormally fragile, as a result of unchecked oxidative radical attack. This may lead to haemolytic anaemia if they are not given supplements of the vitamin.

Experimental animals depleted of vitamin E become sterile. However, there is no evidence that the nutritional status of vitamin E is in any way associated with human fertility, and there is certainly no evidence that vitamin E supplements increase sexual potency, prowess or vigour!

Requirements

It is difficult to establish vitamin E requirements. The requirement depends mainly on the intake of polyunsaturated fatty acids. It is generally accepted that the intake of vitamin E should be 0.4 mg α-tocopherol equivalent/g dietary polyunsaturated fatty acid. This does not present any problem, since all foods which are rich sources of polyunsaturated fatty acids (the plant oils, see Table 2.7, p. 21) are also rich sources of vitamin E.

There is some evidence that higher intakes of vitamin E may have a useful protective effect against the development of ischaemic heart disease. This is because high concentrations of vitamin E inhibit the oxidation of polyunsaturated fatty acids in plasma lipoproteins, and it is this oxidation which is responsible for the initiation of atherosclerosis. The levels that appear to be beneficial are of the order of 17–40 mg α-tocopherol/day, which is above what could be achieved by eating ordinary foods.

Vitamin K

Vitamin K was discovered as a result of investigations into the cause of a bleeding disorder (haemorrhagic disease) of cattle fed on silage made from sweet clover, and of chickens fed on a fat-free diet. The missing factor in the diet of the chickens was identified as vitamin K, while the problem in the cattle was that their diet contained an antagonist of the vitamin.

Since the effect of either deficiency of the vitamin or an excessive intake of the antagonist was severely to impair blood clotting, the antagonist was isolated and tested in smaller amounts as an **anticoagulant**, for use in patients at risk of thrombosis. Although it was effective, the naturally occurring antagonist had unwanted side-effects, and synthetic vitamin K antagonists were developed for clinical use as anticoagulants. The most commonly used of these is Warfarin. Warfarin is also used as a poison to kill rats and mice. In small doses it causes a slight impairment of blood clotting, which is what is required in patients at risk of thrombosis. In excess, it causes a very severe impairment of blood clotting, and the victims suffer from haemorrhage.

Three compounds have the biological activity of vitamin K (see Fig. 11.8):

(a) **phylloquinone**, which is the normal dietary source, being found in green leafy vegetables;

(b) the **menaquinones**, which are a family of closely related compounds synthesized by intestinal bacteria, with differing lengths of the side-chain;

(c) **menadione**, a synthetic compound which can be metabolized to yield phylloquinone.

Metabolic functions

Although it has been known since the 1920s that vitamin K was required for blood clotting, it was not until the 1970s that its precise function was established. It is the cofactor for the carboxylation of glutamate residues in the post-synthetic modification of proteins to form the unusual amino acid γ-**carboxyglutamate** (see Fig. 11.9).

Prothrombin and several other proteins of the blood-clotting system contain between four and six γ-carboxyglutamate residues. This amino acid chelates calcium ions, and so permits the binding of the blood-clotting proteins to lipid membranes. In vitamin K deficiency, or in the presence of an antagonist such as Warfarin, an abnormal precursor of prothrombin containing little or no γ-carboxyglutamate is released into the circulation. This abnormal protein cannot chelate calcium or bind to phospholipid membranes, and it is therefore unable to initiate blood clotting.

Another protein also contains γ-carboxyglutamate, and is dependent on vitamin K for its formation. This is **osteocalcin**, one of the calcium-binding proteins of bone matrix. Infants born to mothers treated with Warfarin are at risk of severe bone deformities (the fetal Warfarin syndrome) as a result of impaired synthesis of osteocalcin.

It can be seen from Figure 11.9 that vitamin K is oxidized to the epox-

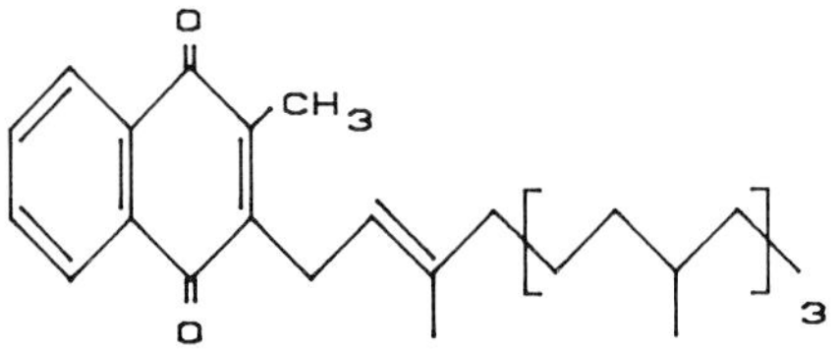

Phylloquinone

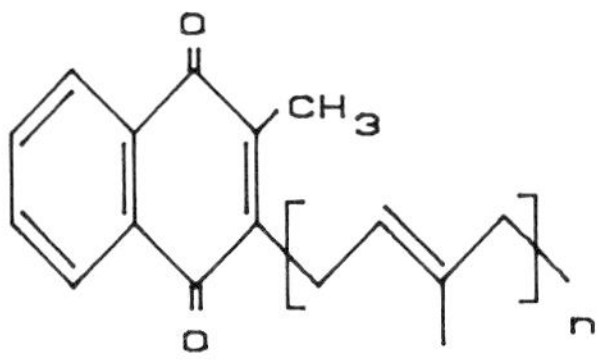

Menaquinone

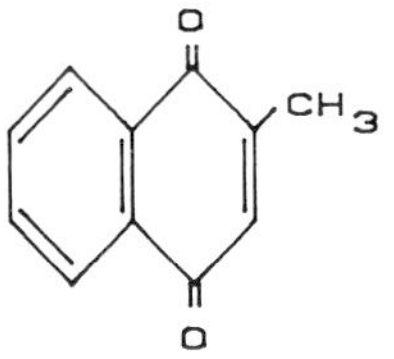

Menadione

Figure 11.8 Vitamin K vitamers
Phylloquinone is the main dietary form of vitamin K, found in a variety of plant foods. Intestinal bacteria produce a variety of menaquinones (with varying lengths of the side-chain) which are absorbed and make some contribution to vitamin K nutrition. Menadione is a synthetic compound which can be converted to phylloquinone in the liver. It is little used nowadays, since the conversion to phylloquinone is relatively slow and unmetabolized menadione can cause liver damage.

ide during the carboxylation of glutamate. Normally the epoxide is reduced back to the active form of the vitamin. It is this reduction which is inhibited by Warfarin. Even in the presence of Warfarin, glutamate carboxylation can proceed more or less normally, provided that enough vitamin K is available to be used just once, then excreted as the epoxide and its metabolites. High doses of vitamin K are used to treat patients who have received an overdose of Warfarin.

It is possible that patients who are being treated with Warfarin could overcome the beneficial effects of their medication if they took supple-

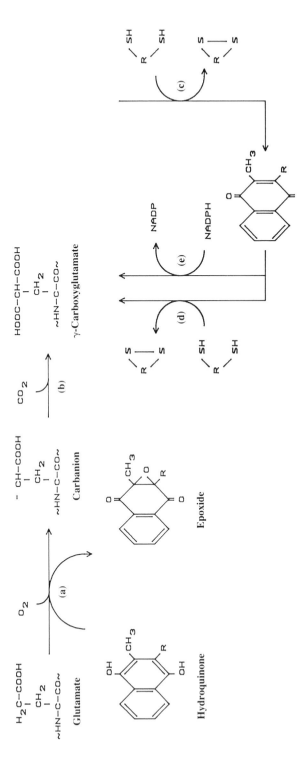

Figure 11.9 The role of vitamin K in the carboxylation of glutamate in proteins

(a) The reduced form of vitamin K (the hydroquinone) removes a hydrogen ion from a glutamate in the protein, forming the glutamate carbanion, and reacting with oxygen to form vitamin K epoxide. (b) The glutamate carbanion reacts with carbon dioxide to form γ-carboxyglutamate. (c) Vitamin K epoxide is reduced to vitamin K quinone in a reaction in which a disulphydryl compound is oxidized to a disulphide. This reaction is inhibited by anticoagulants such as Warfarin. (d) Vitamin K quinone is reduced to the hydroquinone by a similar reaction in which a disulphydryl compound is oxidized to a disulphide. This reaction is also inhibited by anticoagulants such as Warfarin. (e) Vitamin K quinone can also be reduced to the hydroquinone by a Warfarin-insensitive reaction in which NADPH is oxidized to NADP.

ments of vitamin K. The danger would be that if their dose of Warfarin was increased to counteract the effects of the vitamin supplements and they then stopped taking the supplements, they would be receiving considerably too much Warfarin, and would be at risk of haemorrhage. It is most unlikely that a normal diet could provide such an excess of vitamin K; it would need a habitual intake of 250g a day of broccoli or other vitamin K rich vegetables to have any significant effect on Warfarin action.

Requirements

Determination of vitamin K requirements is complicated by the fact that we do not know how important a contribution to intake is made by the menaquinones synthesized by intestinal bacteria. However, a prolonged blood clotting time is observed in volunteers maintained on vitamin K deficient diets, so there is clearly a need for a dietary intake.

Because of the lack of evidence, there is no RNI for vitamin K. An intake of $1 \mu g/kg$ body weight/day is considered safe and adequate, since at this level of intake there is no evidence of any impairment of blood clotting.

A small number of new-born infants have very low reserves of vitamin K, and are at risk of **haemorrhagic disease** of the new-born. It is therefore generally recommended that all new-born infants should be given a single prophylactic dose of vitamin K. This should preferably be given by mouth, rather than by injection, since there is some evidence to suggest a link between injection of vitamin K at birth and an increased risk of leukaemia.

Vitamin B₁ (thiamin)

Thiamin, as the diphosphate (see Fig. 11.10), is the coenzyme for several oxidative decarboxylation reactions. The most important of these are pyruvate dehydrogenase (see Fig. 6.7 on p. 141) in **carbohydrate metabolism** and 2-oxoglutarate dehydrogenase in the **citric acid cycle** (see Fig. 6.8 on p. 142). This means that thiamin has a central rôle in metabolism. In addition, thiamin triphosphate has a rôle in the conduction of nerve impulses, which has not been completely elucidated.

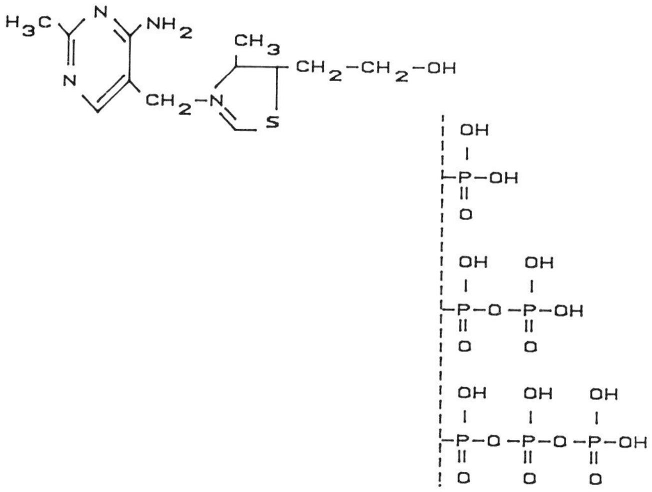

Figure 11.10 Thiamin – vitamin B_1

Thiamin can be esterified with one, two or three phosphates, forming thiamin mono-, di- and triphosphates. The active coenzyme form of thiamin is thiamin diphosphate. Thiamin triphosphate has a rôle in nerve conduction.

Deficiency

Two different diseases are associated with thiamin deficiency: beriberi and the Wernicke–Korsakoff syndrome.

Beriberi is associated with long-term thiamin deficiency, with a generally low food intake but a relatively high intake of carbohydrate. It is mainly a problem in Southeast Asia. There is damage to the peripheral nervous system, with ascending neuritis, which causes muscle weakness and atrophy. This begins with weakness, pain and stiffness in the legs, and spreads upwards: the ankle-jerk reflex is lost, then the muscles of the calf are affected, and the patient is unable to keep either the toes or the whole foot off the ground. The hands and arms may also be affected. Although there is loss of sensation in the affected regions, there is also deep muscle pain.

The heart can also be affected in beriberi, especially in people whose diet is high in carbohydrate. There is **right-sided heart failure**, leading to oedema. In some patients, the oedema and heart failure may occur without the nerve damage being apparent.

In Western countries, thiamin deficiency is seen in alcoholics and narcotic addicts. Here the damage is to the central nervous system. Patients develop **Korsakoff's psychosis**, which is characterized by loss of recent memory, although memory for distant events is normally unimpaired, and what is called confabulation – the making up of wondrous stories. Later there are clinical signs of central nervous system damage: **Wernicke's encephalopathy**. The Wernicke–Korsakoff syndrome is associated with a relatively acute deficiency of thiamin, with a relatively high energy intake. In alcoholics the problem is made worse because alcohol impairs the absorption of thiamin from the gut.

Requirements

The requirement for thiamin depends on energy expenditure. RNIs are based on 95μg thiamin/MJ energy expenditure. The main sources of thiamin in the diet are cereals (it is added to flour and breakfast cereals to replace losses in milling), vegetables and meat. Pork and ham are especially rich sources of thiamin.

Vitamin B$_2$ (riboflavin)

Like thiamin, riboflavin is involved in the metabolism of metabolic fuels, as the coenzyme of a wide variety of enzymes involved in oxidation and reduction reactions (the flavoproteins, see Fig. 5.7 on p. 119). Riboflavin and the flavin coenzymes are shown in Figure 11.11. Flavoproteins are important in the metabolism of carbohydrates, fatty acids and amino acids, as well as in the electron transport chain in mitochondria.

Deficiency

Although riboflavin is involved in all areas of metabolism, and deficiency is widespread on a global scale, deficiency is not fatal. The clinical signs of deficiency are cracking at the edges of the lips (cheilosis) and corners of the mouth (angular stomatitis), painful loss of the normal epithelium of the tongue (glossitis), and skin lesions resembling seborrhoea.

There seem to be two reasons why deficiency is not fatal. One is that although deficiency is common, the vitamin is widespread in foods, and most diets will provide minimally adequate amounts of the vitamin to permit maintenance of central metabolic pathways. The second, more important, reason is that in deficiency there is extremely efficient re-utilization of the riboflavin that is released by the turnover of flavoproteins, so that only a very small amount is metabolized or excreted.

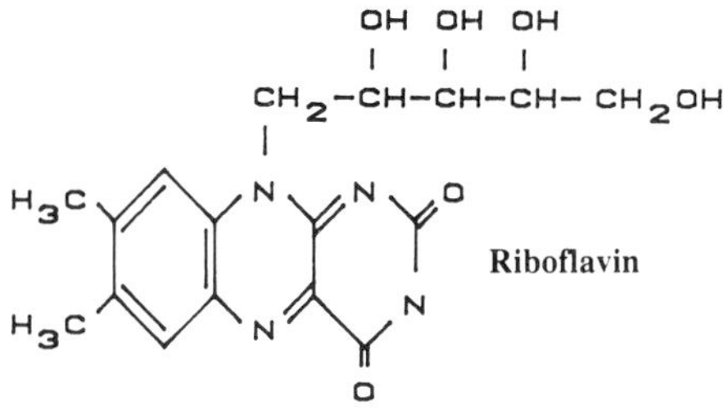

Riboflavin

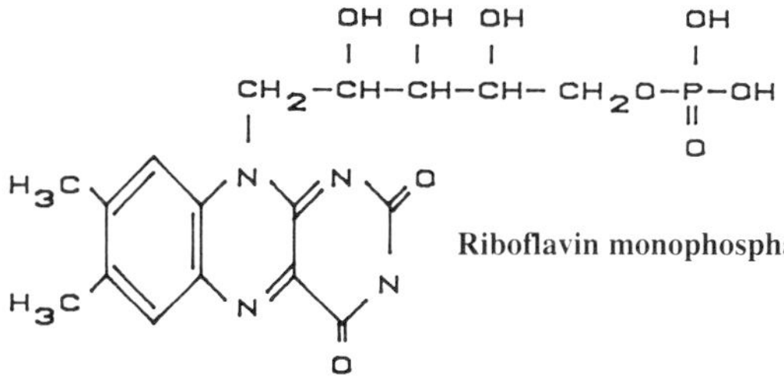

Riboflavin monophosphate

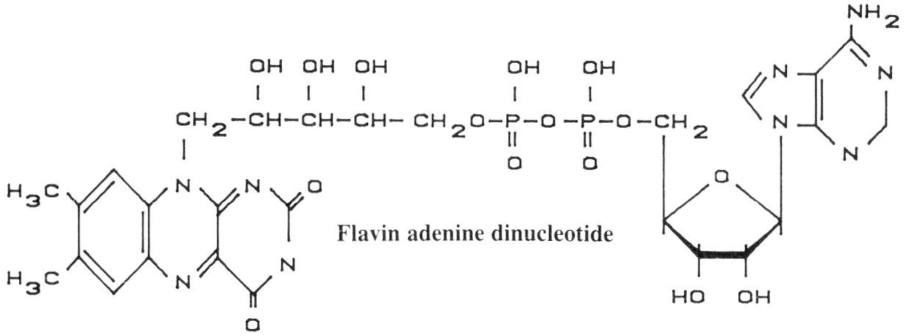

Flavin adenine dinucleotide

Figure 11.11 Riboflavin and the flavin coenzymes
Riboflavin acts as a coenzyme in a wide variety of oxidation and reduction reactions; it may be present in the enzyme as a covalently bound derivative of free riboflavin, or as riboflavin monophosphate (sometimes called flavin mononucleotide) or flavin adenine dinucleotide (FAD). See Figure 5.7 on p. 119 for the rôle of riboflavin and the flavin coenzymes in oxidation and reduction reactions.

Requirements

Estimates of riboflavin requirements are based on depletion/repletion studies to determine the minimum intake at which there is significant excretion of the vitamin. As noted above, in deficiency there is virtually no excretion of the vitamin; as requirements are met, so any excess is excreted in the urine.

A more generous estimate of requirements, and the basis of the RNI, is the level of intake at which there is normalization of the activity of the red cell enzyme **glutathione reductase**; this is a flavoprotein whose activity is especially sensitive to riboflavin nutritional status.

The main sources of riboflavin are milk and milk products, meat (especially liver and kidney) and eggs.

Niacin

Two compounds, nicotinic acid and nicotinamide have the biological activity of niacin (see Fig. 11.12). As discussed below, it can also be synthesized in the body from the essential amino acid tryptophan.

Nicotinic acid   Nicotinamide

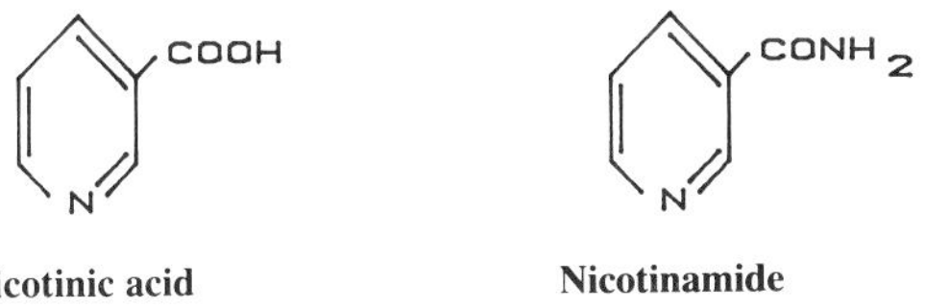

Figure 11.12 The niacin vitamers, nicotinic acid and nicotinamide
Nicotinic acid and nicotinamide can both be incorporated into the nicotinamide nucleotide coenzymes, NAD and NADP, which function in a wide variety of oxidation and reduction reactions (see Fig. 5.6 on p. 117).

Niacin is also involved in the metabolism of metabolic fuels, as the functional nicotinamide part of the coenzymes NAD and NADP (see Fig. 5.6 on p. 117).

Deficiency

Deficiency of niacin results in the disease **pellagra**. This is characterized by a sunburn-like rash in areas of the skin exposed to sunlight, and a depressive psychosis. Untreated pellagra is fatal, and was a major cause of death in the southern United States throughout the first half of the 20th century. It is still an important problem in parts of Africa and India.

Requirements

Determination of requirements for niacin is complicated by the fact that the nicotinamide part of NAD and NADP can be formed from either preformed niacin or by the metabolism of the essential amino acid tryptophan. On average, 60 mg of dietary tryptophan is equivalent to 1 mg of preformed niacin in the diet. It is usual to express niacin intake as **mg niacin equivalents**. This is calculated by adding:

mg preformed niacin (excluding cereals)

+ 1/60 mg tryptophan.

The niacin in cereals is excluded from the calculation of intake because much of it is present in a chemically bound form which is not released during digestion, so that the vitamin is not biologically available.

The average requirement for niacin is 1.3 mg niacin equivalents/MJ energy expenditure, and RNIs are based on 1.6 mg/MJ.

The metabolic pathway that leads to NAD formation from tryptophan is also the main pathway of **tryptophan metabolism**. This means that for an adult in nitrogen balance (see p. 189), an amount of tryptophan equal to the whole of the dietary intake is available for NAD synthesis. Average intakes of tryptophan in Western countries are more than adequate to meet niacin requirements without any need for preformed niacin in the diet.

Toxicity

Nicotinic acid has been used to lower blood triglycerides and cholesterol in patients with hyperlipidaemia. However, relatively large amounts are required (of the order of 1–6 g/day, compared with an RNI of 18–20 mg/day). At this level of intake, nicotinic acid causes dilatation of blood vessels and flushing, with skin irritation, itching and a burning sensation. This effect wears off after a few days.

High intakes of both nicotinic acid and nicotinamide, in excess of 500 mg/day, also cause liver damage, and prolonged use can result in liver failure. This is especially a problem with sustained-release preparations of niacin, which permit a high blood level to be maintained for a relatively long time.

Vitamin B$_6$

Six related compounds have the biological activity of vitamin B$_6$; they are all converted in the body to the metabolically active form, **pyridoxal phosphate** (see Fig. 11.13).

Pyridoxal phosphate is a coenzyme in three main areas of metabolism:

(a) in a wide variety of reactions of amino acids, and especially **transamination**, in which it functions as the intermediate carrier of the amino group (see Fig. 9.3 on p. 200);

(b) as the cofactor of **glycogen phosphorylase** in muscle and liver (see p. 150);

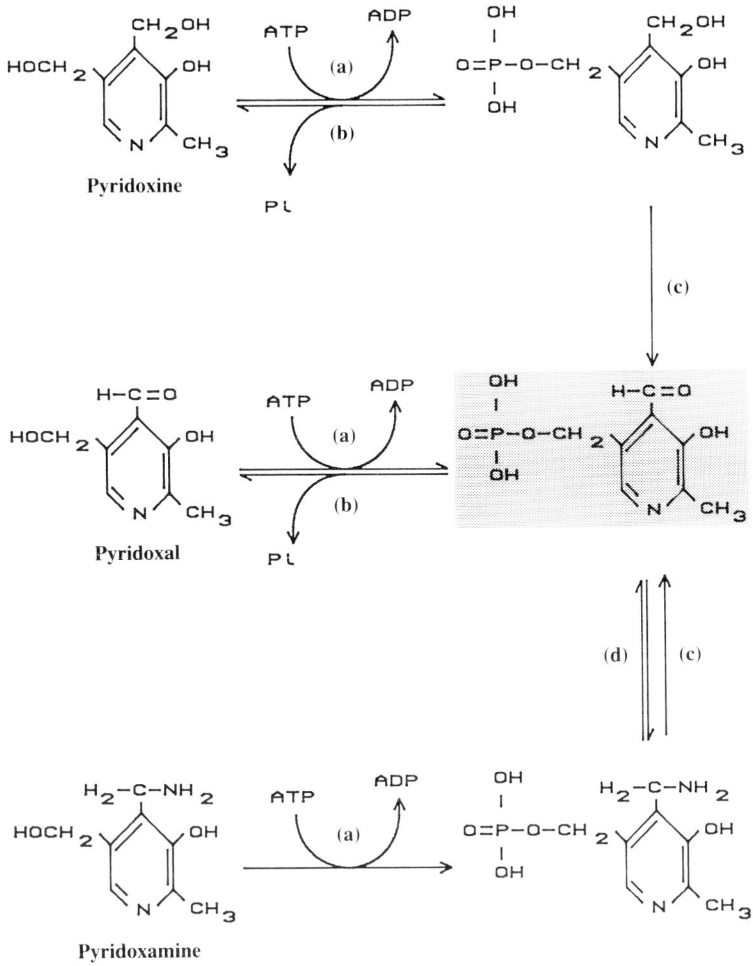

Figure 11.13 The interconversion of the vitamin B₆ vitamers

The metabolically active form of vitamin B_6 is pyridoxal phosphate (shown boxed). Foods may contain pyridoxine (the alcohol), pyridoxal (the aldehyde) or pyridoxamine (the amine) or their phosphates. These can all be converted to pyridoxal phosphate: (a) *Pyridoxine kinase* catalyses the phosphorylation of pyridoxine, pyridoxal or pyridoxamine to the phosphate. (b) *Phosphatase*: pyridoxine phosphate and pyridoxal phosphate can both be dephosphorylated by the action of a variety of phosphatases. This reaction is important for the uptake of pyridoxal phosphate from the bloodstream into tissues, since the phosphate cannot cross cell membranes, while free pyridoxal can. In the liver any surplus pyridoxal phosphate is dephosphorylated to pyridoxal and oxidized to pyridoxic acid, which is excreted. (c) *Pyridoxine phosphate oxidase* oxidizes either pyridoxine phosphate or pyridoxamine phosphate to pyridoxal phosphate. (d) *Transaminases* form pyridoxamine phosphate as part of their reaction and can interconvert pyridoxamine and pyridoxal phosphates.

261

(c) in the regulation of the action of **steroid hormones** (see p. 226). Pyridoxal phosphate acts to remove the hormone-receptor complex from gene enhancers, and so terminate the action of the hormones. In vitamin B_6 deficiency there is increased sensitivity of target tissues to the actions of low concentrations of such hormones as the oestrogens, androgens and cortisol.

Deficiency

Deficiency of vitamin B_6 is extremely rare, and clear deficiency has only been reported in one outbreak, during the 1950s, when babies were fed on a milk preparation which had been severely overheated during manufacture. Many of the affected infants went into convulsions, which responded rapidly to the administration of vitamin B_6.

The cause of the **convulsions** was severe impairment of the activity of the enzyme glutamate decarboxylase, which is dependent on pyridoxal phosphate. The product of glutamate decarboxylase is GABA (γ-aminobutyric acid), which is a regulatory neurotransmitter in the central nervous system.

Moderate vitamin B_6 deficiency results in abnormalities of amino acid metabolism. The metabolism of tryptophan and methionine is especially severely affected, and tests of tryptophan and methionine metabolism are widely used to assess vitamin B_6 nutritional status. The activity of transaminases is also impaired in vitamin B_6 deficiency, and measurement of red blood cell transaminase activity provides an additional way of assessing vitamin B_6 nutritional status.

Requirements

Although most of the body's vitamin B_6 is associated with glycogen phosphorylase in muscle, this is relatively stable and well conserved. The requirement depends not on energy expenditure and glycogen metabolism, but on the intake of protein. The average requirement is 13 μg/g dietary protein; RNIs are based on 15 μg/g protein intake, and the observed intake of protein, which is 15% of energy intake in Western countries.

The main sources of vitamin B_6 are meat, whole-grain cereals, vegetables and nuts.

Vitamin B$_6$, oral contraceptives and the premenstrual syndrome

Studies have suggested that oral contraceptives cause vitamin B$_6$ deficiency. As a result of this, supplements of vitamin B$_6$ of between 50 and 100 mg/day, and sometimes higher, have been suggested to overcome the side-effects of oral contraceptives. Similar supplements have also been recommended for the treatment of the premenstrual syndrome.

All of the studies which have suggested that oral contraceptives cause vitamin B$_6$ deficiency have used the metabolism of tryptophan as a means of assessing vitamin B$_6$ nutritional status. When other biochemical markers of status have also been assessed, they are not affected by oral contraceptive use.

Oral contraceptives do not cause vitamin B$_6$ deficiency. The problem is that both the oestrogens and the progestagens in the contraceptives inhibit the metabolism of tryptophan. This results in the excretion of abnormal amounts of tryptophan metabolites, similar to levels seen in vitamin B$_6$ deficiency, but for quite a different reason. There is no evidence that supplements have any beneficial effect in overcoming the side-effects of oral contraceptive use. There is very little evidence that vitamin B$_6$ supplements have any beneficial effect in the premenstrual syndrome.

Toxicity

Very high intakes of vitamin B$_6$ (several hundreds of mg/day) over a period of several weeks or months cause severe damage to peripheral nerves, resulting in partial paralysis. This is only partially cured by ceasing the vitamin B$_6$ supplements. More modest doses (of the order of 50–100 mg/day, still vastly in excess of requirements) cause less serious nerve damage, and result in a tingling sensation in the fingers and toes. This is reversed on cessation of the supplements.

Vitamin B$_6$ dependency syndromes

Very rarely, children show just one of the biochemical signs of vitamin B$_6$ deficiency: abnormalities of the metabolism of tryptophan or methionine, or another amino acid, or perhaps convulsions due to abnormally low activity of glutamate decarboxylase, despite an adequate intake of the vitamin. In such children, other biochemical indices of vitamin B$_6$ nutritional status are unaffected, but the metabolic abnormalities and clinical signs respond well to the administration of relatively large amounts of vitamin B$_6$.

In these children the problem is a genetic defect of just one enzyme, affecting the coenzyme-binding site. This means that the enzyme can only bind pyridoxal phosphate, and hence have significant activity, in the presence of abnormally high concentrations of the coenzyme. Such conditions are called **vitamin dependency syndromes**.

Vitamin B$_{12}$

Vitamin B$_{12}$ functions in the transfer of methyl groups in a small number of metabolic reactions. Its metabolic function is closely linked with that of folic acid (see p. 266), and indeed the signs of vitamin B$_{12}$ deficiency are due largely to derangements of folic acid metabolism. As shown in Fig. 11.14, vitamin B$_{12}$ contains the metal cobalt – the only known function of cobalt in human metabolism.

The main problem of vitamin B$_{12}$ deficiency is not nutritional, but is due to a failure to absorb the vitamin. Vitamin B$_{12}$ absorption requires a protein secreted by the parietal cells of the stomach, the **intrinsic factor**. The vitamin is liberated from proteins to which it is bound in foods by the action of acid in the stomach, and then bound by intrinsic factor. In the small intestine, the intrinsic factor-vitamin B$_{12}$ complex binds to receptors on the surface of mucosal cells for absorption. Failure of the secretion of intrinsic factor, or lack of secretion of gastric acid (**achlorhydria**), can lead to a failure to absorb vitamin B$_{12}$, and cause deficiency.

Vitamin B$_{12}$ is found only in foods of animal origin, although it is also formed by some bacteria. There are no plant sources of this vitamin. This means that strict vegetarians (vegans) who eat no foods of animal origin are at risk of developing dietary vitamin B$_{12}$ deficiency. Preparations of vitamin B$_{12}$ made by bacterial fermentation which are ethically acceptable to vegans are readily available.

Interestingly, there are claims that yeasts and some plants (especially some algae) contain vitamin B$_{12}$. This seems to be incorrect. The problem is that the officially recognized, and legally required, method of determining vitamin B$_{12}$ in food analysis depends on the growth of micro-organisms for which vitamin B$_{12}$ is an essential growth factor. However, these organisms can also use some compounds which are chemically related to vitamin B$_{12}$, but have no vitamin activity in man. Therefore analysis reveals the presence of something which appears to be vitamin B$_{12}$, but in fact is not the active vitamin, and is useless in human nutrition.

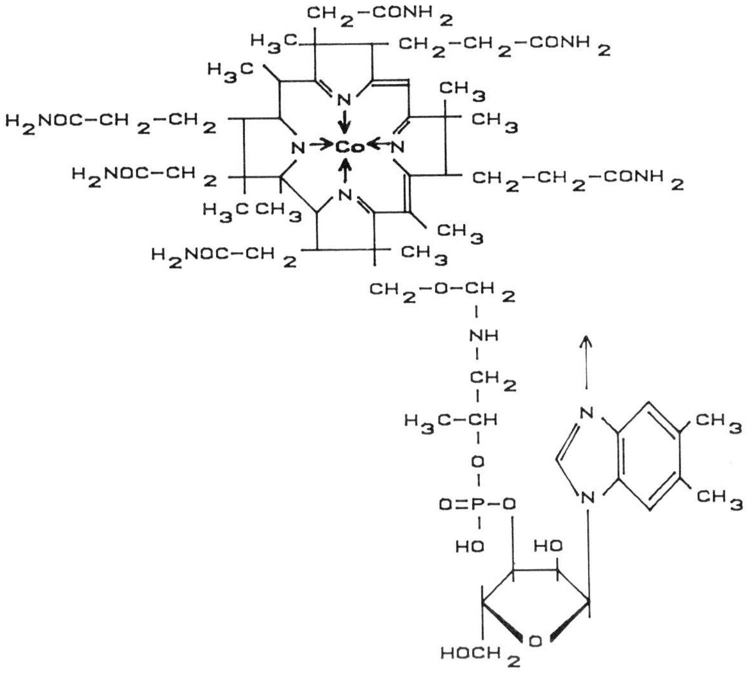

Figure 11.14 Vitamin B$_{12}$
The central cobalt (Co) atom of vitamin B$_{12}$, can be chelated by (share electrons with) six donor atoms in the molecule. Four of the chelation sites are occupied by nitrogen atoms of the central ring structure, shown by the arrows. The fifth site, below the plane of the ring, is occupied by the nitrogen of the side-chain, again shown by an arrow. The sixth site may be occupied by:

a cyanide ion (CN$^-$)   cyanocobalamin
water (H$_2$O)   aquocobalamin
a hydroxyl ion (OH$^-$)   hydroxocobalamin
a methyl group (-CH$_3$)   methylcobalamin

Deficiency

Vitamin B$_{12}$ deficiency causes **pernicious anaemia**. The anaemia is due to the release into the bloodstream of immature precursors of red blood cells **megaloblastic anaemia**. As discussed below (see p. 268), folic acid is required for the synthesis of thymidine for DNA synthesis, and vitamin B$_{12}$ deficiency interferes with the metabolism of folic acid. As a result, the rapid multiplication of red blood cells is disturbed, and immature precursors are released into the circulation.

The other clinical feature of vitamin B$_{12}$ deficiency, which is very

265

rarely seen in folic acid deficiency, is **degeneration of the spinal cord**; hence the name "pernicious" for the anaemia of vitamin B_{12} deficiency. This degeneration of the spinal cord occurs in about one-third of patients with pernicious anaemia due to vitamin B_{12} deficiency, and in about one-third of patients who do not show signs of anaemia.

The commonest cause of pernicious anaemia is a failure of the secretion of intrinsic factor. This may be the result of autoimmune disease, when the patient produces antibodies against either intrinsic factor or the parietal cells of the stomach. It can also result from atrophy of the gastric mucosa, which occurs in the elderly. Obviously, patients who have undergone gastrectomy will also be at risk. Treatment may be by oral administration of intrinsic factor, so permitting more or less normal absorption of vitamin B_{12}, or by injection of relatively large amounts of vitamin B_{12} every few months.

Requirements

Early estimates of vitamin B_{12} requirements were based on the amounts required to maintain normal red blood cell maturation in patients with pernicious anaemia due to lack of intrinsic factor secretion. However, we now know that there is a considerable enterohepatic circulation of vitamin B_{12}. It is secreted in the bile and reabsorbed in the small intestine. However, in patients with defective secretion of intrinsic factor, the vitamin cannot be reabsorbed, but is excreted in the faeces. This means that patients with impaired secretion of intrinsic factor have a very much higher requirement for vitamin B_{12} than normal.

The RNI for vitamin B_{12} is 1 μg/day. The average intake of adults who eat meat and meat products is of the order of 5 μg/day.

Folic acid

Folic acid is involved in a wide variety of metabolic reactions, as a carrier of methyl groups and other "one-carbon" fragments. As shown in Figure 11.15, several different forms of folic acid are found in foods, with different numbers of glutamate residues attached, and carrying different one-carbon fragments. The extent to which the different forms of folate acid can be absorbed varies; on average only about half of the folic acid in the diet is available.

The metabolism of folic acid is closely linked to that of vitamin B_{12}. Methyl-folic acid is a normal intermediate of folic acid metabolism; it can

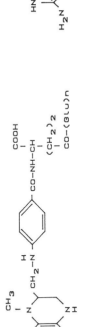

Figure 11.15 Folic acid

There can be a variable number of glutamate residues attached to folic acid, shown as (Glu)ₙ. Folic acid can exist as a variety of derivatives carrying different one-carbon fragments.

only be converted back to free folic acid by the methylation of homocysteine to methionine. This is catalysed by a vitamin B_{12}-dependent enzyme, and in vitamin B_{12} deficiency much of the body's folic acid accumulates as methyl-folate, which cannot now be utilized. Thus, vitamin B_{12} deficiency results in secondary folic acid deficiency, despite an apparently adequate intake of this vitamin.

The administration of folic acid supplements to patients with megaloblastic anaemia due to vitamin B_{12} deficiency can cause the degeneration of the spinal cord, so it is important to eliminate vitamin B_{12} deficiency as a cause of megaloblastic anaemia before treating with folic acid.

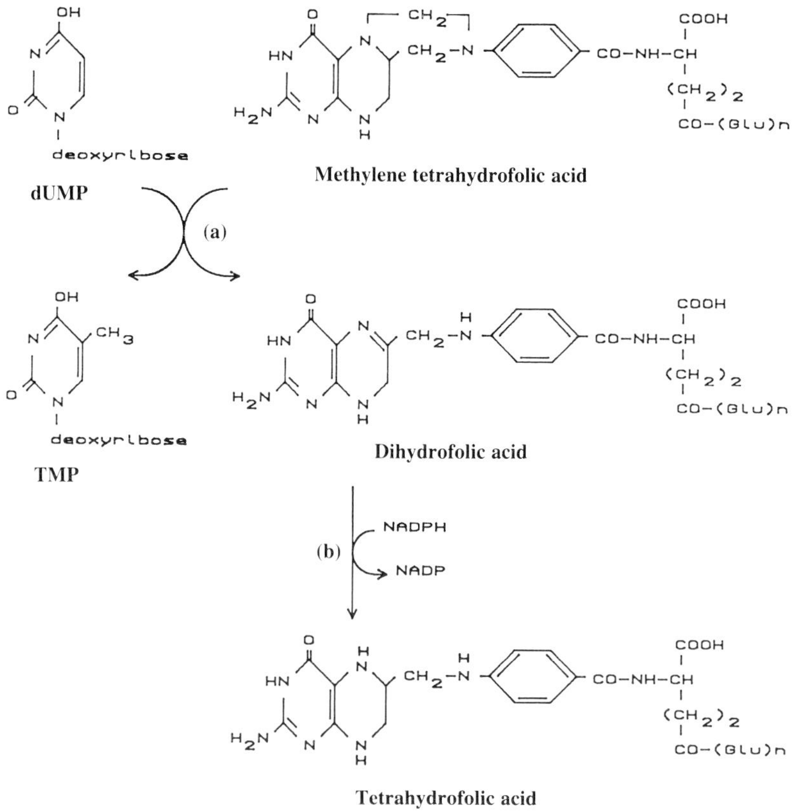

Figure 11.16 The rôle of folic acid in thymidylate synthetase
(a) *Thymidylate synthetase*: methylene tetrahydrofolic acid is the donor; the methylene (=CH$_2$) group is reduced to a methyl group (–CH$_3$) at the expense of the folic acid, which is oxidized to dihydrofolic acid. (b) *Dihydrofolate reductase*: dihydrofolic acid has to be reduced back to tetrahydrofolic acid before it can be re-used.

The other folic acid dependent reaction which is important to an understanding of the basis of the effects of folic acid and vitamin B_{12} deficiency is the formation of thymidine for **DNA synthesis**. As shown in Figure 11.16, this reaction involves the transfer of a methylene ($=CH_2$) fragment from methylene-folic acid onto dUTP, associated with reduction of the methylene group to a methyl group ($-CH_3$). In the process, folic acid is oxidized to dihydrofolic acid. The second step in the reaction involves the reduction of dihydrofolate back to the active form, tetrahydrofolate.

Deficiency

Dietary deficiency of folic acid is not uncommon, and, as noted above, deficiency of vitamin B_{12} also leads to functional folic acid deficiency. In either case, it is cells which are dividing rapidly, and which therefore have a large requirement for thymidine for DNA synthesis, which are most severely affected. These are the cells of the bone marrow which form red blood cells; the cells of the intestinal mucosa, which turn over in about 48h; and the hair follicles. Clinically, folic acid deficiency leads to **megaloblastic anaemia**, the release into the circulation of immature precursors of red blood cells.

Requirements

Folic acid requirements have been estimated in depletion and repletion studies, in which biochemical markers of folic acid deficiency are followed in response to graded intakes of the free vitamin. Allowing for the incomplete absorption of the mixed derivatives of folic acid in foods, the RNI for adults is 200 µg/day.

Rich sources of folic acid are mainly green leafy vegetables, liver and kidney, nuts and whole-grain cereals.

Folic acid and neural tube defects One factor in the development of **spina bifida** and other congenital neural tube defects is inadequate folic acid nutrition of the expectant mother. Folic acid supplements of about 400 µg/day, begun before conception, have a significant effect in reducing the incidence of neural tube defects.

Closure of the neural tube occurs early in embryological development, often before the mother knows that she is pregnant. Folic acid supplements taken after she knows she is pregnant may have no effect on the risk of neural tube defect. It is obviously desirable that all women who may become pregnant should have an adequate intake of folic acid.

Unfortunately, we do not know whether the amount provided by a good diet is adequate to provide protection against neural tube defect in women who are at risk. An intake of 400 μg of free folic acid/day is considerably higher than can be obtained from foods, and there is considerable controversy as to whether or not fortification of foods with folic acid, to ensure high intakes for women of child-bearing age, is desirable, in view of the potential risks associated with excessive intakes of the vitamin, discussed below.

Toxicity

There is no evidence that moderately large supplements of folic acid have any adverse effects. However, there are two potential problems:

(a) Folic acid supplements will mask the megaloblastic anaemia of vitamin B_{12} deficiency, and may hasten the development of the (irreversible) nerve damage. This is especially a problem of the elderly, who may suffer impaired absorption of vitamin B_{12} as a result of gastric atrophy with increasing age.

(b) Some people with epilepsy controlled by anticonvulsants show signs of mild folic acid deficiency. This is the result of an increased rate of metabolism of folic acid, caused by the anticonvulsants. However, antagonism between folic acid and the anticonvulsants is part of the mechanism of action of these drugs. Relatively large supplements of folic acid (in excess of 1,000 μg/day) may antagonize the beneficial effects of the anticonvulsants, and lead to an increase in the frequency of attacks.

Folic acid antagonists in chemotherapy

Since folic acid is required for the synthesis of thymidine for DNA synthesis, rapidly dividing cells are the most susceptible to folic acid deficiency, i.e. the bone marrow, intestinal mucosal cells and hair follicles. Cancer cells also have a very high requirement for DNA synthesis, and are also sensitive to folic acid deficiency. Folic acid antagonists, such as methotrexate, are used in the chemotherapy of cancer.

Bacteria and parasites also have a rapid rate of reproduction, and hence are again sensitive to the folic acid status of the host. The dihydrofolate reductase (see Fig. 11.16) of some bacteria and parasites (such as the malarial parasite) differs from the human enzyme, and can be inhibited by drugs such as trimethoprim, which have little or no effect on human dihydrofolate reductase.

270

Biotin

Biotin is required as the cofactor for a small number of carboxylation reactions; it acts as the carrier for carbon dioxide, as shown in Figure 11.17. The most important of these reactions are the formation of malonyl CoA from acetyl CoA in **fatty acid synthesis** (see Fig. 6.12 on p. 146) and the carboxylation of pyruvate to oxaloacetate for **gluconeogenesis** (see Fig. 6.15 on p. 155).

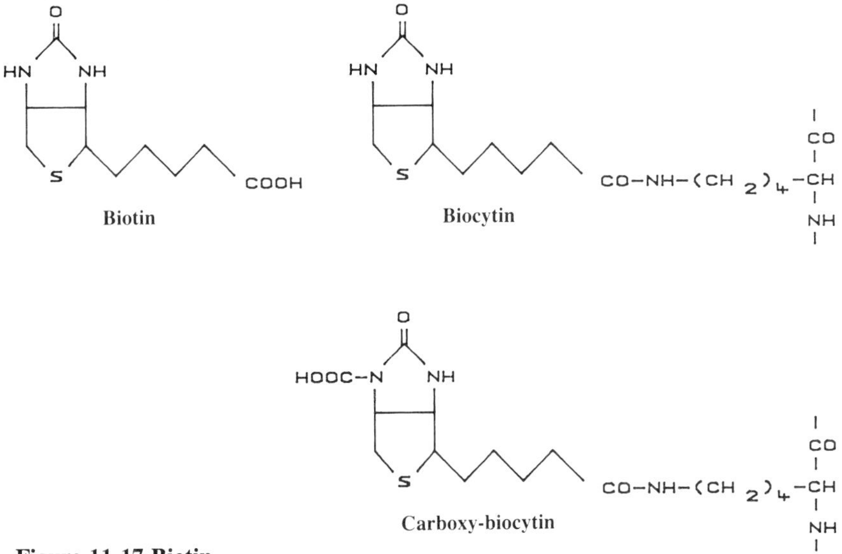

Figure 11.17 Biotin
Biotin is normally bound to the side-chain amino group of lysine in enzymes, forming biocytin. It functions in carboxylation reactions as an intermediate carrier of carbon dioxide for transfer to substrates, for example in the carboxylation of pyruvate to oxaloacetate in gluconeogenesis (see Fig. 6.15 on p. 155) and the carboxylation of acetyl CoA to malonyl CoA in fatty acid synthesis (see Fig. 6.12 on p. 146).

Biotin is widely distributed in foods, and deficiency is unknown, except among people maintained for many months on total parenteral nutrition, and a very small number of people who eat abnormally large amounts of uncooked egg.

There is a protein in egg-white, **avidin**, which binds biotin extremely tightly, and renders it unavailable for absorption. Avidin is denatured by cooking, and then loses its ability to bind biotin. The amount of avidin in uncooked egg-white is relatively small, and problems of biotin deficiency have only occurred in people eating abnormally large amounts – a dozen or more raw eggs a day, for many years.

There is no evidence on which to estimate requirements for biotin. Average intakes are between 10 and 200 μg/day. Since dietary deficiency does not occur, such intakes are more than adequate to meet requirements.

Pantothenic acid

Pantothenic acid is part of CoA and the prosthetic group of the acyl carrier protein of fatty acid synthesis (see Fig. 11.18).

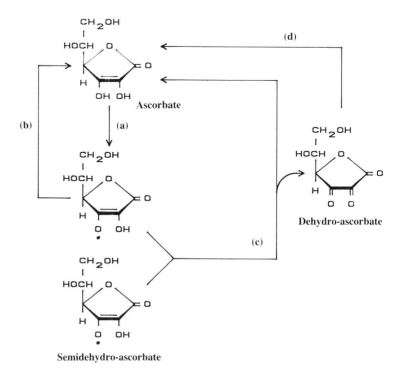

Figure 11.18 Pantothenic acid and coenzyme A (CoA)
Pantothenic acid is a part of both CoA (shown here) and also the acyl carrier protein involved in fatty acid synthesis (see Fig. 6.12 on p. 149). In both CoA and acyl carrier protein, the functionally important part of the molecule is the sulphydryl (–SH) group. This is derived from the amino acid cysteine, not from pantothenic acid.

It is widely distributed in foods; indeed, the name pantothenic acid is derived from the Greek for "from everywhere". There is no good evidence of a specific pantothenic acid deficiency disease, although metabolic abnormalities have been observed in experimental subjects maintained on diets containing no pantothenic acid. Prisoners of war in the Far East at the end of the Second World War suffered from neurological disease involving severe burning pain in the feet (the so-called **burning-foot syndrome**). It was assumed that this was due to pantothenic acid deficiency. However, they were suffering from general malnutrition, and deficiency of a variety of vitamins. Rather than conducting unethical experiments in order to determine whether or not the burning-foot syndrome was the result of pantothenic acid deficiency, these patients were treated with rich sources of all the B vitamins (commonly yeast extract).

There is no evidence on which to estimate pantothenic acid requirements. Average intakes are between 3 and 7 mg/day, and since deficiency does not occur, such intakes are obviously more than adequate to meet requirements.

Vitamin C (ascorbic acid)

Vitamin C is required as the cofactor for a small number of hydroxylation reactions. The most important of these are the hydroxylation of proline and lysine in the post-synthetic modification of collagen and the hydroxylation of dopamine to noradrenaline. It also has a general antioxidant rôle, especially in the reduction of oxidized vitamin E in membranes (see Fig. 11.7). The oxidation and reduction of vitamin C is shown in Figure 11.19.

Deficiency

The vitamin C deficiency disease, **scurvy**, was formerly a common problem at the end of winter, when there had been no fresh fruits and vegetables (the dietary sources of the vitamin) for many months. Sailors on long sea-voyages similarly suffered from scurvy before the protective rôle of fresh fruit and vegetables, or fruit juice, was discovered. On some of the voyages of exploration during the 16th and 17th centuries, up to 90% of the crew died from scurvy.

Almost all of the clinical signs of scurvy can be attributed to impairment of collagen formation, and hence defects of connective tissue. The earliest sign is the development of petechial haemorrhages around hair follicles. This is followed by inflammation of the gums between the teeth, with loss of dental cement, so that the teeth become loose and fall out. Because of the impairment of collagen synthesis, wound healing is much delayed in vitamin C deficiency. In advanced deficiency, the collagen of bones is affected, leading to severe bone pain. The impaired synthesis of adrenaline and noradrenaline leads to depression and irritability.

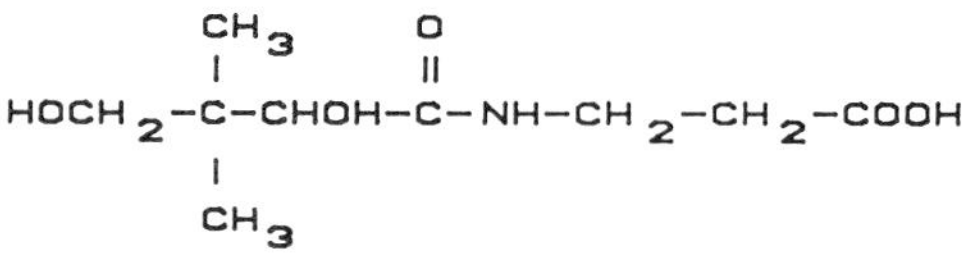

$$CH_3 \quad O$$
$$HOCH_2-C-CHOH-C-NH-CH_2-CH_2-COOH$$
$$CH_3$$

Pantothenic acid

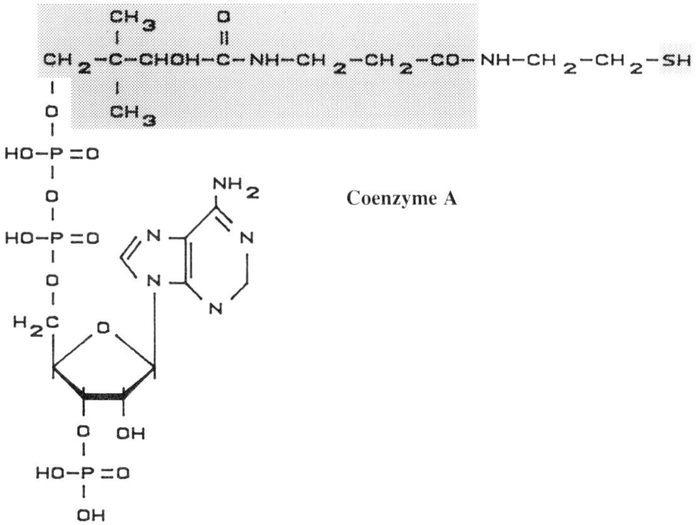

$$CH_3 \quad O$$
$$CH_2-C-CHOH-C-NH-CH_2-CH_2-CO-NH-CH_2-CH_2-SH$$
$$O \quad CH_3$$
$$HO-P=O$$
$$O$$
$$HO-P=O$$

NH$_2$

Coenzyme A

$$H_2C \quad O$$

$$HO-P=O$$
$$OH$$

Figure 11.19 The rôle of vitamin C in oxidation and reduction reactions
(a) Ascorbic acid can be oxidized to the semidehydro-ascorbate radical by a variety of reactions (see for example the rôle of ascorbic acid in vitamin E action in Fig. 11.7). (b) Semidehydro-ascorbate can be reduced back to ascorbic acid by a specific reductase linked to the oxidation of a reduced flavoprotein. (c) Two molecules of semidehydro-ascorbate can react with each other to form one molecule of ascorbic acid and one of dehydro-ascorbate. (d) Dehydro-ascorbate can be reduced to ascorbate by reaction with NADH.

Requirements

Vitamin C illustrates extremely well how different criteria of adequacy, and different interpretations of experimental evidence, can lead to different estimates of requirements, and to reference intakes varying between 30 and 80 mg/day for adults.

The requirement for vitamin C to prevent clinical scurvy is less than 10 mg/day. However, at this level of intake wounds do not heal properly, because of the requirement for vitamin C in the synthesis of collagen in connective tissue. An intake of 20 mg/day is required for optimum wound healing. Allowing for individual variation in requirements, this leads to an RDA for adults of 30 mg/day, which was the British RDA until 1991, and is the United Nations Food and Agriculture Organization/World Health Organization RDA.

The 1991 British RNI for vitamin C is based on the level of intake at which the plasma concentration rises sharply, showing that requirements have now been met, tissues are saturated, and there is spare vitamin C being transported between tissues, available for excretion. This criterion of adequacy gives an RNI of 40 mg/day for adults.

The alternative approach to determining requirements is to estimate the total body content of vitamin C, then measure the rate at which it is metabolized, by giving a test dose of radioactive vitamin. This is the basis of both the US RDA of 60 mg/day for adults and the Netherlands RDA of 80 mg/day. Indeed, it also provides an alternative basis for the RNI of 40 mg/day adopted in Britain in 1991.

The problem lies in deciding what is an appropriate total body content of vitamin C. The American studies were performed on subjects whose total body vitamin C was estimated to be 1,500 mg at the beginning of a depletion study. However, there is no evidence that this is a necessary, or even a desirable, body content of the vitamin. It is simply the body content of the vitamin among a small group of young people eating a self-selected diet rich in fruit. There is good evidence that a total body content of 900 mg is more than adequate. It is three times larger than the body content at which the first signs of deficiency are observed, and will protect against the development of any signs of deficiency for several months on a diet completely lacking vitamin C.

There is a further problem in interpreting the results of this kind of study. The rate at which vitamin C is metabolized varies with the amount consumed. This means that as the experimental subjects become depleted, so the rate at which they metabolize the vitamin decreases. Thus, the rate at which we assume the vitamin is metabolized, and hence the amount which is required to maintain the body content, depends on the way in which we extrapolate from the results obtained during depletion studies to the rate in subjects consuming a normal diet, and on the amount of vitamin C in that diet.

An intake of 40 mg/day is more than adequate to maintain a total body content of 900 mg of vitamin C (the same as the British RNI). At a higher level of habitual intake, 60 mg/day is adequate to maintain a total body content of 1,500 mg (the US RDA). Making allowances for changes in the rate of metabolism with different levels of intake, and allowing for incomplete absorption of the vitamin gives the Netherlands RDA of 80 mg/day.

At intakes between 70 and 100 mg/day the body's capacity to metabolize vitamin C is saturated, and any further intake is excreted unchanged in the urine.

High intakes of vitamin C There are those who argue that intakes of vitamin C very much higher than those discussed above may confer some benefits. Since intakes above about 70–100 mg/day lead to increased excretion of the unchanged vitamin, it is difficult to justify such claims. Certainly there is no good evidence that high intakes of vitamin C either protect against cancer, or provide any benefit to patients suffering from cancer. Equally, there is no evidence from several large studies that vitamin C has any useful effect in treating or preventing the common cold or flu.

The one benefit of a high intake of vitamin C is in aiding the **absorption of iron**. As discussed on p. 285, iron absorption is enhanced by vitamin C present in the gut together with the iron. This means that taking foods rich in vitamin C together with iron-rich foods will increase the absorption of the iron. The best estimate is that optimum iron absorption is achieved with an intake of about 25–50 mg of vitamin C with each meal. Certainly, people who are taking supplements to treat iron-deficiency anaemia should either take vitamin C tablets with them, or should swallow the iron tablets with a glass of fruit juice.

Minerals

The nutritionally important inorganic mineral elements are those which have a function in the body. Obviously, they must be provided in the diet, since elements cannot be interconverted. We can classify the minerals according to their functions, although some minerals have functions which fall into more than one class.

Many of the minerals, even those which are essential, are of little practical nutritional importance, since they are widely distributed in foods, and most people eating a normal mixed diet are likely to receive adequate intakes.

In general, mineral deficiencies are a problem when people live more or less entirely on foods grown in one small region, where the soil may be deficient in some minerals. For people whose diet consists of foods grown in a variety of different regions, mineral deficiencies are extremely unlikely. However, as discussed on p. 284, iron deficiency is a problem in most parts of the world, because if iron losses from the body are relatively high (e.g. from heavy menstrual blood loss), it is difficult to have a large enough intake of iron to replace the losses.

Mineral deficiency is unlikely among people eating an adequate mixed diet. More importantly, many of the minerals, including those which are dietary essentials, are toxic in even fairly modest excess. It is unlikely that the mineral content of foods will be high enough to be a problem, although crops grown in regions where the soil content of selenium is especially high may provide dangerously high levels of intake of this mineral. The problem arises when people whose diet is adequate take inappropriate supplements of minerals, or are exposed to contamination of food and water supplies.

Minerals with a structural function

Calcium, magnesium and phosphate The mineral of bones and teeth is a complex mixture of calcium and magnesium phosphates and carbonates. Calcium nutrition is discussed on p. 282.

Sodium and potassium The maintenance of the normal composition of intracellular and extracellular fluids, and osmotic homeostasis depend largely on the maintenance of relatively high concentrations of potassium inside cells and of sodium outside. There is little or no problem in meeting sodium requirements; indeed, as discussed on p. 25, the main problem with sodium nutrition is an excessive intake, rather than deficiency.

Minerals which function as prosthetic groups in enzymes

Copper Copper provides the essential functional part of several enzymes involved in oxidation and reduction reactions (see p. 55), including dopamine hydroxylase in the synthesis of noradrenaline and adrenaline, and cytochrome oxidase in the electron transport chain (see p. 126).

Iron The most obvious function of iron is in the haem of haemoglobin, the oxygen carrying protein in red blood cells, and myoglobin in muscles. Haem is also important in a variety of enzymes, including the cytochromes (see p. 126), where it is the coenzyme in oxidation and reduction reactions (see p. 55). Some enzymes also contain non-haem iron (i.e. iron bound to the enzyme other than in haem), which is essential to their function. Iron nutrition is discussed on p. 284.

Molybdenum Molybdenum functions as the prosthetic group of a small number of enzymes, including xanthine oxidase (which is involved in the metabolism of purines to uric acid for excretion) and pyridoxal oxidase (which metabolizes vitamin B_6 to the inactive excretory product pyridoxic acid). It occurs in an organic complex, molybdopterin, which is chemically similar to folic acid (see p. 266) but can be synthesized in the body as long as adequate amounts of molybdenum are available.

Molybdenum deficiency has been associated with increased incidence of cancer of the oesophagus, but this seems to be an indirect association. The problem occurs among people living largely on maize grown on soil which is poor in molybdenum. For reasons which are not altogether clear, the resultant molybdenum-deficient maize is more susceptible to attack by fungi which produce carcinogenic toxins. Thus, while the people living on this diet are at risk of molybdenum deficiency, the main problem is not one of molybdenum deficiency in the people, but rather of fungal spoilage of their food.

Selenium Selenium functions in at least two enzymes: glutathione peroxidase and thyroxine deiodinase, which forms the active **thyroid hormone**, tri-iodothyronine, from thyroxine secreted by the thyroid gland. In both cases it is present as the selenium analogue of the amino acid cysteine, **selenocysteine**.

Glutathione peroxidase acts to reduce the oxygen radicals which would otherwise attack polyunsaturated fatty acids, and also to reduce the products of oxidative damage to polyunsaturated fatty acids. Selenium thus has an important rôle in the body's overall antioxidant status, to a great extent in conjunction with vitamin E (see p. 249).

Deficiency is widespread in parts of China, and the soil in some parts of the United States, New Zealand and Finland is so poor in selenium that it is added to fertilizers, in order to increase the selenium intake of the population, and so prevent deficiency.

However, selenium is also extremely toxic even in modest excess. The RNI for selenium for adults is 75 μg/day; signs of poisoning can be seen at intakes above 450 μg/day and the World Health Organization recommends that selenium intakes should not exceed 200 μg/day. In some parts of the world the soil is so rich in selenium that locally grown crops would provide more than this recommended upper limit of selenium intake if they were the main source of food, and it is not possible to graze cattle safely on the pastures in these regions.

Zinc Zinc is the prosthetic group of more than a hundred enzymes, with a wide variety of functions. It is also involved in the receptor proteins for steroid and thyroid hormones, calcitriol and vitamin A. In these proteins, zinc forms an integral part of the region of the protein which interacts with the promoter site on DNA to initiate gene transcription in response to hormone action (see p. 226).

Zinc deficiency occurs only among people living in tropical or subtropical areas whose diet is very largely based on unleavened wholemeal bread. The problem is seen mainly as much-delayed puberty, so that 18–20-year-old males are still prepubertal. This is a result of reduced sensitivity of target tissues to androgens and oestrogens, because of the rôle of zinc in steroid-hormone receptors. Two separate factors contribute to the deficiency:

(a) wheat flour provides very little zinc, and in unleavened wholemeal bread much of the zinc that is present is not available for absorption because it is bound to **phytate** (see p. 282);

(b) sweat contains a relatively high concentration of zinc, and in tropical conditions there can be a considerable loss of zinc in sweat.

Marginal zinc deficiency in developed countries may be associated with poor wound healing, and impairment of the senses of taste and smell.

Minerals which have a regulatory rôle
(in neurotransmission, as enzyme activators or in hormones)

Calcium In addition to its rôle in bone mineral, calcium has a major function in metabolic regulation (see p. 222), nerve conduction and muscle contraction. Calcium nutrition is discussed on p. 282.

Chromium Chromium is involved, as an organic complex called the **glucose tolerance factor**, in the interaction between insulin and cell-surface insulin receptors. Chromium deficiency is associated with impaired glucose tolerance, as is seen in diabetes. However, there is no evidence that increased intakes of chromium have any beneficial effect in diabetes.

Iodine Iodine is required for the synthesis of the thyroid hormones, thyroxine and tri-iodothyronine. Deficiency, leading to goitre, is widespread in inland upland areas over limestone soil. This is because the soil over limestone is thin, and minerals, including iodine, readily leach out, so that locally grown plants are deficient in iodine. Near the coast, sea spray contains enough iodine to replace these losses. Worldwide, many millions of people are at risk of deficiency, and in parts of central Brazil and the Himalayas goitre may affect more than 90% of the population. Because of the rôle of selenium in the metabolism of the thyroid hormones (see p. 278), the effects of iodine deficiency will be exacerbated by selenium deficiency.

In developed countries where there is a risk of iodine deficiency, supplementation of foods is common. Iodized salt may be available, or bread may be baked using iodized salt. In developing countries, such enrichment of foods is not generally possible, and the treatment and prevention of iodine deficiency generally depends on periodic visits to areas at risk by medical teams who give relatively large doses of iodized oil by intramuscular injection.

Magnesium Magnesium is a cofactor for enzymes that utilize ATP and also for several of the enzymes involved in DNA replication (see p. 100) and transcription (see p. 205).

Manganese Manganese functions as the prosthetic group of a variety of enzymes, including superoxide dismutase, a part of the body's antioxidant defence system, pyruvate carboxylase in gluconeogenesis (see p. 153) and arginase in urea synthesis (see p. 203). Deficiency has only been observed in deliberate depletion studies.

Sodium and potassium The normal gradient of sodium and potassium across cell membranes, with a relatively high intracellular concentration of potassium and a relatively low intracellular concentration of sodium, is maintained by active (i.e. ATP-dependent) pumping (see Fig. 6.1 on p. 126). Nerve conduction depends on the rapid reversal of this trans-membrane gradient to create and propagate the electrical impulse, followed by a more gradual restoration of the normal ion gradient.

Minerals known to be essential, but whose function is not known

Silicon Silicon is known to be essential for the development of connective tissue and the bones, although its function in these processes is not known. The silicon content of blood vessel walls decreases with age, and with the development of atherosclerosis. It has been suggested, although the evidence is not convincing, that silicon deficiency may be a factor in the development of atherosclerosis.

Vanadium Experimental animals maintained under very strictly controlled conditions show a requirement for vanadium for normal growth. There is some evidence that vanadium has a rôle in regulation of the activity of sodium/potassium pumps, although this has not been proven.

Nickel and tin There is some evidence, from experimental animals maintained under strictly controlled conditions, that a dietary intake of nickel and tin is required for optimum growth and development, although this remains to be demonstrated conclusively.

Minerals which have effects in the body, but whose essentiality is not established

Fluoride Fluoride has clear beneficial effects in modifying the structure of bone mineral and dental enamel. This strengthens the bones, and protects teeth against decay. The use of fluoride toothpaste, and the addition of fluoride to drinking water in many regions, has resulted in a very dramatic decrease in the incidence of dental decay despite high consumption of sucrose and other extrinsic sugars (see p. 22). These benefits are seen at levels of fluoride of the order of 1 part/million in drinking water. Such concentrations occur naturally in many parts of the world, and this is the concentration at which fluoride is added to water in many areas.

Excessive intake of fluoride leads to brown discoloration of the teeth (dental **fluorosis**). A concentration above about 12 ppm. in drinking water, as occurs in some parts of the world, is associated with excessive deposition of fluoride in the bones, leading to increased fragility (skeletal fluorosis).

Although fluoride has beneficial effects, there is no evidence that it is a dietary essential. Fluoride prevents dental decay, but it is probably not correct to call dental decay a fluoride-deficiency disease.

Lithium Lithium salts are used in psychiatry. They have a beneficial effect in the treatment of manic-depressive disease, by altering the responsiveness of some nerves to stimulation. However, this seems to be a purely pharmacological effect, and there is no evidence that lithium has any essential function in the body, nor that it provides any benefits for healthy people.

Other minerals

In addition to minerals which we know to be dietary essentials, we can consider a number which may be consumed in relatively large amounts, but which have, as far as we know, no function in the body. Indeed, excessive accumulation of these minerals may be dangerous, and several of them are well known as poisons. Such elements include: aluminium, arsenic, antimony, boron, cadmium, caesium, cobalt, germanium, lead, mercury, silver and strontium.

Cobalt is involved in human metabolism only as part of the molecule of vitamin B_{12} (see p. 264). Inorganic cobalt salts have no metabolic function, and can cause damage to heart muscle.

Calcium nutrition and metabolism

The most obvious requirement for calcium in the body is in the mineral of bones and teeth, a complex mixture of calcium carbonates and phosphates (hydroxyapatite) together with magnesium salts and fluorides. An adult has about 1.2kg of calcium in the body, 99% of which is in the skeleton and teeth. This means that calcium requirements are especially high in times of rapid growth, during infancy and adolescence, and in pregnancy and lactation.

Although the major part of the body's calcium is in bones, the most important functions of calcium are in the maintenance of muscle contractility, cell structure and responses to hormones and neurotransmitters (see p. 222). To maintain these essential regulatory functions, bone calcium is mobilized in deficiency, so as to ensure that the plasma and intracellular concentrations are kept within a strictly controlled range. If the plasma concentration of calcium falls, neuromuscular regulation is lost and the patient goes into tetany.

The main sources of calcium are milk and cheese; dietary calcium is absorbed by an active process in the mucosal cells of the small intestine, and is dependent on **vitamin D**. The active metabolite of vitamin D, calcitriol, induces the synthesis of a calcium-binding protein which permits the mucosal cells to accumulate calcium from the intestinal lumen (see p. 244). In vitamin D deficiency the absorption of calcium is seriously impaired.

Not all of the dietary calcium is available for absorption. Some compounds in foods can form complexes with calcium, or can form insoluble calcium salts which cannot be absorbed. Nutritionally, the most important of these is **phytic acid**, which is found in cereal bran and some nuts and pulses. Phytate also inhibits the absorption of other minerals, including iron and zinc.

Chemically, phytic acid is inositol hexaphosphate. It can be dephosphorylated to inositol to a limited extent in the intestinal lumen by the enzyme phytase, and during the leavening of bread dough the phytase of yeast has the same action. It is not clear to what extent a high phytate diet may impair the absorption of calcium and other minerals, although people with a high intake of unleavened whole-grain bread (such as chapattis) absorb a lower proportion of their dietary calcium. However, whole grain cereal products contain more calcium than refined flour unless the flour has been fortified with calcium salts to replace the losses in milling. As discussed on p. 278, a diet based largely on unleavened wholemeal bread is a contributory factor in the development of zinc deficiency.

Although the effect of vitamin D deficiency is impairment of the absorption and utilization of calcium, rickets (see p. 244) does not seem to be simply the result of calcium deficiency. Calcium-deficient children with adequate vitamin D nutritional status do not develop rickets but have a much reduced rate of growth. Nevertheless, as discussed on p. 244, calcium deficiency may be a contributory factor in the development of rickets when vitamin D status is marginal.

Osteoporosis Osteoporosis is a progressive loss of bone mass with increasing age, after the peak bone mass is achieved at the age of about 30. The cause is the normal process of bone turnover, but with reduced replacement of the tissue which has been broken down. Both bone mineral and the organic matrix of bone are lost in osteoporosis, unlike osteomalacia (see p. 246) where there is loss of bone mineral, but the organic matrix is unaffected.

Osteoporosis can occur in relatively young people, as a result of prolonged bed rest – bone continues to be degraded, but without physical activity there is less stimulus for replacement of the lost tissue. More importantly, it occurs as an apparently unavoidable part of the ageing process. Here the main problem is the reduced secretion of oestrogens (in women) and androgens (in men) with increasing age; among other actions, the sex steroids are involved in the stimulation of new bone formation. The problem is especially serious in women, since there is a much more abrupt fall in oestrogen secretion at the menopause than the more gradual (and less severe) fall in androgen secretion in men with increasing age. As a result, very many more elderly women than men suffer from osteoporosis. Post-menopausal hormone replacement therapy with oestrogens has a protective effect against the development of osteoporosis.

Because there is a net breakdown of bone in osteoporosis, considerable amounts of calcium are excreted in the urine. This shows as **negative calcium balance** – excretion is greater than the dietary intake. This has led to suggestions that a high intake of calcium may slow or reverse the process of osteoporosis. However, the negative calcium balance is the result of osteoporosis, not the cause. There is no evidence that higher intakes of calcium have any effect on the development of osteoporosis.

People with higher peak bone mass are less at risk from osteoporosis, since they can tolerate more loss of bone before there are clinically important effects. Therefore, adequate calcium and vitamin D nutrition through adolescence and young adulthood is likely to provide protection against osteoporosis in old age. High intakes of calcium have no beneficial effect once peak bone mass has been achieved. However, high intakes of calcium have no adverse effects either, because of the close regulation of calcium homeostasis. Problems of hypercalcaemia and calcinosis (the calcification of soft tissues) occur as a result of vitamin D intoxication (see p. 247), or other disturbances of calcium homeostasis, not as a result of high intakes of calcium.

High intakes of vitamin D have no beneficial effect on the progression of osteoporosis, although the vitamin will prevent the development of osteomalacia, which can occur together with osteoporosis in the elderly.

Iron nutrition and metabolism

The major function of iron in the body is in the haem part of haemoglobin (the oxygen-carrying protein in red blood cells), myoglobin (the oxygen-carrying protein in muscle) and the cytochromes (see p. 127). Deficiency of iron leads to reduced synthesis of haemoglobin, and hence to a lower than normal amount of haemoglobin in red blood cells. Iron deficiency anaemia is relatively common, especially among women.

Iron deficiency is mainly due to a loss of blood greater than can be replaced by absorption of dietary iron. In developing countries intestinal parasites (especially hookworm), which cause large losses of blood in the faeces, can be a common cause of iron depletion and hence anaemia. In developed countries it is mainly women who are at risk of iron deficiency anaemia, as a result of heavy **menstrual losses** of blood. Pregnancy and lactation place an additional strain on the mother's iron reserves.

Iron in foods occurs in two forms: haem in meat and meat products, and inorganic iron salts in plant foods. Relatively little is known about the absorption of haem, except that it is by a different mechanism from that involved in the absorption of inorganic iron salts. The absorption of haem iron is considerably better than that of inorganic iron salts.

Only between 10 and 15% of the inorganic iron of the diet is absorbed. There are three steps in the absorption of inorganic iron salts:

(a) The iron salts in the intestinal lumen must be reduced from the Fe^{3+} to the Fe^{2+} form. Several compounds will effect this reduction, including fructose and, probably most importantly, vitamin C. However, this is an effect of vitamin C present in the intestinal lumen together with the iron. Quite apart from the requirement for vitamin C to maintain normal health (an RNI of 40 mg/day), discussed on p. 274, an intake of about 25–50 mg with each meal results in optimum absorption of the inorganic iron in that meal.

A high intake of phytate (see p. 282) results in the formation of insoluble complexes of the iron in that meal. These are not well absorbed. There is some evidence that relatively high amounts of calcium inhibit the absorption of iron in the same meal, although the mechanism for this is unknown.

(b) Iron is concentrated in the cells of the intestinal mucosa by binding to the protein ferritin. This means that once the ferritin in the mucosal cells is saturated with iron, no more can be absorbed from the intestinal lumen into the mucosal cells. Once the mucosal cells are saturated with iron, any excess will remain in the faeces and be excreted.

(c) Iron is transferred from the mucosal cells into the bloodstream only by binding to the protein transferrin in plasma. If the transferrin in plasma is saturated with iron, then no more can be absorbed from the mucosal cells into the bloodstream. The excess will remain in the mucosal cells until they are shed into the intestinal lumen from the tip of the villus.

The result of this is that the absorption of iron varies to some extent with the state of the body's iron reserves, and deficient subjects absorb a slightly higher proportion of dietary iron than those who have adequate iron reserves. Nevertheless, people with large iron losses due to blood loss cannot absorb enough to maintain iron balance. It is likely that about 5% of women, with the highest menstrual blood losses, are unable to obtain enough iron from foods to meet those losses, and will have to take iron supplements to prevent the development of iron-deficiency anaemia.

There is little or no excretion of iron from the body, and excessive absorption can lead to the development of abnormally large stores of iron. This can result in the development of **haemosiderosis**, with very large amounts of iron stored inappropriately in tissues. Two factors are commonly associated with such **iron overload**: a relatively high intake of inorganic iron salts together with alcohol, which increases the absorption of iron; and taking excessive supplements of iron, a significant amount of which can then be absorbed passively across the gut wall, bypassing the normal regulation of absorption. This is mainly a problem among young children, who take their mother's iron tablets thinking they are sweets. Iron overload can also occur as a result of repeated blood transfusions, as for example in the treatment of thalassaemia. Here the problem is that the iron released from breakdown of haemoglobin is not excreted from the body, but is added to the body's iron stores.

Iron overload can have two adverse effects:

(a) Transfer of iron between different storage pools in the body involves a vitamin C-dependent reduction reaction. The vitamin is irreversibly oxidized in process, and iron overload is associated with the depletion of body reserves of vitamin C, and the development of scurvy.

(b) Free iron ions catalyse several oxidative reactions, which result in the formation of reactive oxygen radicals, thus adding significantly to the body's burden of radicals and leading to damage to membrane lipids and DNA (see p. 249).

CHAPTER TWELVE

Inborn errors of metabolism

We have seen that the process of DNA replication involves very careful checking, to ensure that the correct bases have been incorporated into the newly synthesized strand of DNA (see p. 100). Nevertheless, there remains a possibility of error, estimated at $1/10^9$ bases incorporated.

More importantly, errors can be caused by such agents as free radicals and the products of free-radical attack on membrane lipids. This means that exposure to ionizing radiation (both environmental exposure to background radioactivity and occupational exposure to radioactivity and X-rays), as well as exposure to compounds which increase free radical generation, will be likely to cause damage to DNA. In addition, a great many chemicals can cause chemical modification of DNA bases. Many of these changes are detected by the DNA repair mechanism, and the abnormal bases are removed and replaced (see p. 101). Nevertheless, some changes to DNA do occur and persist. When such changes occur in germ cells (ova and sperm), a **heritable mutation** has occurred; the modified DNA is inherited by the next generation.

The process of evolution has been due to this process of mutation, with most changes being neutral or deleterious, but some resulting in beneficial changes. The beneficial mutations, which confer an advantage on the individual affected, have survived, while the most deleterious mutations have not.

Individual variation is the result of the different patterns of changes in DNA which we have all inherited; this is the basis of DNA fingerprinting, as discussed on p. 102. We all have a great many differences from each other in the details of our DNA. Some of these result in differences in proteins, sometimes major, sometimes minor. Rarely, the effects are sufficiently serious to cause a loss or severe impairment of enzyme activity, with more or less serious effects on metabolism. Collectively we call such conditions **inborn errors of metabolism**.

Although they are of great interest, and we have learnt a great deal about normal metabolism from studying inborn errors of metabolism, they are extremely rare. Cystic fibrosis is among the commonest, occurring about 1:2000 live births. Other conditions are much less common: phenylketonuria (see p. 292) occurs in 80 per million live births; galactosaemia (see p. 133) in 25 per million; argininosuccinic aciduria (see p. 292) in 4 per million; and maple syrup urine disease (see p. 294) in 3 per million. Other conditions are more rare, and some have only ever been reported in a single family.

It is most unlikely that inborn errors of metabolism seriously affecting enzymes of the central metabolic pathways will ever be discovered, since they would not be compatible with life and fetal development. The conditions which do occur are generally those in which toxic metabolites can be passed across the placenta back into the mother's circulation during uterine development. It is after birth that the infant has problems. Many conditions cause death in early life, and many which are not fatal result in very serious impairment of the normal development of the brain and hence gross impairment of intelligence.

For some of the less rare inborn errors of metabolism, such as phenylketonuria and homocystinuria, infants are screened at or shortly after birth, by looking for abnormal metabolites in blood or urine. This is only worthwhile if there is some means of treating or controlling the condition.

Increasingly, it is also possible to detect genetic diseases *in utero*, by sampling the amniotic fluid and probing for the expression of specific genes. This is done by testing the mRNA from the cells in the amniotic fluid with a genetic probe to see whether or not it contains the message which will bind to a single strand of DNA which is complementary to the mRNA normally produced by transcription of that gene.

The possible effects of mutations in DNA

Mutations having no effect on enzyme activity

Not all changes in DNA lead to changes in enzymes and other proteins. There are three reasons for this:
(a) As discussed on p. 100, only about 10% of human DNA codes for proteins. Apart from the various initiator and promoter regions, much

of the remainder seems to have no function. Obviously, a mutation in a "silent" region of DNA with no function will not have any detectable effects.

(b) It is obvious, from examination of the genetic code (see Tables 9.6 and 9.7 on p. 209) that some changes in DNA will have no effect on the amino acid which is incorporated into a protein, because several different codons code for the same amino acid. Such mutations, like those in silent regions of DNA, will be apparent on DNA fingerprinting, but will have no other detectable effects.

(c) Some changes in DNA which do result in a different amino acid being incorporated into a protein will still have little or no effect on the structure and function of the protein. There are two possible reasons for this:

(i) The change might be a conservative one – the replacement of one amino acid with another which is chemically similar. For example, changing glutamate for aspartate might have very little effect, since both have acidic side-chains. Similarly, changing valine for leucine or isoleucine would have little or no effect; all three have large, branched aliphatic side-chains (see Fig. 4.11 on p. 87).

(ii) Even a radical change in an amino acid (e.g. changing an acidic for a basic amino acid) may have little or no effect on the structure and function of the enzyme if the change is away from the active site, and not in an area where it will affect the secondary or tertiary structure of the protein to any significant extent.

Changes of this type will be detectable on examination of the protein, but again will have no effect on the body's metabolism.

Mutations which affect enzyme activity

Almost all mutations which result in changes in enzyme activity are likely to be deleterious, although it is important to note that evolution has occurred as a result of the accumulation of rare beneficial changes.

The mutation results in low activity of the enzyme Some mutations result in the formation of an enzyme with some activity, but with a low maximum rate of activity, an abnormally high K_m for the substrate (see p. 110) or an impaired ability to bind a coenzyme (see p. 263). Such mutations are generally due to one of two causes:

(a) A change in an amino acid in the active site. This could be a conservative change. For example, if the side-chain carboxyl group of glutamate is involved in the binding of the substrate or coenzyme, or in the catalytic activity of the enzyme, then changing this to aspartate, where the carboxyl group is closer to the peptide backbone of the protein, will result in changed activity of the enzyme. Other changes of amino acids in the active site can also change the shape enough to impair binding or catalytic activity.

(b) A change in an amino acid away from the catalytic site, but in a region which is critical for the correct conformation of the enzyme. Such changes may well affect the conformation of the active site, and cause impaired activity.

Changes of the kinds discussed here may affect not the active site of the enzyme, but a secondary site which binds a regulator. In this case there will be abnormal activity of the enzyme as a result of loss of sensitivity to control. Such effects may result in either increased or decreased activity of the enzyme under normal conditions.

The mutation results in no detectable activity of the enzyme There are three possible reasons why a mutation might result in a complete loss of enzyme activity:

(a) there has been a mutation in the active site or in a structurally important region of the protein, resulting in a change so major that the resultant enzyme has no activity at all;

(b) the mutation has resulted in a change from a codon for an amino acid to a stop codon; this means that only a fragment of the protein will be synthesized, and is most unlikely to have an active site;

(c) the mutation is in the promoter region of the gene, so that the gene is not transcribed.

The treatment of inborn errors of metabolism

Most mutations which lead to loss or severe impairment of enzyme activity result in metabolic disease. However, this is not always so. There are some conditions in which abnormal metabolites are excreted in the urine, as a result of loss of activity of the enzyme which would normally metabolize them, but this has no effect on the health or metabolic integrity of the affected person. An example of such a condition is **idiopathic pentosuria**, the excretion of pentose (five-carbon) sugars in the urine, a biochemical oddity affecting people of north European (Ashkenazi) Jewish origin which has no clinical consequences at all.

Some inborn errors of metabolism are amenable to relatively simple treatment. For example, there are some conditions in which the affinity of one enzyme for the active metabolite of vitamin B_6, pyridoxal phosphate, is very much lower than normal. These are the **vitamin B_6 depend-**

ency diseases (see p. 263). Without treatment the patient develops more or less severe disease, depending on which enzyme is affected. However, in the presence of high concentrations of pyridoxal phosphate the enzyme has more or less normal activity. Here the solution is simple; high intakes of vitamin B_6 (considerably greater than the normal requirement) maintain adequate activity of the affected enzyme, and the patient remains in good health as long as he or she takes the vitamin.

Similar **vitamin dependency syndromes** are known involving other vitamins, including thiamin (vitamin B_1) (some forms of maple syrup urine disease, see below); vitamin B_{12} and biotin.

Some inborn errors of metabolism result in the inability to synthesize a coenzyme which is normally formed in the body. Here, in general, there is a simple treatment. We now have a patient for whom a compound which most people can synthesize readily is, because of a mutation, a dietary essential. Provided that we can synthesize the compound which is required, it can be given to the patient. One very rare variant of phenyl-ketonuria (see below) is of this type; it is due to a failure to synthesize **biopterin**, which is the coenzyme of phenylalanine hydroxylase. Affected patients can be maintained perfectly well by giving them supplements of biopterin.

It is not generally possible to treat a disease due to lack of an enzyme by simply giving the enzyme. Since enzymes are proteins, it is obviously not possible to give them by mouth, they would be digested together with the other dietary proteins. If given by injection, they would almost certainly cause an immune response, and lead to anaphylactic shock, causing the death of the patient. In any case, simple administration of the enzyme into the bloodstream would not be expected to lead to any useful results, since in almost all cases what is lacking is an enzyme inside a cell. There have been some promising results in the treatment of glycogen storage disease due to lack of glucose-6-phosphatase in the liver (see p. 154) in which the enzyme has been given by intravenous injection enclosed in lipid membrane vesicles which are taken up by the liver.

The hope for the future is that we will be able to cure inborn errors of metabolism by introducing into the patient's DNA the gene for the defective or lacking enzyme, in the same way as we can introduce the gene for a human protein into bacteria for the production of human hormones (see p. 216). This has not yet been achieved, but there is great hope that some of the more intractable genetic diseases will be treated in this way in the near future.

For the present, the main means of controlling most inborn errors of metabolism is by dietary modification, in order to reduce as far as possible the burden of compounds which cannot be metabolized. In some cases this is extremely successful; in some cases it is moderately successful; in a few cases it prolongs the child's life, but as yet not for long enough. In all too many cases we cannot offer any treatment.

Glucose-6-phosphate dehydrogenase deficiency: favism

There is an alternative pathway of glucose metabolism, not discussed in Chapter 6, in which glucose-6-phosphate is oxidized to 6-phospho-gluconate, catalysed by the enzyme glucose-6-phosphate dehydrogenase. This reaction occurs in all tissues, but is especially important in the metabolism of red blood cells.

Deficiency of glucose-6-phosphate dehydrogenase is relatively common in people of Mediterranean and African origin. In response to the some drugs (especially antimalarial drugs and sulphonamide antibacterial agents) there is excessive destruction of red blood cells, leading to haemolytic anaemia. Some of the compounds present in broad beans (fava beans) also precipitate the haemolytic crisis, hence the name of the condition, favism.

Affected subjects obviously have to avoid fava beans, and they and their physicians must be aware of which drugs should never be given.

Glycogen storage diseases

Several diseases involve inborn errors of glycogen metabolism. All of them result in the formation of large stores of glycogen in liver and/or muscle, which cannot be mobilized for use in the fasting state because the defect is in one of the enzymes involved in glycogen breakdown: glycogen phosphorylase, the debranching enzyme or glucose-6-phosphatase. This last condition affects only the liver, since muscle normally lacks glucose-6-phosphatase.

The problem with all of these glycogen storage diseases is that glycogen is synthesized normally in the fed state, but it cannot be broken down in the fasting state. Therefore there is a considerable, and increasing, accumulation of glycogen, which causes tissue damage. At present there is no long-term treatment available; all that can be done is to feed the affected child small, frequent meals, so as to minimize the amount of glycogen that is formed after any one meal. In the case of glucose-6-phosphatase deficiency, it is also desirable to avoid conditions that would lead to gluconeogenesis (i.e. the fasting state, see p. 153), since the glucose-6-phosphate formed in the liver cannot be released as free glucose, and therefore will be used for yet more glycogen synthesis.

Inborn errors of the urea synthesis cycle

Several conditions are known, affecting different enzymes of the urea synthesis cycle. In all cases urinary excretion of the substrate of the defective enzyme occurs. More seriously, in response to normal amounts of protein, the child shows signs of ammonia intoxication. Because of the defect in the cycle, the child is unable to metabolize ammonia in the normal way.

Two methods of treatment are used in such conditions:

(a) Feeding a low-protein diet, just the minimum amount required for the maintenance of nitrogen balance and growth (see p. 189). This reduces the burden of ammonia which must be metabolized.

(b) In at least some cases the administration of arginine is beneficial. From the pathway for urea synthesis shown in Figure 9.7 on p. 203, it is obvious that breaking the cycle, for example at argininosuccinase, has two effects: accumulation and excretion of argininosuccinic acid, the substrate of the defective enzyme; and a deficiency of arginine, since it is not being formed from arginosuccinate. In turn, this results in a deficiency of ornithine. Feeding arginine permits the formation of more ornithine, which is then available for the synthesis of carbamyl phosphate, taking up ammonia, and forming argininosuccinic acid, which is excreted. In this way, the broken cyclic pathway can be considered to have been converted to a linear pathway, in which the administered arginine is converted to argininosuccinic acid for excretion, taking with it two nitrogen atoms (one from ammonia and one from aspartate) which would otherwise have contributed to the child's ammonia intoxication.

Phenylketonuria

Phenylketonuria was one of the first inborn errors of metabolism to be investigated. The condition is due to a defect of the enzyme phenylalanine hydroxylase, which catalyses the hydroxylation of phenylalanine to tyrosine (see Fig. 12.1). This is the normal pathway for the metabolism of phenylalanine. When it is defective, the concentration of phenylalanine in the bloodstream rises to very high levels, and some is metabolized by a different pathway, leading to the formation of phenylpyruvate, phenyl-lactate and phenylacetate, which are excreted in the urine. Collectively these three compounds are called phenylketones (although only phenyl-pyruvate is chemically a ketone), hence the name of the condition.

Untreated phenylketonuria has a very major effect on the development of the central nervous system, and affected subjects have very impaired

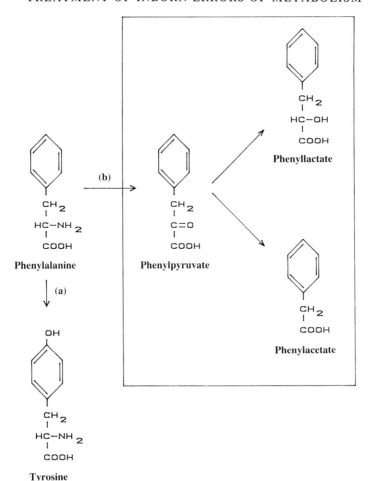

Figure 12.1 The metabolism of phenylalanine in phenylketonuria

(a) *Phenylalanine hydroxylase*: phenylalanine is normally metabolized by way of tyrosine. In phenylketonuria this enzyme is absent or inactive; blood and tissue concentrations of phenylalanine rise to 100-fold greater than normal. (b) *Phenylalanine transaminase* has a high K_m compared with normal concentrations of phenylalanine in tissues, so normally there is little or no transamination of phenylalanine. In phenylketonuria, the tissue concentration of phenylalanine rises high enough for transamination to occur. Phenyl-pyruvate, formed by phenylalanine transaminase, can undergo either reduction to phenyllactate or oxidation and decarboxylation to phenylacetate.

intelligence (an IQ as low as 40–50 in severe cases). However, if the condition is detected early enough, feeding the affected infant a specially formulated diet, which provides only minimally adequate amounts of phenylalanine for growth and the maintenance of nitrogen balance, permits completely normal development of the brain with no impairment of intelligence. All infants born in developed countries are screened for phenylketonuria about a week after birth, when phenylalanine hydroxylase would normally have developed.

The strict dietary restriction on phenylalanine intake can be relaxed when the affected child is aged between about 8 and 12 years. After this stage, when brain development is complete, there seem to be no adverse effects of a high concentration of phenylalanine in the bloodstream. However, if an affected woman wishes to become pregnant, then strict dietary control must again be instituted, before conception. High concentrations of phenylalanine in the mother's blood have a very serious effect on the development of the nervous system of the fetus.

A small proportion of infants with phenylketonuria do not respond to the low phenylalanine diet. The hydroxylation of phenylalanine involves two enzymes, phenylalanine hydroxylase and dihydrobiopterin reductase. The immediate reducing agent in the hydroxylation of phenylalanine is tetrahydrobiopterin, which is oxidized to dihydrobiopterin. This is normally reduced back to the active form by dihydrobiopterin reductase. Many of the patients who do not respond to diet therapy have a defect of dihydrobiopterin reductase, rather than of phenylalanine hydroxylase. At present there is nothing we can do for infants who lack dihydrobiopterin reductase; it is not possible to give them reduced tetrahydrobiopterin, since it is chemically unstable.

A few of the infants with phenylketonuria which does not respond to diet have a different enzyme defect. They are unable to synthesize biopterin. These are the lucky few; biopterin is relatively easy to synthesize in the laboratory, and is chemically stable. Therefore they simply need to receive a daily intake of biopterin. For these infants biopterin is a dietary essential.

Maple syrup urine disease

This is a defect of the metabolism of the branched-chain amino acids, leucine, isoleucine and valine. Abnormal metabolites of the amino acids are excreted in the urine, giving it a sweet smell, similar to maple syrup. Like phenylketonuria, untreated maple syrup urine disease can lead to very severe impairment of brain development. It can also cause acute neurological crises, with convulsions, coma and even death if the concentrations of the branched-chain amino acids and their metabolites in the bloodstream rise too high.

For about half the affected infants, treatment consists of a specially formulated diet which provides only minimally adequate amounts of leucine, isoleucine and valine to permit the maintenance of nitrogen balance and growth. Unlike phenylketonuria, the diet cannot be discontinued when brain development is complete. Older patients are still liable to convulsions and coma if the concentration of these amino acids and their metabolites in the bloodstream rises too high.

The other patients with maple syrup urine disease are more fortunate. Their problem is that the enzyme involved in the metabolism of the oxoacids formed from leucine, isoleucine and valine has low activity because it has a defect in the binding site for its cofactor, thiamin diphosphate. They are able to achieve more or less normal activity of this enzyme if they are provided with very high concentrations of thiamin, i.e. they have a vitamin dependency disease (see p. 290). A modest restriction of protein intake, together with supplements of relatively large amounts of thiamin maintains these children in good health.

APPENDIX I

Units of measurement

	Unit	Symbol
length	metre	m
mass	kilogram	kg
volume	litre	l
time	second	s
amount of substance	mole	mol
energy	joule	J
radioactivity	becquerel	Bq
absorbed dose	gray	Gy
dose equivalent	sievert	Sv

Submultiples and multiples of units

Multiple		Prefix	Symbol
10^9	× 1,000,000,000	giga	G
10^6	× 1,000,000	mega	M
10^3	× 1,000	kilo	k
10^2	× 100	hecto	h
10	× 10	deca	da
10^{-1}	/10	deci	d
10^{-2}	/100	centi	c
10^{-3}	/1,000	milli	m
10^{-6}	/1,000,000	micro	μ
10^{-9}	/1,000,000,000	nano	n
10^{-12}	/1,000,000,000,000	pico	p
10^{-15}	/1,000,000,000,000,000	femto	f
10^{-18}	/1,000,000,000,000,000,000	atto	a

APPENDIX II
The nutrient yields of some common foods

This is a very brief and simplified table of food composition; for more detailed information you are referred to:

- Bender A. E. & D. A. Bender 1986. *Food tables*. Oxford: Oxford University Press.
- Bender A. E. & D. A. Bender 1991. *Food labelling: a companion to food tables*. Oxford: Oxford University Press.
- *McCance & Widdowson's The Composition of Foods*, 5th edn. Cambridge: Royal Society of Chemistry / Ministry of Agriculture, Fisheries and Food, 1991.

- Davies J. & J. W. T. Dickerson 1991. *Nutrient content of food portions*. Cambridge: Royal Society of Chemistry. See also Table 2.7 on page 21.

Breakfast cereals

/100g	Energy kcal	Energy kJ	Protein grams	Fat grams	Carboh grams	Sodium mg	Calcium mg	Iron mg	Vit B₁ mg	Vit B₂ mg	Fibre grams
All-Bran	258	1079	13	2.5	46	1700	85	9	1	1.5	30
Cornflakes	364	1523	8	0.5	82	1200	negl	7	1	1.5	11
Muesli	383	1603	13	7.5	66	180	200	4.5	0.3	0.3	8
Porridge	47	197	1.5	1	8	600	negl	0.5	0.1	0.01	0.7
Puffed Wheat	341	1427	14	1.3	68.5	negl	25	4.6	negl	0.06	9
Ready Brek	409	1712	12	9	70	25	65	5	1.5	0.1	7
Rice Krispies	382	1600	6	0.7	88	1300	negl	7	1	1.5	1
Shredded Wheat	341	1427	10.5	3	68	negl	40	4	0.3	0.05	10
Special K	377	1578	19	1	73	1000	50	13	1.2	1.7	3
Sugar Puffs	367	1540	6	0.8	84	negl	15	2.1	negl	0.03	6
Weetabix	357	1494	11.5	3.5	70	360	30	7.6	1	1.5	12

Baked goods (Baked goods containing butter or margarine will be a modest source of vitamin A).

/100g	Energy kcal	kJ	Protein grams	Fat grams	Carboh grams	Sodium mg	Calcium mg	Iron mg	Vit B$_1$ mg	Vit B$_2$ mg	Fibre grams
Biscuits, chocolate	535	2239	6	27	67	160	110	1.7	0.5	0.15	3
cream crackers	454	1900	9.5	16	68	600	100	1.7	0.15	0.1	6
plain digestive	484	2026	10	20	66	440	110	2	0.15	0.1	5
semi-sweet	481	2013	7	17	75	400	120	2	0.15	0.1	3
shortbread	520	2176	6	26	66	270	100	1.5	0.15	negl	3
wafer	554	2319	5	30	66	70	70	1.6	0.1	0.1	2
water biscuits	460	1925	11	12.5	76	470	120	1.6	0.1	0.03	3
Bread, brown	235	984	9	2.2	45	550	100	2.5	0.25	0.05	5
malt	255	1067	8	3	49	280	90	3.5	negl	negl	3
white	246	1030	7.8	1.7	50	540	100	1.7	0.2	0.03	3
wholemeal	227	950	8.8	2.7	42	540	25	2.5	0.3	0.08	7.5
Currant buns	320	1339	7	8	55	100	90	2.5	0.2	0.03	3
Cake, fruit	347	1452	4	11	58	170	75	1.8	0.1	0.1	3
Madeira	405	1695	5	17	58	400	40	1	0.05	0.1	2
sponge	481	2013	6.5	27	53	350	140	1.4	negl	0.1	1
iced	427	1787	4	15	69	250	45	1.5	negl	0.05	2
Chapattis	349	1461	8	13	50	130	70	2.3	0.25	0.05	7
Crispbread, rye	340	1423	9.5	2	71	220	50	4	0.3	0.15	12
wheat	395	1653	45	7.5	37	600	60	5.5	0.15	0.1	5
Pastry, flaky	572	2394	6	40	47	500	90	1.5	0.1	negl	2
shortcrust	540	2260	7	32	56	500	100	2	0.2	negl	1
Scones	389	1628	7.5	15	56	800	600	1.5	negl	0.1	2

Fruit The fat content of fruits is negligible, apart from bananas (0.3 g/100g); the sodium content is also negligible.

/100g	Energy kcal	Energy kJ	Protein grams	Carboh grams	Calcium mg	Iron mg	Vit A µg	Vit B_1 mg	Vit B_2 mg	Vit C mg	Fibre grams
Apples	36	150	0.2	9	negl	0.2	negl	0.03	0.02	2	2
Apricots	30	125	0.6	7	negl	0.4	250	0.04	0.05	10	2
Bananas	86	360	1	20	negl	0.4	200	0.04	0.07	10	3
Bilberries	58	243	0.5	14	negl	0.7	15	0.02	0.02	20	7
Blackberries	30	125	1.5	6	60	1	15	0.03	0.04	20	7
Black currants	32	134	1	7	60	1.5	30	0.03	0.06	200	9
Cherries	42	176	0.5	10	negl	0.3	15	0.04	0.06	5	2
Cranberries	18	75	0.5	4	15	1	negl	0.03	0.02	10	4
Gooseberries	16	67	1	3	30	0.3	30	0.04	0.03	40	3
Grapefruit	22	92	0.5	5	negl	0.3	negl	0.05	0.02	40	0.5
canned in syrup	66	276	0.5	16	negl	0.7	negl	0.04	0.01	30	0.3
Grapes black	54	226	0.5	13	negl	0.3	negl	0.04	0.02	negl	0.5
white	62	260	0.6	15	20	0.3	negl	0.04	0.02	negl	0.5
Lemons	16	67	1	3	100	0.4	negl	0.05	0.04	80	0.5
Loganberries	18	75	1	3.5	40	1.5	negl	0.02	0.03	0	6
Mangoes	62	260	0.5	15	negl	0.5	1000	0.03	0.04	0	2
Melon	22	92	0.5	5	negl	0.5	1000	0.05	0.03	5	1
Nectarines	48	200	1	11	negl	0.4	500	0.02	0.05	10	2
Oranges	40	167	1	9	40	0.3	50	0.1	0.03	50	2
Orange juice	38	159	0.6	9	negl	0.3	50	0.08	0.02	50	2
Peaches	34	142	0.5	8	negl	0.3	70	0.02	0.04	10	1
Pears	32	134	0.2	8	negl	negl	negl	0.02	0.02	0	2
Pineapple	50	210	0.5	12	negl	0.4	negl	0.08	0.02	5	1
canned in syrup	81	339	0.3	20	negl	0.4	negl	0.05	0.02	0	1
Plums	42	176	0.5	10	negl	0.4	30	0.05	0.03	negl	2
Prunes	84	352	1	20	negl	1.5	80	0.04	0.08	negl	8
Raspberries	28	117	1	6	40	1.2	15	0.02	0.03	25	8
Rhubarb	42	176	0.5	10	80	0.3	negl	negl	0.03	5	2
Satsumas	36	150	1	8	40	0.3	15	0.07	0.02	30	2
Strawberries	26	109	0.5	6	20	0.7	5	0.02	0.03	60	2
Tangerines	36	150	1	8	40	0.3	15	0.07	0.02	30	2

Sweets and desserts

/100g	Energy kcal	Energy kJ	Protein grams	Fat grams	Carboh grams	Sodium mg	Calcium mg	Iron mg	Vit A μg	Vit B$_1$ mg	Vit B$_2$ mg
Chocolate, milk	538	2252	8	30	59	120	220	1.6	negl	0.1	0.2
plain	541	2265	5	29	65	negl	40	2.5	negl	0.1	0.1
Custard	120	502	4	4	17	80	140	negl	40	0.05	0.2
Dairy ice cream	179	749	4	7	25	80	140	0.2	negl	0.04	0.2
Egg custard	122	510	6	6	11	80	130	0.5	60	0.05	0.3
Fruit pie	384	1607	4	16	56	200	50	1	negl	0.05	negl
Non-dairy ice cream	168	703	3	8	21	70	120	0.3	negl	0.04	0.15
Pancakes	312	1306	6	16	36	50	120	1	40	0.1	0.2
Rice pudding	96	402	3.5	2.5	15	50	100	0.2	30	0.03	0.15

Nuts

/100g	Energy kcal	Energy kJ	Protein grams	Fat grams	Carboh grams	Sodium mg	Calcium mg	Iron mg	Vit B$_1$ mg	Vit B$_2$ mg	Fibre grams
Almonds	570	2386	17	54	4	negl	250	4	0.2	1	14
Barcelona nuts	640	2679	11	64	5	negl	170	3	0.1	0.1	10
Brazil nuts	604	2528	12	60	4	negl	180	2.8	1	0.12	9
Chestnuts	180	753	2	2.7	37	negl	50	1	0.2	0.2	7
Coconut	352	1473	3	36	4	negl	negl	2	negl	negl	14
Peanuts	582	2436	24	50	9	negl	60	2	1	0.1	8
salted	582	2436	24	50	9	450	60	2	0.2	0.1	8
Walnuts	532	2227	11	52	5	negl	60	2.5	0.3	0.15	5

Vegetables

/100g	Energy kcal	Energy kJ	Protein grams	Fat grams	Carboh grams	Sodium mg	Calcium mg	Iron mg	Vit A µg	Vit B$_1$ mg	Vit B$_2$ mg	Vit C mg	Fibre grams
Asparagus	8	33	1.7	negl	0.5	negl	negl	0.5	50	0.05	0.04	negl	1
Aubergine	14	57	0.7	negl	3	negl	negl	0.4	negl	0.05	0.03	5	2
Avocados	204	854	4	20	2	negl	15	1.5	15	0.1	0.1	5	2
Beans, baked	64	268	5	0.5	10	480	45	1.4	negl	0.07	0.05	negl	7
broad	49	205	4	0.6	7	20	20	1	40	0.1	0.04	15	4
butter	98	410	7	0.3	17	negl	20	1.7	negl	0.1	negl	negl	5
French	7	29	0.8	negl	1	negl	40	0.6	80	0.04	0.07	5	3
haricot	98	410	6.6	0.5	17	negl	70	2.5	negl	0.2	0.05	negl	7
mung (dahl)	104	435	6	4	11	820	35	2.6	negl	0.1	0.04	negl	5
red kidney	283	1185	22	1.7	45	40	140	6.7	negl	0.5	0.2	negl	25
runner	21	88	2	0.2	3	negl	25	0.7	60	0.03	0.07	5	3
Beetroot	47	197	1.8	negl	10	65	30	0.4	negl	0.02	0.04	5	4
Broccoli	18	75	3	negl	1.6	negl	80	1	500	0.06	0.2	35	4
Brussels sprouts	18	75	3	negl	1.7	negl	25	0.5	60	0.06	0.1	40	3
Cabbage	8	33	1	negl	1	negl	30	0.5	100	0.03	0.03	25	2
white	22	92	2	negl	3.5	negl	45	0.4	negl	0.06	0.05	40	3
Carrots	22	92	0.7	negl	5	100	50	0.6	12000	0.06	0.05	5	3
Cauliflower	14	59	2	negl	1.5	negl	negl	0.5	5	0.1	0.1	60	2
Celery	9	38	1	negl	1.3	140	50	0.6	negl	0.03	0.03	7	2
Chickpeas	149	624	8	3.3	22	850	65	3.1	90	0.1	0.05	3	5
Chicory	9	38	0.8	negl	1.5	negl	negl	0.7	negl	0.05	0.05	4	2
Cucumber	10	42	0.6	negl	2	negl	25	0.3	negl	0.04	0.04	8	0.5
Leeks	27	113	1.8	negl	5	negl	60	2	negl	0.07	0.03	15	2.5
Lentils	104	435	8	0.5	17	negl	negl	2.4	negl	0.1	0.04	negl	4
Lettuce	8	33	1	negl	1	negl	25	0.9	200	0.07	0.08	15	1.5
Marrow	7	29	0.4	negl	1.4	negl	negl	0.2	5	negl	negl	2	1
Mushrooms	13	54	2	0.6	negl	negl	negl	1	negl	0.1	0.4	3	negl
Onions	24	100	1	negl	5	negl	30	0.3	negl	0.03	0.05	10	1
Parsnips	52	218	2	negl	11	negl	60	0.6	negl	0.1	0.08	4	2.5
Peas	71	297	6	0.4	11	negl	negl	2	50	0.3	0.2	25	5
Peppers	15	63	1	0.4	2	negl	negl	0.4	40	negl	0.03	100	1
Potato, baked	88	368	2	negl	20	negl	negl	0.6	negl	0.1	0.03	10	2

/100g	Energy kcal	Energy kJ	Protein grams	Fat grams	Carboh grams	Sodium mg	Calcium mg	Iron mg	Vit A µg	Vit B₁ mg	Vit B₂ mg	Nicotinic acid mg	Vit C mg
Spaghetti	122	511	4	0.3	26	negl	negl	0.4	negl	0.01	0.01	2	negl
Spinach	30	126	5	0.5	1.5	120	600	4	1000	0.15	0.15	6	25
Swedes	20	84	1	negl	4	negl	40	0.3	negl	0.03	0.03	3	20
Tomatoes	16	67	1	negl	3	negl	13	0.4	15	0.05	0.05	1.5	20
Turnips	10	42	0.7	negl	2	30	60	0.4	negl	0.04	0.04	2	20
Watercress	14	59	3	negl	0.7	60	220	1.6	500	0.1	0.1	3	60

Milk and dairy produce

/100g	Energy kcal	Energy kJ	Protein grams	Fat grams	Carboh grams	Sodium mg	Calcium mg	Iron mg	Vit A µg	Vit B₁ mg	Vit B₂ mg
Butter	740	3097	0.5	82	negl	870	15	0.2	1000	negl	negl
Cheese, soft	299	1252	23	23	negl	1400	400	1	250	0.05	0.6
Cheddar	410	1716	26	34	negl	600	800	0.4	400	0.04	0.5
cottage	66	276	14	0.5	1.5	450	60	0.1	30	0.02	0.2
cream	435	1821	3	47	negl	300	100	0.1	450	0.02	0.15
Danish blue	353	1478	23	29	negl	1400	580	0.2	300	0.03	0.6
Edam	303	1268	24	23	negl	1000	750	0.2	300	0.04	0.4
Parmesan	410	1716	35	30	negl	750	1200	0.4	400	0.02	0.5
processed	313	1310	22	25	negl	1400	700	0.5	250	0.02	0.3
Stilton	464	1942	26	40	negl	1200	350	0.5	450	0.07	0.3
Cream, double	446	1867	1.5	48	2	30	50	0.2	400	0.02	0.1
single	212	887	2.4	21	3	40	80	0.3	250	0.03	0.1
sterilized	229	959	2.6	23	3	60	80	0.3	200	0.01	0.1
whipping	332	1389	1.9	35	2.5	30	60	0.3	300	0.02	0.1
Egg	147	615	12.3	11	negl	140	50	2	140	0.1	0.5
Margarine	729	3051	negl	81	negl	800	negl	negl	1000	negl	negl
Milk, full cream	66	276	3.3	3.8	4.7	50	120	negl	50	0.05	0.2
skimmed	34	142	3.4	0.1	5	50	130	negl	negl	0.04	0.2
Channel Islands	76	318	3.6	4.8	4.7	50	120	negl	50	0.05	0.2
evaporated, whole	160	670	8.6	9	11.3	180	280	negl	100	0.06	0.5
Yoghurt, flavoured	85	356	5	1	14	60	170	negl	negl	0.05	0.25
plain	53	222	5	1	6	80	180	negl	negl	0.05	0.3

Meat and meat products

/100g	Energy kcal	Energy kJ	Protein grams	Fat grams	Carboh grams	Sodium mg	Calcium mg	Iron mg	Vit A µg	Vit B$_1$ mg	Vit B$_2$ mg
Bacon rashers	420	1758	15	40	negl	1500	negl	1	negl	0.4	0.15
Beef	248	1038	17	20	negl	70	negl	1.5	negl	0.05	0.15
corned beef	216	904	27	12	negl	1000	negl	3	negl	negl	0.2
sausages	304	1272	10	24	12	800	50	1.4	negl	0.03	0.1
steak	202	845	19	14	negl	50	negl	2.3	negl	0.08	0.26
stewing	170	712	20	10	negl	70	negl	2.1	negl	0.06	0.23
Black pudding	310	1298	13	22	15	1200	35	20	negl	0.1	0.1
Chicken	145	607	25	5	negl	80	negl	0.8	negl	0.1	0.2
Cornish pastie	336	1406	8	20	31	600	60	1.5	negl	0.1	0.1
Duck	190	795	25	10	negl	100	negl	2.7	negl	0.3	0.5
Gammon	271	1134	25	19	negl	1000	negl	1.3	negl	0.4	0.15
Goose	314	1314	29	22	negl	150	negl	4.6	negl	negl	negl
Haggis	318	1331	11	22	19	800	30	5	2000	0.2	0.2
Ham	117	490	18	5	negl	1200	negl	1.2	negl	0.5	0.3
Hamburger	269	1126	15	21	5	600	25	2.5	negl	0.04	0.2
Heart	112	469	19	4	negl	100	negl	5	negl	0.5	1
Kidney	95	398	17	3	negl	220	negl	7	100	0.5	1.8
Lamb breast	383	1603	17	35	negl	100	negl	1.3	negl	0.08	0.17
chops	375	1569	15	35	negl	60	negl	1.2	negl	0.1	0.15
cutlets	384	1607	15	36	negl	60	negl	1.2	negl	0.1	0.15
leg	243	1017	18	19	negl	50	negl	1.7	negl	0.14	0.25
shoulder	316	1323	16	28	negl	70	negl	1.2	negl	0.1	0.2
Liver	151	632	20	7	2	90	negl	8	1500	0.2	3.1
Pork pie	383	1603	10	27	25	700	50	1.4	negl	0.2	0.1
chops	334	1398	16	30	negl	50	negl	0.8	negl	0.6	0.15
luncheon meat	315	1319	13	27	5	1000	15	1	negl	0.07	0.1
leg	275	1151	17	23	negl	60	negl	0.8	negl	0.7	0.2
sausages	372	1557	11	32	10	750	40	1.1	negl	0.04	0.1
Salami	489	2047	19	45	2	2000	negl	1	negl	0.2	0.2
Turkey	106	444	22	2	negl	50	negl	0.8	negl	0.1	0.15
Veal	111	465	21	3	negl	110	negl	1.2	negl	0.1	0.25

Fish and sea foods

/100g	Energy kcal	Energy kJ	Protein grams	Fat grams	Carboh grams	Sodium mg	Calcium mg	Iron mg	Vit A µg	Vit B₁ mg	Vit B₂ mg
Cod	74	310	17	1	negl	80	20	0.3	negl	0.1	0.1
Crab	125	523	20	5	negl	400	30	1.3	negl	0.1	0.2
Fish fingers	183	766	13	7.5	16	320	45	0.7	negl	0.1	0.1
Halibut	94	393	18	2.5	negl	85	85	negl	0.5	negl	0.1
Herring	239	1000	17	19	negl	70	35	0.8	50	negl	0.2
Kipper	203	849	26	11	negl	1000	70	1.4	50	negl	0.2
Lemon sole	80	335	17	1.4	negl	100	negl	0.5	negl	0.1	0.1
Lobster	120	502	22	3.5	negl	330	60	0.8	negl	0.1	0.1
Mackerel	220	921	19	16	negl	130	25	1	45	0.1	0.35
Mussels	66	276	12	2	negl	300	100	6	negl	negl	negl
Pilchards in tomato	123	515	19	5	0.7	400	300	2.7	negl	0.02	0.3
Plaice	91	381	18	2	negl	120	50	0.3	negl	0.3	0.1
Prawns	110	460	23	2	negl	1600	150	1.1	negl	negl	negl
Salmon	180	753	18	12	negl	100	30	0.7	negl	0.2	0.15
canned	152	636	20	8	negl	600	100	1.4	100	0.04	0.2
smoked	145	607	25	5	negl	2000	negl	0.6	negl	0.2	0.2
Sardines in oil	222	929	24	14	negl	650	550	2.9	negl	0.04	0.4
in tomato	182	762	18	12	0.5	700	460	4.6	negl	0.02	0.3
Shrimps	118	493	24	2.5	negl	4000	300	1.8	negl	0.03	0.03
Trout	136	569	24	4.5	negl	90	40	1	negl	negl	negl
Tuna in brine	100	420	24	0.6	negl	320	negl	1	negl	0.02	0.1
in oil	190	790	27	9	negl	290	negl	1.6	negl	0.02	0.1

GLOSSARY

In addition to the brief glossary here, the following small and reasonably priced reference books will be useful:

Bender, A. E. 1990. *Dictionary of nutrition and food technology*, 6th edn. London: Butterworths.
Bingham, S. 1987. *The Everyman companion to food and nutrition*. London: Dent.
Concise dictionary of biology 1990. Oxford: Oxford University Press.
Concise dictionary of chemistry 1990. Oxford: Oxford University Press.
Penguin dictionary of biology 1990. London: Penguin.
Penguin dictionary of chemistry 1990. London: Penguin.
Yudkin, J. 1985. *The Penguin encyclopedia of nutrition*. London: Penguin.

In addition, most reference libraries have one or more large medical dictionaries, encyclopedias of medicine and biology, etc.

acceptable daily intake (ADI) The total amount of a food additive or contaminant judged to be safe and hence the maximum amount permitted in foods, allowing for the average pattern of consumption of different foods. Normally 1/100 of the lowest dose at which any adverse effect can be detected. For a compound with *ADI not specified* there is no evidence of any adverse effect at any dose tested.

acesulphame K A non-nutritive sweetener, about 200 times as sweet as sucrose.

acid A compound which, when dissolved in water, dissociates to yield hydrogen ions (H^+).

acidosis A condition in which the pH of blood plasma falls below the normal value of 7.4. A fall to pH 7.2 is life-threatening.

activation Increase in the activity of existing molecules of enzyme in a cell, with no change in the amount of enzyme protein present.

acyl group In an ester or other compound, the part derived from a fatty acid is called an acyl group.

ADI Acceptable daily intake of food additives and contaminants.

ADP Adenosine diphosphate.

alanine A non-essential amino acid.

alcohol A compound with an –OH group attached to an aliphatic carbon chain. Also used generally to mean ethanol (ethyl alcohol), the commonly consumed alcohol in beverages.

aldehyde A compound with an HC=O group attached to a carbon atom.

aliphatic A compound with chains of carbon atoms (straight or branched), rather than rings. Aliphatic compounds may be saturated or unsaturated.

alkali A compound which, when dissolved in water, gives an alkaline solution, i.e. one with a pH above 7.

alkalosis A condition in which the pH of blood plasma rises above the normal value of 7.4.

alkane A saturated hydrocarbon, of general formula $C_nH_{(2n+2)}$.

alkene An unsaturated hydrocarbon with a carbon–carbon double bond (C=C), of the general formula C_nH_{2n}.

alkyne An unsaturated hydrocarbon with a carbon–carbon triple bond (C≡C), of

306

general formula $C_nH_{(2n-2)}$.

amide The product of a condensation reaction between a carboxylic acid and ammonia, a $-CONH_2$ group.

amine A compound with an amino $(-NH_2)$ group attached to a carbon atom.

amino acid A compound with both an amino $(-NH_2)$ and a carboxylic acid $(-COOH)$ group attached to the α-carbon.

AMP Adenosine monophosphate.

amylopectin The branched-chain structure of starch.

amylose The straight-chain structure of starch.

anabolism Metabolic reactions resulting in the synthesis of more complex compounds from simple precursors. Commonly linked to the hydrolysis of ATP to ADP and phosphate.

anaerobic Occurring in the absence of oxygen.

anion An ion which has a negative electric charge and therefore migrates to the anode (positive pole) in an electric field. The ions of non-metallic elements are anions.

anorexia Loss of appetite; hence appetite-suppressant drugs are known as anorectic agents.

anorexia nervosa A psychological disturbance resulting in a refusal to eat, or restriction to a very limited range of foods.

anti-codon The three-base region of transfer RNA which recognizes and binds to the codon on messenger RNA.

antioxidant nutrients Those micronutrients which are important in preventing tissue damage due to free-radical action. The principal dietary antioxidants are vitamins E, C and carotene, and the minerals selenium and copper.

arginine A non-essential amino acid. The capacity for arginine synthesis in infants is not adequate enough to meet requirements, and for infants it is an essential amino acid.

aromatic A cyclic compound in which the ring consists of alternating single and double bonds.

ascorbic acid Vitamin C.

asparagine A non-essential amino acid. The amide of aspartic acid.

aspartame A non-nutritive sweetener,

chemically ß-methylaspartyl-phenylalanine; about 180–200 times as sweet as sucrose.

aspartic acid A non-essential amino acid.

atherosclerosis The deposition of lipids on the inner wall of blood vessels, leading to narrowing of the arteries.

atom The smallest particle of an element which can exist as an entity. The atom consists of a nucleus containing protons, neutrons and other uncharged particles, surrounded by a cloud of electrons.

atomic mass The mass of the atom of any element, relative to that of carbon $=$ 12. 1 unit of atomic mass $=$ 1.660×10^{-27} kg.

atomic number The number of protons in the nucleus of an atom (and hence the number of electrons surrounding the nucleus) determines the atomic number of that element.

ATP Adenosine triphosphate.

basal metabolic rate The energy expenditure by the body at complete rest, but not asleep, in the post-prandial state, measured under strictly controlled conditions of thermal neutrality.

base Chemically, an alkali. Also used as a general term for the purines and pyrimidines in DNA and RNA.

biotin A vitamin, sometimes called vitamin H.

body mass index (BMI) The ratio of body weight (in kg)/height^2 (in m). A person having a BMI greater than 25 is considered to be overweight; and above 30, obese.

branched-chain amino acid Three amino acids, leucine, isoleucine and valine, have a branched aliphatic side-chain.

buffer A solution of a weak acid and its salt which can prevent changes in pH as the concentration of H^+ ions changes, by shifting the equilibrium between the dissociated and undissociated acid. Any buffer system only acts around the pH at which the acid is half dissociated.

cachexia The state of undernutrition and extreme emaciation seen in patients with advanced cancer.

calciferol Vitamin D.

calcitriol The active metabolite of vitamin D.

calorie An (obsolete) unit of heat or energy. The amount of heat required to raise 1g of water through 1°C. Nutritionally the kcal is sometime used; 1 kcal = 1,000 cal. 1 cal = 4.186 Joules, 1 Joule = 0.239 cal.

calorimetry The measurement of energy expenditure by heat output; indirect calorimetry estimates heat output from oxygen consumption.

carbohydrate Compounds composed of carbon, hydrogen and oxygen in the ratio $C_nH_{2n}O_n$. The dietary carbohydrates are sugars, starches and non-starch polysaccharides.

carboxylic acid A compound with a –COOH group attached to a carbon atom.

carcinogen A compound that can cause the development of cancer.

catabolism Metabolic reactions resulting in the breakdown of complex molecules to simpler products; commonly, oxidation to carbon dioxide and water, linked to the phosphorylation of ADP to ATP.

catalyst Something which increases the rate at which a chemical reaction achieves equilibrium, without itself being consumed in, or altered by, the reaction.

cation A positively charged ion which migrates to the cathode (negative pole) in an electric field. The ions of metallic elements are cations.

cell The structural and functional unit of all living organisms. A cell is bounded by a lipoprotein membrane, and contains a nucleus, mitochondria, ribosomes, lysosomes and other subcellular organelles. Cells in different organs are differentiated (i.e. specialized in their structure and function).

cellulose A polymer of glucose, linked by ß-1,4 glycoside links, which are not digested by human enzymes.

chemical score A method of expressing the nutritional value of a protein by comparing its content of the limiting essential amino acid with that in egg protein.

cholecalciferol Vitamin D.

cholesterol A steroid which is required for cell-membrane formation and as the precursor for the steroid hormones.

chromosome The DNA in the nucleus of a cell is organized into a number of chromosomes, which consist of DNA and a variety of proteins, collectively known as nucleoproteins. Human cells contain 46 chromosomes; 2 of each of 22 different chromosomes, and two which are known as the sex chromosomes – these may be the same (X-chromosomes) in females, or different (one X and one Y) in males. Ova and spermatozoa are haploid, i.e. they contain only one copy of each chromosome. Ova always have an X sex chromosome; spermatozoa may contain an X or a Y.

codon A sequence of three nucleic acid bases in DNA or mRNA which specify an individual amino acid.

coenzyme A non-protein organic compound which is required for an enzyme reaction. Coenzymes may be loosely or tightly associated with the enzyme protein, and may be covalently bound to the enzyme, in which case they are known as prosthetic groups.

condensation A chemical reaction in which water is eliminated from two compounds to result in the formation of a new compound. The formation of esters, peptides and amides are condensation reactions.

covalent bond A bond between two atoms in which electrons are shared between the atoms.

cyclamate A non-nutritive sweetener, about 30–40 times as sweet as sucrose.

cysteine A non-essential amino acid, derived metabolically from the essential amino acid methionine. It has a sulphydryl (–SH) group on the side-chain.

cystine The product of the oxidation of the sulphydryl groups of two cysteine molecules, to form a disulphide (–S–S–) bridge.

cytoplasm The gel of proteins which fills the cell outside the nucleus; the subcellular organelles are suspended in the cytoplasm.

deoxyribose A pentose (five-carbon) sugar in which one hydroxyl (–OH) group has been replaced by hydrogen. The sugar of DNA.

dextrose An alternative name for glucose.

diet-induced thermogenesis The increase in heat output or energy expenditure after a meal, associated with the digestion and processing of food. Also known as the specific dynamic action of food.

dietary fibre The residue of plant cell walls after extraction and treatment with digestive enzymes. Chemically a mixture of lignin and a variety of non-starch polysaccharides, including cellulose, hemicellulose, pectin, gums and mucilages.

disaccharide A sugar consisting of two monosaccharides linked by a glycoside bond. The common dietary disaccharides are sucrose (cane or beet sugar), lactose, maltose and isomaltose.

dissociation The process whereby a molecule separates into ions on solution in water.

DNA Deoxyribonucleic acid.

double bond A covalent bond in which two pairs of electrons are shared between the participating atoms.

e On food labels the prefix e before the size indicates that this is a standard-size package which has been registered with the appropriate authorities of the European Community.

E- On food labels, additives may be listed either by name or by number; the prefix E- before the number means that this is the number in the list of additives approved for use throughout the European Community.

electrolyte A compound which undergoes partial or complete dissociation into ions when dissolved, and so is capable of transporting an electric current. In clinical chemistry, electrolyte is normally used to mean the major inorganic ions in body fluids.

electron The smallest unit of negative electric charge. The fundamental particles which surround the nucleus of an atom.

electron transport chain The system of cytochromes and other coenzymes in the mitochondrial membrane which transport electrons (and hydrogen ions) from reduced coenzymes to react with oxygen (forming water), linked to the phosphorylation of ADP to ATP.

electronegative An electronegative atom exerts greater attraction for the shared electrons in a covalent bond than does its partner, so developing a partial negative charge.

electropositive An electropositive atom exerts less attraction for the shared electrons in a covalent bond than does its partner, so developing a partial positive charge.

element A substance which cannot be further divided or modified by chemical means. The basic substances from which compounds are formed.

enzyme A protein which acts as a catalyst in a metabolic reaction.

epinephrine North American name for adrenaline.

essential amino acid Eight amino acids, required for protein synthesis, which cannot be synthesized at all in the body, but must be provided in the diet: lysine, methionine, phenylalanine, tryptophan, threonine, valine, leucine, isoleucine. In addition, histidine cannot be synthesized in adequate amount to meet requirements without some dietary intake, and arginine is similarly essential in infants.

essential fatty acids Those polyunsaturated fatty acids which cannot be synthesized in the body and must be provided in the diet. Linoleic and linolenic acids are the only two that are dietary essentials, since the other polyunsaturated fatty acids can be synthesized from them.

ester The product of a condensation reaction between an alcohol and a carboxylic acid.

exons Those regions of DNA which code for proteins, as opposed to the introns, which are non-coding regions inserted between exons in a gene.

fat Triacylglycerols, esters of glycerol with three fatty acids; fats are generally considered to be those triacylglycerols which are solid at room temperature, while oils are triacylglycerols which are liquid at room temperature.

fatty acid Aliphatic carboxylic acids (i.e. with a –COOH group). The metabolically important fatty acids have between 2 and 24 carbon atoms (always an even number) and may be completely saturated or have one (mono-unsaturated) or more (polyunsaturated) C=C double bonds in the carbon chain.

fermentation Anaerobic catabolism by micro-organisms. Commonly used to describe the formation of ethanol from carbohydrates by yeast, but including a variety of catabolic pathways in different organisms.

fibre Crude fibre is a term used in food analysis for the residue after food has been extracted successively with petroleum ether, dilute sulphuric acid and sodium hydroxide, minus the mineral ash. Not related to dietary fibre, nor to non-starch polysaccharide.

flavin A derivative of the vitamin riboflavin, normally acting as an electron-carrying coenzyme or prosthetic group in oxidation and reduction reactions.

flavoprotein A protein with a flavin prosthetic group.

folic acid A vitamin.

galactose A hexose (six-carbon) monosaccharide.

gene A region of DNA which carries the information for a single protein or poly-peptide chain.

genetic code The sequence of triplets of the nucleic acid bases (purines and pyrimidines) which specifies the individual amino acids.

gluconeogenesis The metabolic reactions involved in the synthesis of glucose from non-carbohydrate precursors (mainly amino acids) in the fasting state.

glucose A monosaccharide; a hexose (six-carbon) sugar, of empirical formula $C_6H_{12}O_6$.

glutamic acid (glutamate) A non-essential amino acid.

glutamine A non-essential amino acid, the amide of glutamic acid.

glycerol A trihydric alcohol to which three fatty-acid molecules are esterified in the formation of triacylglycerols (fats and oils). Glycerol has a sweet taste, and is hygroscopic (attracts water); it is commonly used as a humectant in food processing.

glycine A non-essential amino acid.

glycogen A branched-chain polymer of glucose, linked by α-1,4 links, with branch points provided by α-1,6 links. The storage carbohydrate of mammalian liver and muscle.

glycolysis The metabolic pathway by which glucose is oxidized to pyruvate. Anaerobic glycolysis in micro-organisms is also called fermentation.

gums Soluble non-starch polysaccharides in plant extracts and exudates, including guar, acacia and carob gums, gum Arabic and gum tragacanth.

hemicelluloses Branched polymers of pentose (five-carbon) and hexose (six-carbon) monosaccharides.

heterocyclic A cyclic organic compound in which one or more atoms in the ring is of an element other than carbon (commonly nitrogen, oxygen or sulphur in biologically important compounds).

hexose A monosaccharide with six carbon atoms, and hence the empirical formula $C_6H_{12}O_6$. The nutritionally important hexoses are glucose, galactose and fructose.

histidine An amino acid which is partially essential, in that it cannot be synthesized in adequate amounts to meet the requirement for protein synthesis; some has to be provided in the diet.

hormone A compound synthesized in one organ (an endocrine or ductless gland) and released into the bloodstream, where it circulates, acting only on cells which have receptors for that hormone. Hormones are important in the integration and regulation of metabolic processes.

hydrocarbon A compound of carbon and hydrogen only. Hydrocarbons may have linear, branched or cyclic structures, and may be saturated or unsaturated.

hydrogen bond The attraction between a partial positive charge on a hydrogen atom attached to an electronegative atom and a partial negative charge associated with an electronegative atom in another molecule or region of the same macromolecule.

hydrolysis The process of splitting a chemical bond between two atoms by the introduction of water, usually adding –H to one side of the bond and –OH to the other, resulting in the formation of two separate product molecules. The digestion of proteins to amino acids, poly-saccharides and disaccharides to monosaccharides and triacylglycerols to glycerol and fatty acids are all hydrolysis reactions.

hydrophilic A compound which is soluble in water, or a region of a macromolecule which can interact with water molecules.

hydrophobic A compound which is insoluble in water, but soluble in lipids, or a region of a macromolecule which cannot interact with water, although it does interact with lipids.

hypertension Raised blood pressure, high enough above the normal range to be clinically important and possibly life-threatening.

hypoglycaemia A fall in the plasma concentration of glucose to below about 3 mmol/l.

induction The initiation of new synthesis of an enzyme or other protein by activation of the transcription of the gene for the protein. Inducers are commonly metabolic intermediates or hormones. Induction results in an increase in the amount of enzyme protein in the cell.

inhibition Decrease in the activity of an enzyme, with no effect on the amount of enzyme protein present in the cell.

inorganic Any chemical compound other than those carbon compounds which are considered to be organic.

inositol A cyclic hexahydro-alcohol, important in cell membrane phospholipids. Not a dietary essential for man.

insoluble fibre Lignin and non-starch polysaccharides in plant cell walls (cellulose and hemicellulose).

international units (IU) Before vitamins and other substances were purified, their potency was expressed in arbitrary, but standardized, units of biological activity. Now obsolete, but vitamins A, D and E are sometimes still quoted in IU.

intron Regions of DNA between those parts of a gene which code for the protein. They may be control regions, or may have no known function.

inulin A polymer of fructose, which is the storage carbohydrate of Jerusalem artichoke and some other tubers. Not digestible by human enzymes, and

therefore a part of non-starch polysaccharide or dietary fibre.

ion An atom or group of atoms which has lost or gained one or more electrons and thus has an electric charge.

isoleucine An essential amino acid.

isomaltose A disaccharide, composed of two glucose molecules linked by an α-1,6 glycoside bond.

isomers Forms of the same chemical compound, but with a different spatial arrangement of atoms or groups in the molecule. D- and L-isomerism refers to the arrangement of four different substituents around a carbon atom relative to the arrangement in the triose sugar D-glyceraldehyde. *R*- and *S*-isomerism refers to the arrangement of four different substituents around a carbon atom according to a set of systematic chemical rules. *Cis*- and *trans*-isomerism refers to the arrangement of groups adjacent to a carbon–carbon double bond.

isotope Different forms of the same chemical element (i.e. having the same number of protons in the nucleus and the same number of electrons surrounding the nucleus as each other) differing in the number of neutrons in the nucleus, and hence in the relative atomic mass.

joule The SI unit of energy. 1 joule is the work done when the point of application of a force of 1 newton moves 1 metre in the direction of the force. 1 joule = 0.239 cal, 1 cal = 4.186 joule.

ketone A compound with a carbonyl (C=O) group attached to two aliphatic groups.

ketone bodies Acetoacetate and ß-hydroxybutyrate (not chemically a ketone) formed in the liver from fatty acids in the fasting state and released into the circulation as metabolic fuels for use by other tissues. Acetone is also formed non-enzymically from acetoacetate, circulates in the bloodstream, but cannot be metabolized as a metabolic fuel.

ketosis An elevation of the plasma concentrations of acetoacetate, hydroxybutyrate and acetone, as occurs in the fasting state.

Kjeldahl determination A method for determining the nitrogen content of organic compounds, by catalytic conversion to ammonia and determination of the ammonia. Commonly used for protein determination; for most proteins nitrogen is 16% of the mass of the molecule, so nitrogen $\times$ 6.25 = total (crude) protein.

K_m The Michaelis constant of an enzyme; the concentration of substrate which gives half the maximum rate of formation of product.

kwashiorkor A disease of protein–energy malnutrition in which there is oedema masking the severe muscle wastage, fatty infiltration of the liver and abnormalities of hair structure and hair and skin pigmentation.

lactose The sugar of milk. A disaccharide composed of glucose and galactose.

lecithin Phospholipids containing choline, phosphatidylcholine. Commonly used as emulsifying agents in food manufacture. Not a dietary essential.

lectins Toxic compounds found in many legumes which cause red blood cells to agglutinate (hence they are also called phytohaemagglutinins). Destroyed by rapid boiling for several minutes.

leucine An essential amino acid.

lignin A non-carbohydrate component of plant cell walls, one of the constituents of dietary fibre. Chemically a polymer of aromatic alcohols.

lipid A general term including fats and oils (triacylglycerols), phospholipids and steroids.

lipogenesis The metabolic pathway for synthesis of fatty acids from acetyl CoA, then the synthesis of triacylglycerols by esterification of glycerol with fatty acids.

lipolysis The hydrolysis of triacylglycerols to yield fatty acids and glycerol.

Lower Reference Nutrient Intake (LRNI) An intake of a nutrient below which it is unlikely that physiological needs will be met or metabolic integrity be maintained.

lysine An essential amino acid.

macromolecule A term used to describe the large molecules of, for example, proteins, nucleic acids and polysaccharides.

maltose A disaccharide composed of two molecules of glucose linked by an α-1,4 glycoside bond.

marasmus A disease of protein–energy malnutrition in which there is extreme emaciation as a result of catabolism of adipose tissue and protein reserves.

menadione A synthetic compound which has vitamin K activity.

menaquinone Vitamin K.

metabolic fuel Those dietary components which are oxidized as a source of metabolic energy: fats, carbohydrates, proteins and alcohol.

metabolism The processes of interconversion of chemical compounds in the body.

methionine An essential amino acid.

mineral Inorganic salts, so-called because they can be obtained by mining.

mitochondrion A subcellular organelle which contains the enzymes of the citric acid cycle, fatty acid oxidation and the electron transport chain for oxidative phosphorylation of ADP to ATP.

mol Abbreviation for mole, the SI unit for the amount of material. The relative molecular mass of a compound, expressed in grams. 1 mol of any compound contains 6.0223×10^{23} molecules.

molecular mass The mass of a molecule of a compound, relative to that of carbon = 12; the sum of the relative atomic masses of the atoms which comprise the molecule.

molecule The smallest particle of a compound that can exist in a free state.

monosaccharide A simple sugar, the basic units from which disaccharides and polysaccharides are composed. The nutritionally important monosaccharides are the pentoses (five-carbon sugars) ribose and deoxyribose, and the hexoses (six-carbon sugars) glucose, galactose and fructose.

M_r Abbreviation for (relative) molecular mass.

mucilages Soluble non-starch polysaccharides extracted from seaweed and other algae, including agar, alginates and carrageenin.

mutagen A compound that can cause mutations, i.e. changes in DNA which will be inherited by future generations.

NAD Nicotinamide adenine dinucleotide, a coenzyme derived from the vitamin niacin.

NADP Nicotinamide adenine dinucleotide phosphate, a coenzyme derived from the vitamin niacin.

neurotransmitter A compound synthesized in one neurone and secreted into the synaptic cleft in response to electrical conduction in the neurone. It activates receptors on the post-synaptic neurone, and thereby propagates nervous transmission across the synapse.

neutron One of the fundamental particles in the nucleus of an atom. Neutrons have no electric charge, and a mass approximately equal to that of a proton. Differences in the number of neutrons in atoms of the same element account for the occurrence of isotopes.

niacin A vitamin; the two vitamers of niacin are nicotinamide and nicotinic acid.

nitrogen balance The difference between the intake of nitrogenous compounds (mainly protein) and the output of nitrogenous products from the body. Positive nitrogen balance occurs in growth, when there is a net increase in the body content of protein; negative nitrogen balance means that there is a loss of protein from the body.

non-essential amino acid Those amino acids which are required for protein synthesis, but can be synthesized in the body in adequate amounts to meet requirements, and therefore do not have to be provided in the diet. The non-essential amino acids are: glycine, alanine, serine, proline, glutamic acid, aspartic acid, glutamine, asparagine and arginine. In addition, tyrosine can be synthesized in the body, but only from the essential amino acid phenylalanine, and cysteine can be synthesized, but only from the essential amino acid methionine. Arginine is essential for infants, and histidine is partially essential for infants and adults, because although these two amino acids can be synthesized in the body, the capacity for their synthesis is not adequate to meet requirements without some dietary intake.

non-shivering thermogenesis A metabolic process for increasing body temperature without muscle contraction. Largely due to partial uncoupling of oxidative phosphorylation from electron transport in the mitochondria of brown adipose tissue.

non-starch polysaccharides A group of polysaccharides other than starch, which occur in plant foods. They are not digested by human enzymes, although they may be fermented by intestinal bacteria. They provide the major part of dietary fibre. The main non-starch polysaccharides are cellulose, hemicellulose (insoluble non-starch polysaccharides) and pectin and the plant gums and mucilages (soluble non-starch polysaccharides).

norepinephrine North American name for noradrenaline.

nucleic acid DNA and RNA – polymers of nucleotides which carry the genetic information of the cell (DNA in the nucleus) and information from DNA for protein synthesis (RNA).

nucleotides Phosphate esters of purine or pyrimidine bases with ribose (ribonucleotides) or deoxyribose (deoxyribonucleotides).

nucleus Chemically, the central part of an atom, containing protons, neutrons and a variety of other subatomic particles. Biologically, the subcellular organelle which contains the genetic information, as DNA, arranged in chromosomes.

obesity Excessive body weight due to accumulation of adipose tissue. Obesity is generally considered to be a **body mass index** greater than 30; a value of between 25 and 30 indicates that the person is overweight.

oil Triacylglycerols, esters of glycerol with three fatty acids; oils are those triacylglycerols which are liquid at room temperature, while fats are solid. Mineral oil and lubricating oil are chemically completely different, and are mainly long-chain hydrocarbons.

oligopeptide A chain of 2–10 amino acids linked by peptide bonds. Longer chains of amino acids are known as polypeptides (up to about 50 amino acids) or proteins.

oligosaccharide A general term for

polymers of sugars containing about 3–10 monosaccharides.

orbital An allowed energy level for an electron around the nucleus of an atom, or of two atoms in a molecule.

organic Chemically, all compounds of carbon, other than simple carbonate and bicarbonate salts, are called organic, since they were originally discovered in living matter. Also used to describe foods grown under specified conditions without the use of fertilizers, pesticides, etc.

overweight Body weight relative to height greater than is considered desirable (on the basis of life expectancy), but not so much as to be considered obesity.

oxidation A chemical reaction in which the number of electrons in a compound is decreased. In organic compounds this is generally seen as a decrease in the proportion of hydrogen, an increase in the number of carbon–carbon double bonds or an increase in the proportion of oxygen in the molecule.

oxidative phosphorylation The phosphorylation of ADP to ATP, linked to the oxidation of metabolic fuels in the mitochondrial membrane.

pantothenic acid A vitamin, the functional part of coenzyme A and acyl carrier protein.

pectin A complex polysaccharide of a variety of methylated monosaccharides. Not digestible by human enzymes, and therefore a part of soluble non-starch polysaccharide or dietary fibre.

pentose A monosaccharide sugar with five carbon atoms, and hence the empirical formula $C_5H_{10}O_5$. The most important pentose sugars are ribose and deoxyribose (in which one hydroxyl group has been replaced by hydrogen).

peptide bond The link between amino acids in a protein. Formed by condensation between the carboxylic acid group (–COOH) of one amino acid and the amino group (–NH$_2$) of another to give a –CO–NH– link between the amino acids.

pH A measure of the acidity (or alkalinity) of a solution. A neutral solution has pH = 7.0; lower values are acid, higher values are alkaline. pH stands for

potential hydrogen, and is the negative logarithm of the concentration of hydrogen ions (H$^+$) in the solution.

phenol A compound with an –OH group attached to a carbon atom in an aromatic ring.

phenylalanine An essential amino acid.

phospholipid A lipid in which glycerol is esterified to two fatty acids, but the third hydroxyl group is esterified to phosphate, and through the phosphate to one of a variety of other compounds. Phospholipids are both hydrophilic and hydrophobic, and have a central rôle in the structure of cell membranes.

phosphorolysis The cleavage of a bond between two parts of a molecule by the introduction of phosphate, yielding two product molecules. The breakdown of glycogen, to yield glucose-1-phosphate, proceeds by way of sequential phosphorolysis reactions.

phosphorylation The addition of a phosphate group to a compound.

phylloquinone Vitamin K.

physical activity level (PAL) Energy expenditure, averaged over 24h, expressed as a ratio of the basal metabolic rate. The sum of the physical activity ratio × time spent for each activity during the day.

physical activity ratio (PAR) Energy expenditure in a given activity, expressed as a ratio of the basal metabolic rate.

polypeptide A chain of amino acids, linked by peptide bonds. Generally up to about 50 amino acids constitute a polypeptide, while a larger polypeptide would be called a protein.

polysaccharide A polymer of monosaccharide units linked by glycoside bonds. The nutritionally important polysaccharides can be divided into starch and glycogen, and the non-starch polysaccharides.

polyunsaturated Fatty acids with two or more carbon-carbon bonds in the molecule, separated by a methylene (–CH$_2$–) group.

PRI Population reference intake of a nutrient, a term introduced in the 1993 EC tables of nutrient requirements. An intake of the nutrient two standard deviations above the observed mean requirement, and hence greater than the requirements of 97.5% of the population.

proline A non-essential amino acid.

prostaglandins A group of related compounds synthesized from polyunsaturated fatty acids which act as local hormones, having a variety of regulatory rôles in the body.

prosthetic group A non-protein part of an enzyme which is essential for the catalytic activity of the enzyme, and which is covalently bound to the protein.

protein A polymer of amino acids joined by peptide bonds.

proton The positively charged subatomic particle in the nucleus of atoms. The number of protons in the nucleus determines the atomic number of the element. The hydrogen ion (H^+) is a proton.

purine Two of the bases in nucleic acids (DNA and RNA) are purines: adenine and guanine.

pyridoxine Vitamin B_6.

pyrimidine Three of the bases in nucleic acids are pyrimidines: cytosine and thymine in DNA; cytosine and uracil in RNA.

Quetelet's index Alternative name for the body mass index, the ratio of body weight (in kg)/height^2 (in m).

racemic The mixture of D- and L-isomers of a compound.

radical A free radical is a highly reactive molecule with an unpaired electron.

RDA Recommended daily (or dietary) allowance (or amount) of a nutrient. An intake of the nutrient two standard deviations above the observed mean requirement, and hence greater than the requirements of 97.5% of the population.

RDI Recommended daily (or dietary) intake of a nutrient; equivalent to RDA.

reducing sugar A sugar which has a free aldehyde (–HC=O) group, which can therefore act as a chemical reducing agent. Glucose, galactose, maltose and lactose are all reducing sugars.

reduction A chemical reaction in which the number of electrons in a compound is increased. In organic compounds this is generally seen as an increase in the proportion of hydrogen, a decrease in the number of carbon–carbon double bonds or a decrease in the proportion of oxygen

in the molecule. The opposite of oxidation.

repression Decreased synthesis of an enzyme or other protein, as a result of blocking the transcription of the gene for that enzyme. Metabolic intermediates, end-products of pathways and hormones may act as repressors.

resistant starch Starch which is resistant to digestion in the small intestine, either because it is still enclosed in plant cell walls, or because of its crystalline structure. A proportion may be fermented by colonic bacteria.

respiratory quotient (RQ) The ratio of carbon dioxide produced / oxygen consumed in the metabolism of metabolic fuels. The RQ for carbohydrates = 1.0; for fats, 0.71; and for proteins, 0.8.

resting metabolic rate The energy expenditure of the body at rest, but not measured under the strict conditions required for determination of basal metabolic rate.

retinol Vitamin A.

riboflavin Vitamin B_2.

ribose A pentose (five-carbon) sugar.

ribosome The subcellular organelle on which the message of messenger RNA is translated into protein. The organelle on which protein synthesis occurs.

RNI Reference nutrient intake, a term introduced in the 1991 UK tables of dietary reference values (Department of Health 1991). An intake of the nutrient two standard deviations above the observed mean requirement, and hence greater than the requirements of 97.5% of the population.

saccharin A non-nutritive sweetener, about 300–550 times as sweet as sucrose.

salt The product of a reaction between an acid and an alkali. Ordinary table salt is sodium chloride.

satiety The state of satisfaction of hunger or appetite.

saturated An organic compound in which all carbon atoms are joined by single bonds, as opposed to unsaturated compounds with carbon–carbon double bonds. A saturated compound contains the maximum possible proportion of hydrogen.

serine A non-essential amino acid.

soluble fibre Non-starch polysaccharides which are soluble in water; pectin and the plant gums and mucilages.

sorbitol The alcohol formed by reduction of glucose; slowly absorbed and metabolized in the liver, so that it does not lead to a sharp increase in the blood concentration of glucose. Widely used in food preparations for diabetics.

specific dynamic action The increase in energy expenditure and body temperature after a meal, associated with the metabolic cost of digestion and processing of the nutrients. Also known as diet-induced thermogenesis.

starch A polymer of glucose units. Amylose is a straight-chain polymer, with α-1,4 glycoside links between the glucose units. In amylopectin there are also branch points, where chains are linked through an α-1,6 glycoside bond.

steroids Compounds derived from cholesterol (itself also a steroid), most of which are hormones.

stevioside A non-nutritive sweetener, about 300 times as sweet as sucrose.

substrate The substance or substances upon which an enzyme acts.

sugar Chemically, a monosaccharide or small oligosaccharide. Cane or beet sugar is sucrose, a disaccharide of glucose and fructose.

teratogen A compound which can cause congenital defects in the developing fetus.

thaumatin A non-nutritive sweetener, about 3000–4000 times as sweet as sucrose.

thiamin Vitamin B_1.

threonine An essential amino acid.

tocopherol Vitamin E.

transcription The process whereby a copy of the region of DNA containing the gene for a single protein is copied to give a strand of messenger RNA.

translation The process of protein synthesis, whereby the message of messenger RNA is translated into the amino acid sequence.

triacylglycerol The main type of dietary lipid, and the storage lipid of adipose tissue. Glycerol esterified with three molecules of fatty acid. Also known as triglycerides.

triglyceride Alternative (and chemically incorrect) name for triacylglycerol.

tryptophan An essential amino acid, which is also a precursor for the synthesis of the nicotinamide ring of the coenzymes NAD and NADP.

tyrosine An essential amino acid, which is also the precursor for the synthesis of adrenaline, noradrenaline and the thyroid hormones.

unsaturated An organic compound containing one or more carbon–carbon double bonds, and therefore less than the possible maximum proportion of hydrogen.

urea The main excretory end-product of amino acid metabolism.

valency The number of bonds which an atom must form to other atoms in order to achieve a stable electron configuration.

valine An essential amino acid.

van der Waals forces Individually weak forces between molecules depending on transient charges due to transient inequalities in the sharing of electrons in covalent bonds.

vegan A strict vegetarian who will eat no foods of animal origin.

vegetarian One who does not eat meat and meat products. An ovolactovegetarian will eat milk and eggs, but not meat or fish; a lactovegetarian, milk but not eggs; a **vegan** will eat only foods of vegetable origin.

vitamer Related chemical forms of a vitamin which have the same biological activity.

vitamin An organic compound required in small amounts for the maintenance of normal growth, health and metabolic integrity. Deficiency of a vitamin results in the development of a specific deficiency disease, which can be cured or prevented only by that vitamin.

V_{max} The maximum rate at which an enzyme can act when it is saturated with its substrate.

xylitol The sugar alcohol formed by reduction of the pentose sugar xylose. Of interest because it has an action to reduce or prevent dental caries.

zymogen An inactive precursor of an enzyme, which is activated on or after secretion.

BIBLIOGRAPHY

Sources of more detailed information and suggestions for further reading.

General reference books

The Academic Press encyclopedia of food science, food technology and nutrition 1993. London: Academic Press.

Bender, A. E. 1990.*Dictionary of nutrition and food technology*, 6th edn. London: Butterworths.

Bingham, S. 1987. *The Everyman companion to food and nutrition*. London: Dent.

Concise dictionary of biology 1990. Oxford: Oxford University Press.

Concise dictionary of chemistry 1990. Oxford: Oxford University Press.

Penguin dictionary of biology 1990. London: Penguin.

Penguin dictionary of chemistry 1990. London: Penguin.

Yudkin, J. 1985. *The Penguin encyclopedia of nutrition*. London: Viking, Penguin.

General textbooks of nutrition

Bender, A. E. & D. A. Bender 1982. *Nutrition for medical students*. Chichester: John Wiley.

Herbert, V. & G. J. Subak-Sharpe (eds) 1990. *The Mount Sinai School of Medicine complete book of nutrition*. New York: St Martin's Press.

Passmore, R. & M. A. Eastwood 1986. *Davidson and Passmore: human nutrition and dietetics*, 8th edn. Edinburgh: Churchill Livingstone.

General textbooks of biochemistry

Conn, E. E., P. K. Stumpf, G. Bruenning & R. H. Doi 1987. *Outlines of biochemistry*, 5th edn. New York: John Wiley.

Devlin, T. M. (ed.) 1990. *Textbook of biochemistry with clinical correlations*. Chichester: John Wiley.

Lehninger, A. L. 1982. *Principles of biochemistry*. New York: Worth.

Montgomery, R., T. W. Conway, A. A. Spector 1990. *Biochemistry: a case-oriented approach*. St Louis: Mosby.

318

Paterson, C. R. 1983. *Essentials of human biochemistry*. Edinburgh: Churchill Livingstone.

Stryer, L. 1988. *Biochemistry*. New York: W. H. Freeman.

Zubay, G. 1988. *Biochemistry*. New York: Macmillan.

Sources of information on patterns of food consumption and nutrient intake

Barker, M. E., S. McClean, P. G. McKenna, N. G.Reid, J. J. Srain, K. A. Thompson, A. P. Williamson, M. E. Wright 1988. *Diet, lifestyle and health in Northern Ireland*. Centre for Applied Health Studies, University of Ulster, Coleraine.

Department of Health and Social Security Report on Health and Social Subjects 1979. No. 16: *Nutrition and health in old age*. London: HMSO.

Department of Health Report on Health and Social Subjects 1989. No. 36: *The diets of British schoolchildren*. London: HMSO.

Gregory, J., K. Foster, H. Tyler, M. Wiseman 1990. *The dietary and nutritional survey of British adults*. Office of Population Censuses and Surveys, Social Survey Division. London: HMSO.

Ministry of Agriculture, Fisheries and Food. *Household food consumption and expenditure: annual reports of the National Food Survey Committee*. London: HMSO. (Annual publication)

Food composition tables

Bender, A. E. & D. A. Bender 1986. *Food tables*. Oxford: Oxford University Press.

Bender, A. E. & D. A. Bender 1991. *Food labelling, a companion to food tables*. Oxford: Oxford University Press.

Davies, J. & J. W. T. Dickerson 1991. *Nutrient content of food portions*. Cambridge: Royal Society for Chemistry.

McCance & Widdowson's The composition of foods, 5th edn, 1991. Royal Society of Chemistry/Ministry of Agriculture, Fisheries and Food.

Diet and health, reference nutrient intakes

Anderson, D. (ed.) 1986. *A diet of reason: sense and nonsense in the healthy eating debate*. London: Social Affairs Unit.

British Medical Association 1986. *Diet, nutrition and health: report by the Board of Science and Education*. London: BMA.

Department of Health and Social Security Report on Health and Social Subjects 1984. No. 28: *Diet and cardiovascular disease*. London: HMSO.

Department of Health Report on Health and Social Subjects 1989. No. 37: *Dietary sugars and human disease*. London: HMSO.

Department of Health Report on Health and Social Subjects 1991. No. 41: *Dietary reference values for food enegy and nutrients for the United Kingdom*. London: HMSO.

Gibney, M. J. 1986. *Nutrition, diet and health*. Cambridge: Cambridge University Press.

National Research Council 1989. *Recommended dietary allowances*, 10th edn. Washington DC: National Academy Press.

Oliver, M. E. 1981. Diet and coronary heart disease. *British Medical Bulletin* **37**, 49–58.

World Health Organisation 1985. *Energy and protein requirements*. WHO Technical reports Series no. 724. Geneva: WHO.

World Health Organisation 1990. *Diet, nutrition and the prevention of chronic diseases*. WHO Technical Reports Series no. 797. Geneva: WHO.

Energy balance, obesity, and anorexia nervosa

Bender, A. E. & L. J. Brookes (eds) 1987. *Body weight control: the physiology, clinical treatment and prevention of obesity*. Edinburgh: Churchill Livingstone.

Bray, G. A. 1985. Complications of obesity. *Annals of Internal Medicine* **103**, 1052–62.

Crisp, A. H. 1980. *Anorexia nervosa: let me be*. London: Academic Press.

Crisp, A. H. 1983. Anorexia nervosa. *British Medical Journal* **287**, 855–8.

Garrow, J. S. 1988. *Obesity and related disorders*, 2nd edn. Edinburgh: Churchill Livingstone.

James, W. P. T. & E. C. Schofield 1990. *Human energy requirements*. Oxford: FAO/Oxford University Press.

Royal College of Physicians of London 1983. Obesity. *Royal College of Physicians of London, Journal* **17**, 1–58.

Vitamins

Barker, B. M. & D. A. Bender (eds) 1980. *Vitamins in medicine*, Vol. 1. London: Heinemann.

Barker, B. M. & D. A. Bender (eds) 1982. *Vitamins in medicine*, Vol. 2. London: Heinemann.

Bender, D. A. 1992. *Nutritional biochemistry of the vitamins*. Cambridge: Cambridge University Press.

Diplock, A. T. (ed.) 1985. *Fat soluble vitamins*. London: William Heinemann Medical Books.

Friedrich, W. F. 1988. *Vitamins*. Berlin: de Gruyter.

Gaby, S. K., A. Bendich, V. N. Singh, L. J. Machlin 1991, *Vitamin intake and health*. New York: Marcel Dekker.

Marks, J. 1968. *The vitamins in health and disease: a modern reappraisal*. London: J. & A. Churchill.

Clinical nutrition

Dickerson, J. W. T. & E. M. Booth 1985. *Clinical nutrition for nurses, dietitians and other health care professionals*. London: Faber & Faber.

Francis, D. E. M. 1974. *Diets for sick children*. Oxford: Blackwell Scientific.

Leeds, A. R., P. Judd, B. Lewis 1990. *Nutrition matters for practice nurses: a handbook on dietary advice for use in the community*. London: John Libbey.

Food intolerance and allergy

Brostoff, J. & S. J. Challacombe 1987. *Food allergy and intolerance*. London: Baillière Tindall.

Metcalfe, D. P., H. A. Sampson, R. A. Simon 1991. *Food allergy: adverse reactions to foods and food additives*. Boston: Blackwell Scientific.

Research reviews on nutritional topics

Advances in Nutrition Research. New York: Plenum Press.

Annual Reviews of Nutrition. Palo Alto, California: Annual Reviews.

Nutrition Abstracts and Reviews. Oxford: CAB International.

Nutrition Research Reviews. Cambridge: Cambridge University Press.

Nutrition Reviews. New York: The Nutrition Foundation.

Proceedings of the Nutrition Society. Cambridge: Cambridge University Press.

World Review of Nutrition and Dietetics. Basel: Karger.

INDEX

INDEX

Computer-aided learning exercises

The following computer-aided learning exercises are available to accompany this book:

The foods you eat
A program giving the nutrient content of 470 foods. The nutrients listed are: energy, protein, fat, carbohydrate, fibre, vitamins A, B_1, B_2, niacin and C, sodium, iron and calcium. Meals or diets can be compared with the 1991 UK reference nutrient intakes (Department of Health Report on Health and Social Subjects 1991).

Diet and menu planner
A program which permits reverse use of food composition tables, so that you can plan diets and menus which are especially rich or low in specific nutrients. The nutrients listed are the same as in *The foods you eat*.

Understanding nutrient requirements
Simulated experiments to determine energy and protein requirements, the effects of varying physical activity on energy requirements and of varying energy intake on body weight.

Biochemical simulations
Five programs which are computer simulations of laboratory exercises in biochemistry. The areas covered by the simulations are: enzyme activity, the synthesis of urea, the sequencing of a biologically active peptide, studies of oxidative phosphorylation using the oxygen electrode, and radio-immunoassay of oestradiol.

For further information on these programs, please write to the author:
Dr D. A. Bender, Department of Biochemistry and Molecular Biology, University College London, Gower Street, London WC1E 6BT.